Leishmaniasis: Pathogenesis and Management

Leishmaniasis: Pathogenesis and Management

Editor: Jake Morrison

⊕ MURPHY & MOORE
www.murphy-moorepublishing.com

www.murphy-moorepublishing.com

ⓂMURPHY & MOORE

Cataloging-in-Publication Data

Leishmaniasis : pathogenesis and management / edited by Jake Morrison.
   p. cm.
Includes bibliographical references and index.
ISBN 978-1-63987-340-1
1. Leishmaniasis. 2. Leishmaniasis--Pathogenesis. 3. Leishmaniasis--Diagnosis. 4. Leishmaniasis--Treatment.
5. Protozoan diseases. I. Morrison, Jake.
RC153 .L45 2022
616.936 4--dc23

Murphy & Moore Publishing,
1 Rockefeller Plaza,
New York City, NY 10020, USA

ISBN 978-1-63987-340-1 (Hardback)

Contents

Preface

This book has been an outcome of determined endeavour from a group of educationists in the field. The primary objective was to involve a broad spectrum of professionals from diverse cultural background involved in the field for developing new researches. The book not only targets students but also scholars pursuing higher research for further enhancement of the theoretical and practical applications of the subject.

Leishmaniasis refers to a number of medical conditions which are caused by the Leishmania parasite. It is transferred to humans through sandflies belonging to the genus Phlebotomus. Leishmania is broadly classified into three types, cutaneous, mucocutaneous and visceral. Cutaneous leishmania causes skin ulcers while mucocutaneous leishmania causes ulcers in the mouth, nose and skin. Visceral leishmania begins with skin ulcers, which can then develop into fever and enlargement of the liver and spleen. It can be diagnosed in a hematology laboratory, through the direct visualization of the amastigotes. This disease can be prevented by spraying animal shelters and houses with insecticides. The topics covered in this book offer the readers new insights on the evaluation and management of leishmaniasis. Those with an interest in the study of these medical conditions would find it helpful. This book will serve as a valuable source of reference for graduate and post graduate students.

It was an honour to edit such a profound book and also a challenging task to compile and examine all the relevant data for accuracy and originality. I wish to acknowledge the efforts of the contributors for submitting such brilliant and diverse chapters in the field and for endlessly working for the completion of the book. Last, but not the least; I thank my family for being a constant source of support in all my research endeavours.

Editor

Transmission to Humans

Miroslava Avila-García, Javier Mancilla,
Enrique Segura-Cervantes and
Norma Galindo-Sevilla

1. Introduction

Tissue parasites such as *Leishmania* are transmitted from host to host through a vector species, and transmission can be from human to vector to animal or vice versa (zoonotic transmission), which occurs in rural and periurban environments or from human to vector to human (anthroponotic transmission), which occurs in urban environments. *Lutzomyia* and *Phlebotomus* species have long been known as the primary transmitters of leishmaniasis. However, in recent decades, evidence has been building for the existence of alternative transmission pathways. These pathways involve direct contact with infected tissues, such as may be encountered during surgical/therapeutic procedures, biological/reproductive activities, certain work-related practices and by unsafe drug use, all of which are reviewed below.

2. Transmission forms

2.1. The life cycle of *Leishmania* spp.: the vector transmission

Leishmania spp. is a parasite with a dimorphic life cycle that is controlled by the passage from vector to host [1]. As such, the parasite has developed novel adaptations to survive within the vector [2]. The vector phase of the life cycle begins when the vector ingests blood containing the parasites. Following ingestion, the parasites eventually reach the midgut, where they are held for approximately 4 hours in the peritrophic matrix. There, the amastigote cells differentiate into small, motile cells with short flagella, a form known as the procyclic promastigote. Next, *Leishmania* initiates the first stage of the vector life cycle, which occurs over the following 24-48 hours. The body of the parasite elongates in the next 72 hours to form the nectomonad promastigote, and the microorganism then breaks down the peritrophic matrix to reach the midgut lumen and migrate into the thoracic region of the vector. Once there, the promastigotes differentiate into leptomonad promastigotes by decreasing in size and changing the location of their flagella, which is followed by a second replication cycle during days 5-7. This process produces a massive infection in the anterior portion of the midgut, where the parasites differentiate into metacyclic promastigotes within the stomodeal valve, ensuring a large number of parasites for the purpose of infection. To protect the metacyclic promastigotes, the leptomonads also differentiate into gel-producing promastigotes, which surround the leptomonad and metacyclic promastigotes. The latter cell type is considered to be the infective form of the parasite because it possesses an elongated flagellum, which allows for motility and resistance to complement-mediated lysis. When metacyclic promastigotes differentiate into haptomonad promastigotes, they form parasitic rings that plug the stomodeal valve, eventually leading to its degeneration. Finally, this process allows the parasites to pass into the proboscis [2], where they can inoculate the host during feeding of the vector.

Upon entering the host, the parasite first encounters a host immune reaction following activation of the complement system. With respect to this process, four distinct activation pathways have been identified: the classical pathway, the alternative pathway, the lectin pathway and the extrinsic pathway [3]. In humans, the parasite can evade the immune response by inhibiting complement-mediated lysis, which occurs within the phagolysosomes of macrophages. This protective effect is conferred by the membrane protease gp63, or leishmanolysin, which inhibits attacks against the parasite cell membrane by adhering to complement components [4]. Promastigote-stage parasites differentiate into small, round cells 3-5 μm in size that lack flagella, known as amastigotes. This form can be readily observed within host cells by microscopy, where they are referred to as Leishman-Donovan [5] bodies. Finally, when multiplication of the parasites exceeds the holding capacity of the phagocytic cell, cell lysis occurs, releasing the parasites to infect new cells.

By some conservative estimates, a vector might release between 1-1000 metacyclic promastigotes into the host during feeding [6-7]. However, other estimates based on molecular biology techniques indicate that a vector might release as many as 600 to 100,000 metacyclic promastigotes during a feeding period and that this number varies as function of feeding time. In addition, it is known that large numbers of parasites actually increase vector feeding time, as the parasites physically obstruct proper functioning of the proboscis [8]. Therefore, based on these findings, between 100 and 100,000 metacyclic parasites are commonly used to inoculate the footpads or pinnae of animals in *in vivo* models of infection [8-10].

2.2. Organ transplants, blood transfusions and hemodialysis

Therapeutic advances in a wide variety of medical fields have dramatically improved overall quality of life and life expectancy in modern societies. This has partly been achieved through the development of techniques such as organ transplantation, hemodialysis, and blood transfusion, which are particularly useful for the treatment of chronic disease. However, the transmission of infectious diseases during such procedures must account for and avoided. Furthermore, human migration can easily transport diseases transmitted by vectors from endemic locations to non-endemic locations, as often happens with protozoan parasites of the blood, such as *Leishmania* [11-12], *Trypanosoma* and *Plasmodium* [3].

During organ transplantations, there are several possible ways in which microorganisms such as *Leishmania* can be transmitted, including reactivation of dormant parasites in the recipient following treatment with immunosuppressants, infection by parasites derived from the donor, transmission of parasites through blood transfusions during the surgical procedure and *de novo* transmission [11-12]. *Leishmania* infections have been observed in individuals who have undergone kidney [13-16] and liver [17-18] transplants, as well as in patients that have undergone heart [17, 19-23], lung [24], pancreas [25], stem cell [26-27] and bone-marrow transplants, although these are less common. Overall, the number of leishmaniasis cases resulting from organ transplants is estimated to be fewer than 100 in total [11, 13-16], which were mainly associated with kidney transplants. A primary risk factor for transmission is whether the donor had lived in an area where leishmaniasis was endemic. However, this subject is not commonly addressed during screening processes, and relevant laboratory tests are not usually carried out on organ donors [28]. Therefore, it is important to generate and review epidemiological data concerning leishmaniasis, as the number of infected individuals who are asymptomatic could be even greater than the number of those showing clinical symptoms [17]. There have also been reports of organ donors who were asymptomatic before surgery but who died of leishmaniasis several months after the transplantation procedure. Furthermore, there has been at least one case in which an organ recipient developed leishmaniasis symptoms two years after the transplantation procedure [29]. In cases where individuals show symptoms approximately one month after transplantation, transmission is generally considered to be due to the reactivation of dormant parasites within the recipient [30]. On the other hand, in cases where leishmaniasis symptoms are observed approximately 18 months after receiving a new organ, transmission is generally considered to be due to the *de novo* acquisition of parasites [11-12, 16]. In either case, the suggested course of treatments to favour transplant survival includes corticosteroids [24], immunosuppressants [13-14], or monoclonal antibodies [11], which favor the development of leishmaniasis.

Infrequent or atypical symptoms can cause delayed diagnosis of leishmaniasis. The primary clinical signs and symptoms related to *Leishmania* infections due to organ transplantation are fever, splenomegaly, hepatomegaly, leukopenia and hypoalbuminemia [14, 31-32]. Unfortunately, the therapeutic responses to such cases are often insufficient to save the patient's life, which can be ascribed to late diagnoses, particularly severe infections and other health complications [13] due to prolonged immunosuppressive regimens [16, 24].

Blood volume loss or deficiencies in specific blood components are indicators that a transfusion of blood or blood-derivatives from a donor to a recipient may be necessary. Blood transfusions are frequently performed during or after surgical interventions, and in the case of leishmaniasis patients with a history of organ transplantation and blood transfusion, the disease is generally considered to be a complication of the transplantation process [15, 32-33]. In patients without such a background, infections are generally considered to have occurred through the transfusion of blood or blood-derived products. The first case of *Leishmania* transmission via a blood transfer was documented in China in 1948, when two girls were given 20 mL of blood intramuscularly to stimulate passive immunity against measles and rubella. The blood came from their mother, who was hospitalized days later with symptoms suggestive of visceral leishmaniasis; this diagnosis was made one month after her being hospitalized. Therefore, due to the medical history of the mother, the girls were monitored over the subsequent months. Both girls developed leishmaniasis 9-10 months after the blood transfer [34]. Although this case was not due to blood transfusion *per se*, it is the first documented case in which the use of blood components for therapeutic purposes resulted in the contraction of leishmaniasis.

In general, the causative agents of visceral leishmaniasis belong to the *donovani* complex of species, although there have also been reports of visceralization in species more typically related to the mucocutaneous and cutaneous clinical presentations of the disease. These types of clinical presentations have primarily been observed in individuals with compromised immune systems, such as HIV-positive patients. However, there has been a single reported case of a patient with these characteristics who also had a history of kidney transplantation and blood transfusions. Furthermore, there was no history of vector exposure as the patient was not living in an endemic region. The infection hypothesis was ruled out by searching for signs of *Leishmania* in the blood by PCR and by searching for *Leishmania*-specific antibodies in the donor and in the recipient of the second kidney. The patient's death was caused by complications due to the presence of *T. cruzi*, *S. aureus* and *L. mexicana*. Although the patient's transfusion donors could not be evaluated, based on analysis of other possible transmission pathways, it was concluded that the most likely pathway of infection was through blood transfusion [35].

Among other notable cases of secondary leishmaniasis due to blood products and transfusions, there was the case of a patient with an autoimmune disease, idiopathic thrombocytopenic purpura. The patient was transfused with concentrated platelets on multiple occasions over the 2-3 year period prior to the development of leishmaniasis, a diagnosis that was confirmed by bone marrow aspiration [36].

Another case involved an infant who received a blood transfusion within 7 days of birth due to integument pallor with a subsequent diagnosis of myelofibrosis. The blood donor was a relative who died three months after the donation, after developing hepatosplenomegaly, pyrexia and a fever of unknown origin; the diagnosis was made *postmortem* after the detection of Leishman-Donovan bodies. The infant began to show abdominal distension, fever and integument pallor one month after the transfusion. At 5 months of age, visceral leishmaniasis was diagnosed from a spleen aspirate that scored positive for Leishman-Donovan bodies. Leishmaniasis treatment was initiated without improvement, and two months later, the infant was rehospitalized with anemia, respiratory distress, hepatomegaly and splenomegaly. A liver biopsy revealed changes consistent with steatohepatitis with necrotic foci and lipid granulomas. Furthermore, the biopsy was positive for anti-*Leishmania* antibodies (rK-39), whereas the infant's family members were negative for these antibodies. Due to a severe anemic syndrome, the infant was given a blood transfusion. Despite treatment with antimonials, the infant showed no improvement and indeed worsened with the development of septicemia caused by *Staphylococcus*, *Klebsiella* and *Pseudomonas*. A change of drugs to Amphotericin B only deteriorated the infant's health further, and it died one month after admission [37].

In a case involving an elderly patient, a 77-year-old woman with a history of chronic atrial fibrillation, hypertension and chronic kidney disease with hemodialysis treatment underwent surgery due to cholecystitis, during which time she received two units of blood. A month and a half later, she presented with fever, diaphoresis and chills during a hemodialysis session and over the next 24 hours; she also showed occasional diarrhea and weight loss. These symptoms did not improve despite treatment with antibiotics. In the intensive care unit following hemodialysis, the patient showed thrombocytopenia and hypotension with good ventricular systolic function, requiring volume recovery and vasopressor therapy; hydrocortisone was also included in the treatment. A bone marrow aspirate confirmed the presence of intracellular amastigotes and numerous extracellular promastigotes, although these were not observed in the peripheral blood. Treatment with Amphotericin B increased her platelet numbers, although hemodynamic deterioration continued until the patient's death. Cultures begun previous to death showed the presence of *Acinetobacter baumannii*, a bacterium that is resistant to multiple types of antibiotics. During a *postmortem* examination, the presence of *Leishmania* parasites in the bile was tested for due to prior gastrointestinal symptoms. The transmission of *Leishmania* through the blood was confirmed when one of her donors (to the source of the units transfused during the cholecystectomy) tested positive for *Leishmania*-specific antibodies [38].

Seven U.S. military groups assigned to Operation Desert Storm in the 1990s developed atypical clinical presentations of *L. donovani* infection that were suggestive of Kala-azar. The symptoms included stiffness, nonproductive cough, diffuse abdominal tenderness, diarrhea, nausea, headache, myalgia, and arthralgia without organomegaly. One of the patients was asymptomatic, whereas two had diseases that compromised their immune systems: renal carcinoma and HIV. The diagnoses were performed using an immunofluorescent antibody test (IFAT). In all cases, the onset of symptoms occurred 1-14 months after their time in Saudi Arabia, and none showed lesions that may have aided in the diagnosis of leishmaniasis [39]. These clinical cases led U.S. authorities to recommend that all candidates who had visited the Persian Gulf be rejected as blood donors. This situation was further complicated by the fact that the conditions under which the *Leishmania* parasite might survive in blood products in bank bloods were unknown. As a result, *in vitro* assays were performed on parasites isolated from the soldiers. The *Leishmania* parasites that were isolated from the individuals participating in Operation Desert Storm included *L. tropica*, *L. major* and *L. donovani*. These parasites were maintained in log-phase culture and used to inoculate donated blood samples, which were then stored at 4ºC for 35 days or at 24ºC for 5 days. It was observed that in whole-blood units stored under these common blood-bank conditions, *L. tropica* intracellular parasites within monocytes could survive up to 30 days at 4ºC and up to 5 days at 24ºC, in contrast to promastigotes in stationary phase or free amastigotes that does not. With respect to fresh frozen plasma, it was observed that intracellular parasites could survive inside monocytes for 25 days at 4ºC and for at least 5 days in the platelet fraction at 24ºC. For erythrocyte fractions frozen with glycerol, survival time of the parasite was 35 days at 4ºC [40]. It is clear that *Leishmania* shows low-temperature resistance, highlighting the very real possibility of parasite transmission from infected individuals, either in the preclinical or asymptomatic phase, to immunocompromised individuals via blood products.

Transmission of *Leishmania* via blood transfusions has been demonstrated in domestic animals [41] and model organisms, and these typically present symptoms following treatment with either infected human blood or blood from experimentally infected animals [40, 42-43]. For example, blood transfusions can be carried out in rodents by transferring 0.1-1.0 mL blood via tail-vein [40] or intracardiac injection [43]. In a study involving hamsters, all groups that received infected blood showed symptoms between 90-120 days following transfusion [43]. It was found that 22.1% of the transfused hamsters scored positive for *Leishmania* by PCR analysis, and 14.75% remained positive when the test was performed again after 12 months. All of the monocyte cultures were negative. Furthermore, it was demonstrated that 29.5% of the transfused hamsters tested positive by at least one of the techniques, with PCR being the most sensitive assay [44].

There have also been various clinical studies carried out on individuals attending blood banks in which the presence of the parasite was assessed for using techniques such as ELISA (enzyme-linked immunosorbent assay) [45], IFAT [46], Western blotting, culturing and PCR [44-45]. ELISA experiments showed that 2.4% of the individuals had *Leishmania*-specific antibodies, whereas 3.5% scored positive by Western blotting analysis; both tests showed a seroprevalence of 7.6%.

Furthermore, questioning may be insufficient to exclude donors that have visited endemic areas within the last 12 months or that have had clinical diagnoses of leishmaniasis, as recommended by the WHO publication *Blood donor selection: guidelines on assessing donor suitability for blood donation*. Therefore, there is a clear need to develop laboratory techniques to identify this microorganism in blood or derivatives, and indeed, several studies have been carried out to detect the presence of *Leishmania*-specific antibodies in healthy individuals who have donated blood.

In cutaneous species, such as those belonging to the *L. mexicana* complex, it is unknown whether the parasite can be transmitted through blood in humans under the same conditions as the visceral species. However, as was previously mentioned, it should be noted that there are cases of HIV patients that have developed visceral leishmaniasis when infected with cutaneous species [35].

In individuals with chronic kidney disease, hemodialysis is a therapy that can greatly improve patient prognosis and prolong and improve their quality of life. However, like many other therapeutic procedures, hemodialysis can have adverse effects, including bacteremia and sepsis due to poor aseptic techniques during treatment [47]. Indeed, it has been documented that if proper care is not taken to sterilize hemodialysis equipment, including the cleaning and replacement of disposable parts, there is high risk of acquiring infectious/contagious diseases [47], including parasitic infections. Unlike with the situation with *Toxoplasma*, [48] *Leishmania* has not been directly linked to hemodialysis patients, although large assays for *Leishmania*-specific antibodies have been performed [49-50] that found the parasite in 9-25% of patients in endemic areas [50]. Despite the fact that no studies directly link *Leishmania* infection to hemodialysis treatment, perhaps because most patients with kidney disease who are treated with hemodialysis also have a clinical history of immunosuppressive blood treatment, organ transplantation and multiple blood transfusions [38, 50-51]. All of these conditions increase the possibility of acquiring leishmaniasis and negatively affect patient health, making the analysis of causal factors difficult.

2.3. Sexual transmission

2.3.1. Leishmaniasis in sexual organs in humans

Cases of leishmaniasis of the sexual organs have been reported, manifesting as lesions on the genitals, and such cases have been reported in both humans [52-56] and in animals [57-58]. Three possible mechanisms for the development of leishmaniasis of the sexual organs and genitals have been suggested: (1) local infection derived from a wider systemic infection; (2) infection due to exposure of the genitals to a vector in an endemic area; and (3) infection due to direct contact of the genitals with an ulcerated lesion during intercourse [59].

By questioning patients, such cases of genital leishmaniasis in humans could not always be directly linked to either intercourse [52-53] or to sleeping naked in endemic areas [55]. However, in cases where the lesions were observed on the vulvar regions [53], direct vector-mediated infection can be ruled out, leaving open the possibility for localized infection of systemic origin or from intercourse with a previously infected individual.

It should be noted that genital ulcers can have numerous causes, and thorough diagnoses should be conducted in all cases to avoid confusion with other diseases, such as squamous cell carcinoma or primary syphilis [55]. Likewise, the presence of other types of infectious microorganisms should also be ruled out [59].

2.3.2. Leishmaniasis in sexual organs in animals

Among animals, domestic dogs are considered to be the main reservoir of *Leishmania*, and this parasite has been detected in canine sexual organs as well [57-58]. In females, the absence of exposed genitals and internal sex organs suggests that infections are either systemic in origin or sexually transmitted, which is especially true in non-endemic areas [60-61].

It has been observed that when *L. chagasi* infects sexual organs (e.g., the testis, epididymis and prostate) and genitals (e.g., the glans and foreskin), it can induce an inflammatory response. In addition, macrophages infested with parasites accompanied by neutrophils in the foreskin have also been observed in dogs. In one study involving dog semen, the presence of the parasite was detected by PCR in 8 out of 22 samples analyzed [57], a finding which suggests the possibility of sexual infection between animals. Indeed, when 12 serologically negative females were mated to males that tested serologically positive for *L. chagasi*, 165 days after mating, 3 out of the 12 females were serologically positive and 6 out of the 12 females scored positive by PCR [62]. Although the external genitals and the vulva are the most commonly affected areas in symptomatic and asymptomatic females, females that scored positive for *Leishmania* by PCR also showed effects in at least one other region of the reproductive system. Histological changes included perifollicular lymphocytic infiltration with intracellular parasites as well as inflammatory infiltration in the vulvar dermis [58]. Other trials have been carried out in which male and female dogs infected with *Leishmania* were mated to observe vertical transmission.

However, it remains unclear whether sexual transmission plays an important role in vertical transmission [63].

2.4. Congenital transmission

2.4.1. Congenital leishmaniasis in humans

Vertical transmission is defined as the congenital transmission of a pathogenic microorganism, condition, or characteristic from one generation to the next via the placenta, hematogenous, the birth canal, or nursing at the maternal breast [64]. Vertical transmission has been demonstrated for visceral leishmaniasis caused by *L. donovani* and *L. infantum*. The first case of vertical transmission in leishmaniasis was reported in 1926 in a pregnant woman who began to show symptoms suggestive of leishmaniasis during her first trimester. The treatment for visceral leishmaniasis was administered upon the exclusion of malaria and typhoid fever as differential diagnoses by laboratory results. Upon treatment, the symptoms disappeared, and the pregnancy continued to term. The birth took place without complications via the vaginal canal, and the neonate was of normal weight. However, both mother and neonate exhibited a general state of deterioration immediately postpartum. Visceral leishmaniasis was not suspected, and the symptoms were fever, diarrhea, and abdominal pain. Due to the state of the mother, nursing did not occur. The child was tracked during its first year and presented with anemia and splenomegaly. A biopsy of the spleen revealed the presence of Leishman-Donovan bodies [65], indicating that vertical transmission of leishmaniasis had occurred.

The epidemiological antecedents of leishmaniasis are crucial when pediatric patients or those of childbearing age develop symptoms suggestive of leishmaniasis. A mother who was diagnosed with *L. infantum* by ELISA had been on a farm when she was between 28 and 30 weeks pregnant. The child was born by elective caesarean at 38 weeks in a non-endemic zone in the Ukraine. At the age of eight months, the nursing child suddenly exhibited a fever, decreased appetite, weakness, pallor of the integuments, bruising, hepatosplenomegaly, tachypnea, and lymphadenopathy. An aspirate of the bone marrow revealed ovoid cells of 3-5 µm that were identified as Leishman-Donovan bodies [66].

In Germany, there have been two reported cases of leishmaniasis involving mothers who visited endemic zones prior to their pregnancies. The first case involved a 16-month-old pediatric patient with visceral leishmaniasis whose mother had traveled to endemic zones two years earlier [67]. The second case was a 15-month-old child with visceral leishmaniasis whose mother was on a farm in an endemic zone between 20 and 22 weeks of pregnancy [68].

Chronic visceral leishmaniasis has been linked to premature birth and materno-fetal deaths. [69] A histological analysis of the placenta and an aspirate of the lymphatic ganglion revealed the presence of thrombotic, vascular changes in the placenta of a fetus at five months of gestation in a mother that had been infected with leishmaniasis for two months [70]. Neonates carried to term from infected mothers have remained asymptomatic during the first weeks or months of life. However, Leishman bodies have ultimately been detected in the bone marrow, and anti-*Leishmania* antibodies have also been detected, corroborating the diagnosis of leishmaniasis [65, 69, 71].

Leishmaniasis can be accompanied by concomitant infections by organisms from similar genera. During the second trimester, a pregnant patient was initially treated for leishmaniasis and showed improvement at 30 days. The baby was born vaginally at 36 weeks without complications and weighed 1,700 grams. He was readmitted three days later for deterioration due to probable malaria and tuberculosis, but he did not show improvement following treatment. Amastigotes were detected in an aspirate of the lymphatic ganglion of the mother. In addition, IgG antibodies were detected in the baby; these antibodies were attributed to passive transplacental transfer of parasite-specific antibodies from the mother to the fetus, negating the need for treatment. He was admitted once more at seven months old for symptoms suggestive of *Plasmodium falciparum,* and he did not show improvement upon treatment. A bone marrow aspirate revealed *Leishmania*. However, despite treatment, the infant died. An autopsy revealed that the presence of abundant *Leishmania* parasites in the kidneys, spleen, thymus, bone marrow, liver, and lungs and *Candida* spp. in the respiratory tract [70].

Individuals, whether mother or offspring, in endemic zones can be infected for months or years prior to the onset of symptoms. For example, a woman visited an endemic zone and became pregnant two years later. She did not experience any symptoms during her pregnancy or postpartum while in the non-endemic zone nor was there evidence of the existence of the vector in the geographic area. While the mother remained asymptomatic, the infant exhibited symptoms of possible visceral leishmaniasis, which was confirmed by various laboratory tests [67].

There is evidence that cutaneous leishmaniasis is associated with perinatal health problems, as has been observed in Brazil, where women with *L. braziliensis*-mediated cutaneous leishmaniasis developed vegetative or atypical lesions at the 18th week of pregnancy. Of these patients, 10% delivered prematurely and the fetus died in another 10% of the cases. A biopsy of one of the fetuses revealed intense inflammatory exudates predominated by neutrophils, and parasites were detected by electrophoresis [72].

2.4.2. Congenital leishmaniasis in animals

In Brazil, a trial was performed with asymptomatic and symptomatic mixed-breed dogs that were infected with *L. donovani* and *L. infantum*. There were four dogs in each group, and the livers, spleens, lymph nodes, bone marrow, kidneys, and hearts of their offspring were analyzed by PCR for infection. The numbers of offspring obtained from symptomatic or asymptomatic mothers (26 vs. 27) were nearly identical. The placentas and the offspring were analyzed by PCR, and 13 of the 26 placentas and 9 of the 26 offspring of the symptomatic mothers were positive for the parasite, while 13 of the 27 placentas and 8 of the 27 offspring from the asymptomatic mothers were positive. Furthermore, it was noted that PCR was more sensitive for parasite detection in comparison to immunohistochemistry and hematoxylin and eosin staining [73]. Another study in Italy involved seven female dogs that had been diagnosed with leishmaniasis by serology, microscopy, and PCR. Two of the seven were treated with N-methylglucamine prior to pregnancy, and one of the seven was treated during pregnancy. The pups were examined between 3 and 30 days of age. The parasite was detected in 8 of the 31 pups in both groups, and only 2 of the 8 pups developed symptoms [74].

2.4.3. Experimental models of congenital transmission

In a murine model of visceral leishmaniasis, twenty 12-week -old female BALB/c mice were infected with *L. infantum*. They were mated 8 weeks later with healthy males, and the females were sacrificed at days 13 and 18 of gestation. The offspring were sectioned in half for PCR analysis. In 15 of the 20 pregnant mice, the parasite was detected by PCR in the spleen. In the offspring, 3 of the 88 placentas and 4 of the 88 pups tested positive for *Leishmania* by PCR [75]. In studies to determine vertical transmission of *Leishmania* in beagles, parasitemia was detected in the liver, spleen, and bone marrow of the offspring [63].

In experimental model in which hamsters were infected with 10^6 parasites/mL of *L. panamensis* during the first week of pregnancy, 24 of 93 (25.8%) of the offspring from infected mothers were PCR positive to *Leishmania*, 2 months after the birth [76]. Furthermore, mice infected with high inoculums of *L. mexicana* strain, known as cause of cutaneous leishmaniasis, showed that all female and their placentas were positive to PCR analysis, and revealed that the infection was present in 39 of 110 offspring of infected mothers, also fetal deaths and resorptions were observed [77]. Then is important to be aware to the fact that leishmaniasis could be transmitted transplacentally and causes fetal resorption, death, and reduction in offspring body weight.

2.5. Other factors related to substance abuse and work environment

2.5.1. Drug use

In cases of leishmaniasis infection due to fomites, such as sharp, contaminated objects, the most vulnerable population are illicit drug users. In a Spanish study of syringes used for recreational drug use, it was reported that 32-52% of the syringes were contaminated by *Leishmania*, as determined by PCR. Moreover, 3 different genotypes were identified in multiple samples, confirming that the individuals had shared syringes. Therefore, programs that limit the sharing of needles should decrease the infection rate among vulnerable individuals [78-79].

2.5.2. Work environment transmission

As described above, *Leishmania* spp. can be transmitted through fluids such as blood and by contact with animals or even contaminated objects. In all cases, there must be an entry route, which is usually a wound. In staffs dedicated to clinical, diagnostic or medical research, it is not uncommon to find reported cases of *Leishmania* infection, although many such likely go unrecognized [80]. Infections due to accidental exposure can be affected by a variety of factors, including kinematics (e.g., the path and characteristics of exposure and the amount of inoculum), parasite characteristics (e.g., pathogenicity, virulence, viability and infective dose) and host characteristics (e.g., immune status, barrier status and actions following the accident) [80]. However, the possibility of infection due to vector exposure in an endemic region should not be ruled out when performing questioning [81]. The first case of work-related leishmaniasis was reported in 1930, and to date, there have been 12 reported cases of *Leishmania* infection due to accidents at work; these have included 6 different *Leishmania* species, with *L. donovani* being implicated in half of the affected individuals. In these cases, the incubation period ranged from 3 weeks to 8 months after the accident. Although the United States is not considered to be an endemic region, it has had more than half of reported leishmaniasis cases of laboratory transmission, with the parenteral route being the most frequent means of exposure, followed by animal bites, primarily from experimental animals. In one affected population, the average age of leishmaniasis cases due to work-related accidents was 30, and four of the affected individuals were students [80].

According to the CDC, the *Leishmania* parasite is considered to be a Biosafety Level 2 (BSL-2) organism, which implies that the individual transmission rate is moderate, and low in the case of a community. Therefore, *Leishmania* can cause disease in humans or animals without being considered a serious risk for laboratory staff. Although exposure can lead to serious infection, effective treatments are available and the risk is limited [82]. Potentially infectious parasites can be found in blood, tissues, exudates and infected arthropods, and they can be transmitted through wounds, micro-abrasions, accidental parenteral inoculation or transmission by arthropods [80]. Therefore, it is recommended that all staff having contact with potentially infectious material use protective equipment and that the handling of potentially infectious waste be carried out in accordance with appropriate regulations and good clinical/laboratory practices [80, 82]. In the case of staff with compromised immune systems, it is recommended that they avoid work with live organisms [82].

3. Conclusions

The *Leishmania* parasite can survive in a wide range of temperatures and pH conditions, which has allowed it to adapt to the diverse conditions encountered within different vector and host species. In recent years, transmission pathways other than those based on vector species have been described, including invasive procedures for therapeutic purposes, sexual practices, pregnancy, drug practices and work-related accidents among health/research staff members, all of which have led to an increase in the number of reported leishmaniasis cases. However, considering that the latency period of the parasite within the host can last up to one year, there are likely more infected individuals than those that have been reported. Because leishmaniasis is not considered to be a disease that can be transmitted between individuals without the intervention of a vector species, laboratory tests for the presence of these parasites to rule out prospective donors are not carried out prior to in most invasive therapeutic procedures. However, in the case of patients with immunodeficiency, the possibility of contracting the disease is significantly increased. Furthermore, during pregnancy, changes to the immune system can allow for the transmission of the parasite from the mother to the fetus. It should also be noted that maternal-fetal infection can also be of sexual origin. Among drug addicts, it was demonstrated that syringe sharing is a significant source of infection. Finally, in addition to populations exposed in endemic areas, staff working in the health or research sectors should also be considered as populations at risk of acquiring this disease.

Taken together, there is a clear need for the health system to reevaluate the global situation concerning leishmaniasis transmission and to implement strategies to reduce the exposure of individuals to *Leishmania* infections.

Acknowledgements

Financial support: The chapter was sponsored by Instituto Nacional de Perinatologia (212250-22701). Primary investigator: Dr. Norma Galindo-Sevilla.

Author details

Miroslava Avila-García, Javier Mancilla, Enrique Segura-Cervantes and Norma Galindo-Sevilla*

National Institute for Perinatology, Department of Infectious Diseases and Perinatal Immunology, Mexico City, Mexico

References

[1] Rosal Rabes Td, Baquero-Artigao F, García Miguel MJ. Leishmaniasis cutánea. Pediatría Atención Primaria. 2010;12:263-71.

[2] Kamhawi S. Phlebotomine sand flies and Leishmania parasites: friends or foes? Trends Parasitol. 2006;22:439-45.

[3] Huber-Lang M, Sarma JV, Zetoune FS, Rittirsch D, Neff TA, McGuire SR, et al. Generation of C5a in the absence of C3: a new complement activation pathway. Nat Med. 2006;12:682-7.

[4] Handman E. Cell biology of Leishmania. Adv Parasitol. 1999;44:1-39.

[5] Wheeler RJ, Gluenz E, Gull K. The cell cycle of Leishmania: morphogenetic events and their implications for parasite biology. Mol Microbiol. 2011;79:647-62.

[6] Warburg A, Schlein Y. The effect of post-bloodmeal nutrition of Phlebotomus papatasi on the transmission of Leishmania major. Am J Trop Med Hyg. 1986;35:926-30.

[7] Rogers ME, Ilg T, Nikolaev AV, Ferguson MA, Bates PA. Transmission of cutaneous leishmaniasis by sand flies is enhanced by regurgitation of fPPG. Nature. 2004;430:463-7.

[8] Kimblin N, Peters N, Debrabant A, Secundino N, Egen J, Lawyer P, et al. Quantification of the infectious dose of Leishmania major transmitted to the skin by single sand flies. Proc Natl Acad Sci U S A. 2008;105:10125-30.

[9] Lira R, Doherty M, Modi G, Sacks D. Evolution of lesion formation, parasitic load, immune response, and reservoir potential in C57BL/6 mice following high- and low-dose challenge with Leishmania major. Infect Immun. 2000;68:5176-82.

[10] Quiñones-Diaz L M-RJ, Avila-García M, Ortiz-Avalos J, Berrón A, Gonzalez S, Paredes Y, Galindo-Sevilla N. Effect of Ambient Temperature on the Clinical Manifestations of Experimental Diffuse Cutaneous Leishmaniasis in a Rodent Model. VECTOR-BORNE AND ZOONOTIC DISEASES. [Original Research Manuscript]. 2012;12.

[11] Coster LO. Parasitic infections in solid organ transplant recipients. Infect Dis Clin North Am. 2013;27:395-427.

[12] Miro JM, Blanes M, Norman F, Martin-Davila P. Infections in solid organ transplantation in special situations: HIV-infection and immigration. Enferm Infecc Microbiol Clin. 2012;30 Suppl 2:76-85.

[13] Basset D, Faraut F, Marty P, Dereure J, Rosenthal E, Mary C, et al. Visceral leishmaniasis in organ transplant recipients: 11 new cases and a review of the literature. Microbes Infect. 2005;7:1370-5.

[14] Oliveira CM, Oliveira ML, Andrade SC, Girao ES, Ponte CN, Mota MU, et al. Visceral leishmaniasis in renal transplant recipients: clinical aspects, diagnostic problems, and response to treatment. Transplant Proc. 2008;40:755-60.

[15] Oliveira RA, Silva LS, Carvalho VP, Coutinho AF, Pinheiro FG, Lima CG, et al. Visceral leishmaniasis after renal transplantation: report of 4 cases in northeastern Brazil. Transpl Infect Dis. 2008;10:364-8.

[16] Gontijo CM, Pacheco RS, Orefice F, Lasmar E, Silva ES, Melo MN. Concurrent cutaneous, visceral and ocular leishmaniasis caused by Leishmania (Viannia) braziliensis in a kidney transplant patient. Mem Inst Oswaldo Cruz. 2002;97:751-3.

[17] Antinori S, Cascio A, Parravicini C, Bianchi R, Corbellino M. Leishmaniasis among organ transplant recipients. Lancet Infect Dis. 2008;8:191-9.

[18] Barsoum RS. Parasitic infections in organ transplantation. Exp Clin Transplant. 2004;2:258-67.

[19] Frapier JM, Abraham B, Dereure J, Albat B. Fatal visceral leishmaniasis in a heart transplant recipient. J Heart Lung Transplant. 2001;20:912-3.

[20] Golino A, Duncan JM, Zeluff B, DePriest J, McAllister HA, Radovancevic B, et al. Leishmaniasis in a heart transplant patient. J Heart Lung Transplant. 1992;11:820-3.

[21] Iborra C, Caumes E, Carriere J, Cavelier-Balloy B, Danis M, Bricaire F. Mucosal leishmaniasis in a heart transplant recipient. Br J Dermatol. 1998;138:190-2.

[22] Larocca L, La Rosa R, Montineri A, Iacobello C, Brisolese V, Fatuzzo F, et al. Visceral leishmaniasis in an Italian heart recipient: first case report. J Heart Lung Transplant. 2007;26:1347-8.

[23]   Zorio Grima E, Blanes Julia M, Martinez Ortiz de Urbina L, Almenar Bonet L, Peman Garcia J. [Persistent fever, pancytopenia and spleen enlargement in a heart transplant carrier as presentation of visceral leishmaniasis]. Rev Clin Esp. 2003;203:164-5.

[24]   Morales P, Torres JJ, Salavert M, Peman J, Lacruz J, Sole A. Visceral leishmaniasis in lung transplantation. Transplant Proc. 2003;35:2001-3.

[25]   Colomo Rodriguez N, De Adana Navas MS, Gonzalez Romero S, Gonzalez Molero I, Reguera Iglesias JM. [Visceral leishmaniasis in a type 1 diabetic patient with isolated pancreas transplant]. Endocrinol Nutr. 2011;58:375-7.

[26]   Agteresch HJ, van 't Veer MB, Cornelissen JJ, Sluiters JF. Visceral leishmaniasis after allogeneic hematopoietic stem cell transplantation. Bone Marrow Transplant. 2007;40:391-3.

[27]   Sirvent-von Bueltzingsloewen A, Marty P, Rosenthal E, Delaunay P, Allieri-Rosenthal A, Gratecos N, et al. Visceral leishmaniasis: a new opportunistic infection in hematopoietic stem-cell-transplanted patients. Bone Marrow Transplant. 2004;33:667-8.

[28]   Chongo AG, ER. Leishmaniasis y transfusión. Artículo de revisión. Rev Mex Med Tran. 2010;3:5.

[29]   Munoz P, Valerio M, Puga D, Bouza E. Parasitic infections in solid organ transplant recipients. Infect Dis Clin North Am. 2010;24:461-95.

[30]   Veroux M, Corona D, Giuffrida G, Cacopardo B, Sinagra N, Tallarita T, et al. Visceral leishmaniasis in the early post-transplant period after kidney transplantation: clinical features and therapeutic management. Transpl Infect Dis. 2010;12:387-91.

[31]   Berenguer J, Gomez-Campdera F, Padilla B, Rodriguez-Ferrero M, Anaya F, Moreno S, et al. Visceral leishmaniasis (Kala-Azar) in transplant recipients: case report and review. Transplantation. 1998;65:1401-4.

[32]   Sagnelli C, Di Martino F, Coppola N, Crisci A, Sagnelli E. Acute liver failure: a rare clinical presentation of visceral leishmaniasis. New Microbiol. 2012;35:93-5.

[33]   Cummins D, Amin S, Halil O, Chiodini PL, Hewitt PE, Radley-Smith R. Visceral leishmaniasis after cardiac surgery. Arch Dis Child. 1995;72:235-6.

[34]   Dey A, Singh S. Transfusion transmitted leishmaniasis: a case report and review of literature. Indian J Med Microbiol. 2006;24:165-70.

[35]   Mestra L, Lopez L, Robledo SM, Muskus CE, Nicholls RS, Velez ID. Transfusion-transmitted visceral leishmaniasis caused by Leishmania (Leishmania) mexicana in an immunocompromised patient: a case report. Transfusion. 2011;51:1919-23.

[36]   Mathur P, Samantaray JC. The first probable case of platelet transfusion-transmitted visceral leishmaniasis. Transfus Med. 2004;14:319-21.

[37] Dey A, Singh S. Transfusion transmitted leishmaniasis: A case report and review of literature2006.

[38] Mpaka MA, Daniil Z, Kyriakou DS, Zakynthinos E. Septic shock due to visceral leishmaniasis, probably transmitted from blood transfusion. J Infect Dev Ctries. 2009;3:479-83.

[39] Magill AJ, Grogl M, Gasser RA, Jr., Sun W, Oster CN. Visceral infection caused by Leishmania tropica in veterans of Operation Desert Storm. N Engl J Med. 1993;328:1383-7.

[40] Grogl M, Daugirda JL, Hoover DL, Magill AJ, Berman JD. Survivability and infectivity of viscerotropic Leishmania tropica from Operation Desert Storm participants in human blood products maintained under blood bank conditions. Am J Trop Med Hyg. 1993;49:308-15.

[41] de Freitas E, Melo MN, da Costa-Val AP, Michalick MS. Transmission of Leishmania infantum via blood transfusion in dogs: potential for infection and importance of clinical factors. Vet Parasitol. 2006;137:159-67.

[42] Palatnik-de-Sousa CB, Paraguai-de-Souza E, Gomes EM, Soares-Machado FC, Luz KG, Borojevic R. Transmission of visceral leishmaniasis by blood transfusion in hamsters. Braz J Med Biol Res. 1996;29:1311-5.

[43] Paraguai de Souza E, Esteves Pereira AP, Machado FC, Melo MF, Souto-Padron T, Palatnik M, et al. Occurrence of Leishmania donovani parasitemia in plasma of infected hamsters. Acta Trop. 2001;80:69-75.

[44] Riera C, Fisa R, Udina M, Gallego M, Portus M. Detection of Leishmania infantum cryptic infection in asymptomatic blood donors living in an endemic area (Eivissa, Balearic Islands, Spain) by different diagnostic methods. Trans R Soc Trop Med Hyg. 2004;98:102-10.

[45] Scarlata F, Vitale F, Saporito L, Reale S, Vecchi VL, Giordano S, et al. Asymptomatic Leishmania infantum/chagasi infection in blood donors of western Sicily. Trans R Soc Trop Med Hyg. 2008;102:394-6.

[46] Colomba C, Saporito L, Polara VF, Barone T, Corrao A, Titone L. Serological screening for Leishmania infantum in asymptomatic blood donors living in an endemic area (Sicily, Italy). Transfus Apher Sci. 2005;33:311-4.

[47] Al-Said J, Pagaduan AC. Infection-free hemodialysis: can it be achieved? Saudi J Kidney Dis Transpl. 2009;20:677-80.

[48] Tong DS, Yang J, Xu GX, Shen GQ. [Serological investigation on Toxoplasma gondii infection in dialysis patients with renal insufficiency]. Zhongguo Xue Xi Chong Bing Fang Zhi Za Zhi. 2011;23:144, 53.

[49] Souza RM, de Oliveira IB, Paiva VC, Lima KC, dos Santos RP, de Almeida JB, et al. Presence of antibodies against Leishmania chagasi in haemodialysed patients. Trans R Soc Trop Med Hyg. 2009;103:749-51.

[50] Luz KG, da Silva VO, Gomes EM, Machado FC, Araujo MA, Fonseca HE, et al. Prevalence of anti-Leishmania donovani antibody among Brazilian blood donors and multiply transfused hemodialysis patients. Am J Trop Med Hyg. 1997;57:168-71.

[51] Mirzabeigi M, Farooq U, Baraniak S, Dowdy L, Ciancio G, Vincek V. Reactivation of dormant cutaneous Leishmania infection in a kidney transplant patient. J Cutan Pathol. 2006;33:701-4.

[52] Symmers WS. Leishmaniasis acquired by contagion: a case of marital infection in Britain. Lancet. 1960;1:127-32.

[53] Blickstein I, Dgani R, Lifschitz-Mercer B. Cutaneous leishmaniasis of the vulva. Int J Gynaecol Obstet. 1993;42:46-7.

[54] Cain C, Stone MS, Thieberg M, Wilson ME. Nonhealing genital ulcers. Cutaneous leishmaniasis. Arch Dermatol. 1994;130:1313, 5-6.

[55] Cabello I, Caraballo A, Millan Y. Leishmaniasis in the genital area. Rev Inst Med Trop Sao Paulo. 2002;44:105-7.

[56] Schubach A, Cuzzi-Maya T, Goncalves-Costa SC, Pirmez C, Oliveira-Neto MP. Leishmaniasis of glans penis. J Eur Acad Dermatol Venereol. 1998;10:226-8.

[57] Diniz SA, Melo MS, Borges AM, Bueno R, Reis BP, Tafuri WL, et al. Genital lesions associated with visceral leishmaniasis and shedding of Leishmania sp. in the semen of naturally infected dogs. Vet Pathol. 2005;42:650-8.

[58] Silva FL, Rodrigues AA, Rego IO, Santos RL, Oliveira RG, Silva TM, et al. Genital lesions and distribution of amastigotes in bitches naturally infected with Leishmania chagasi. Vet Parasitol. 2008;151:86-90.

[59] Rosen T, Brown TJ. Genital ulcers. Evaluation and treatment. Dermatol Clin. 1998;16:673-85.

[60] Gaskin AA, Schantz P, Jackson J, Birkenheuer A, Tomlinson L, Gramiccia M, et al. Visceral leishmaniasis in a New York foxhound kennel. J Vet Intern Med. 2002;16:34-44.

[61] Harris MP. Suspected transmission of leishmaniasis. Vet Rec. 1994;135:339.

[62] Silva FL, Oliveira RG, Silva TM, Xavier MN, Nascimento EF, Santos RL. Venereal transmission of canine visceral leishmaniasis. Vet Parasitol. 2009;160:55-9.

[63] Rosypal AC, Troy GC, Zajac AM, Frank G, Lindsay DS. Transplacental transmission of a North American isolate of Leishmania infantum in an experimentally infected beagle. J Parasitol. 2005;91:970-2.

[64] Mosby's Medical Dictionary. 8th ed: Elsevier; 2009.

[65] Low G, Cooke WE. A CONGENITAL CASE OF KALA-AZAR. The Lancet. [doi: 10.1016/S0140-6736(01)05214-X]. 1926;208:1209-11.

[66] Zinchuk A, Nadraga A. Congenital visceral leishmaniasis in Ukraine: case report. Ann Trop Paediatr. 2010;30:161-4.

[67] Meinecke CK, Schottelius J, Oskam L, Fleischer B. Congenital transmission of visceral leishmaniasis (Kala Azar) from an asymptomatic mother to her child. Pediatrics. 1999;104:e65.

[68] Bogdan C, Schonian G, Banuls AL, Hide M, Pratlong F, Lorenz E, et al. Visceral leishmaniasis in a German child who had never entered a known endemic area: case report and review of the literature. Clin Infect Dis. 2001;32:302-6.

[69] Figueiro-Filho EA, El Beitune P, Queiroz GT, Somensi RS, Morais NO, Dorval ME, et al. Visceral leishmaniasis and pregnancy: analysis of cases reported in a central-western region of Brazil. Arch Gynecol Obstet. 2008;278:13-6.

[70] Eltoum IA, Zijlstra EE, Ali MS, Ghalib HW, Satti MM, Eltoum B, et al. Congenital kala-azar and leishmaniasis in the placenta. Am J Trop Med Hyg. 1992;46:57-62.

[71] Nyakundi PM, Muigai R, Were JB, Oster CN, Gachihi GS, Kirigi G. Congenital visceral leishmaniasis: case report. Trans R Soc Trop Med Hyg. 1988;82:564.

[72] Morgan DJ, Guimaraes LH, Machado PR, D'Oliveira A, Jr., Almeida RP, Lago EL, et al. Cutaneous leishmaniasis during pregnancy: exuberant lesions and potential fetal complications. Clin Infect Dis. 2007;45:478-82.

[73] Pangrazio KK, Costa EA, Amarilla SP, Cino AG, Silva TM, Paixao TA, et al. Tissue distribution of Leishmania chagasi and lesions in transplacentally infected fetuses from symptomatic and asymptomatic naturally infected bitches. Vet Parasitol. 2009;165:327-31.

[74] Masucci M, De Majo M, Contarino RB, Borruto G, Vitale F, Pennisi MG. Canine leishmaniasis in the newborn puppy. Vet Res Commun. 2003;27 Suppl 1:771-4.

[75] Rosypal AC, Lindsay DS. Non-sand fly transmission of a North American isolate of Leishmania infantum in experimentally infected BALB/c mice. J Parasitol. 2005;91:1113-5.

[76] Osorio Y, Rodriguez LD, Bonilla DL, Peniche AG, Henao H, Saldarriaga O, et al. Congenital transmission of experimental leishmaniasis in a hamster model. Am J Trop Med Hyg. 2012;86:812-20.

[77] Avila-Garcia M, Mancilla-Ramirez J, Segura-Cervantes E, Farfan-Labonne B, Ramirez-Ramirez A, Galindo-Sevilla N. Transplacental Transmission of Cutaneous Leishmania mexicana Strain in BALB/c Mice. Am J Trop Med Hyg. 2013;89:354-8.

[78] Cruz I, Morales MA, Noguer I, Rodriguez A, Alvar J. Leishmania in discarded syringes from intravenous drug users. Lancet. 2002;359:1124-5.

[79] Pineda JA, Martin-Sanchez J, Macias J, Morillas F. Leishmania spp infection in injecting drug users. Lancet. 2002;360:950-1.

[80] Herwaldt BL. Laboratory-acquired parasitic infections from accidental exposures. Clin Microbiol Rev. 2001;14:659-88.

[81] Knobloch J, Demar M. Accidental Leishmania mexicana infection in an immunosuppressed laboratory technician. Trop Med Int Health. 1997;2:1152-5.

[82] Chosewood LC, Wilson DE, Centers for Disease Control and Prevention (U.S.), National Institutes of Health (U.S.). Biosafety in microbiological and biomedical laboratories. 5th ed. Washington, D.C.: U.S. Dept. of Health and Human Services, Public Health Service, Centers for Disease Control and Prevention, National Institutes of Health; 2009.

2

Otorhinolaryngologic Manifestations in Leishmaniasis

Luiz Alberto Alves Mota and
Roberta Correia Ribeiro Ferreira de Miranda

1. Introduction

Leishmaniasis is considered by the World Health Organization (WHO) as one of the five endemic infectious and parasitic diseases of greatest importance and as a world-wide public health problem [1]. It is an infectious disease that evolves chronically and is caused by a protozoon of the genus *Leishmania*, which may appear as a clinical form which is visceral, cutaneous, mucocutaneous, mucousal and rarely diffuse [2]. The term Leishmaniasis refers to the infection of vertebrate hosts *Leishmania*, which, like the other trypanosomatids of the order Kinetoplastida, characteristically present an extranuclear DNA in its cytoplasm in a mito-chondrial organelle, the kinetoplast. This genus is characterized by having two ways of evolving during its biological cycle in host organisms: amastigote, which is an obligatory intracellular parasite in vertebrates, and promastigote, which develops in the digestive tube of invertebrate vectors or in axenic culture media [3].

In 1903, the agent of the disease was first described and separately by Leishman and Donovan. It is a protozoon identified in splenic tissue from two patients resident in India affected by a fatal disease [4]. It is primarily a zoonotic infection of wild animals, and more rarely pets, including marsupials, carnivores and even primates, with humans being accidental hosts.

All species of *Leishmania* are transmitted by the bite of female mosquitoes called phlebotominae of the genera *Lutzomyia* and *Phlebotomus*, this transmission being made by inoculation of promastigotes into the skin of the vertebrate host [5]. In larynegeal Leishmaniasis, contamination generally occurs starting with high lesions of the nasal cavities and oropharynx by contiguity. It is rare for parasites to be found inside the lesions [6].

The incubation period ranges from 2 weeks to several months [13]. Mucosal involvement is dependent on the combination of the virulence of the parasite and the immune cell response of the host. Within the population of infected individuals, 1-10% experience mucosal involvement [15]. Risk factors for the development of mucosal Leishmaniasis are: the presence of lesions above the pelvis, large skin ulcers and inadequate treatment of cutaneous Leishmaniasis [3].

For the diagnosis of mucosal Leishmaniasis, the clinical history and typical cutaneous scars have been considered as important clinical markers to corroborate the diagnosis of LM in patients with non-specific nasal/ oral granulomatous lesions [20].

In the Americas, pre-Colombus pottery, made by the Indians of Peru, has been found, dating from 400 to 900 AD. These show mutilations of lips and noses, characteristics of espundia, today known as muco-cutaneous leishmaniosis. Subsequently, through studies in paleomedicine, mummies with skin lesions and mucosas characteristic of Leishmaniasis were found [9]. Historical findings suggest that American Cutaneous Leishmaniasis (ACL) already affected the peoples of America before contact with Europeans and Africans. It is assumed that it may have originated in the western Amazon region during archeological times by means of human migrations and later ascended to the high jungle and then to the hot inter-Andean lands across the frontiers of Bolivia and of Peru with Brazil [5].

In the Old World (Asia, Africa and Europe) written accounts of the disease date from the first century AD. About two thousand years later, in 1903, the agent of the disease is described for the first time and separately by LEISHMAN and DONOVAN. The disease was visceral Leishmaniasis and its agent, the species now known as *Leishmania donovani* [4].

The first reference to American Tegumentary Leishmaniasis (ATL) in Brazil is in the document of the Religious Political-Geographical Pastoral 1827, quoted in Tello's book entitled "Antiguidad de la Syfilis en el Peru", where he recounts the journey of Friar Don Hipólito Sanches de Fayas y Quiros de Tabatinga (AM) to Peru, which crossed the regions of the Amazon basin [9]. In 1911, GASPAR VIANNA gave the parasite found by Lindenberg the name *Leishmania brasiliensis*, because he considered it morphologically different from *Leishmania* tropica. This characterized, from then on, the etiological agent of the disease being referred to as "Bauru ulcer", "angry angry" or "tapir-nose" [5].

In the 80s, the ATL was noted in 19 Federative Units (i.e. states), its geographical expansion being verified when, in 2003, autochthony was confirmed in all Brazilian states. It is seen to be widespread and, in some areas there is an intense concentration of cases, while in others, there are isolated cases [7]. The disease has been described in almost all American countries, from the extreme South of the United States to the North of Argentina, with the exception of Chile and Uruguay [22].

2. Epidemiology

Leishmaniasis is the second most common parasitic disease in the world, with an estimated 600,000 new cases per year [6]. It can also be considered an occupational disease, since it has affected workers in mining areas, geologists, scientific expeditions, military personnel in training [2]. It has been documented in several countries, with an estimated prevalence of 12 million worldwide [3]. More than 20 *Leishmania* species pathogenic to man have been described.

Until the 1990s, the classification of these species was based primarily on clinical and geographic criteria, taking into account on the one hand, the distinction between Old and New World, and, on the other, the clinical forms of the disease. This type of classification which has been progressively replaced by phylogenetic classification, is seen to be increasingly less tight and more superficial [4].

Leishmaniasis species are widely distributed and have been documented in Africa, Europe, Asia and America. In the Old World, *L. tropica*, *L. major* and *L. aethiopica*, which cause tegumentary Leishmaniasis, are identified as causal agents of the disease. In the Americas, several species of *Leishmania* are capable of causing tegumentary *Leishmania*sis, such as *L. braziliensis* (LVB), *L. amazonensis*, *L. guianensis*, *L. pananmensis* and *L. Mexicana*.

The characterization of *Leishmania* species that was initially made, considering the behavior of the parasite in the vector, today has biochemical and imminological and molecular biology techniques, by isoenzyme analysis, reactivity with monoclonal antibodies and analysis of the DNA of kinetoplast [3]. In the Americas, 11 dermotropic species of *Leishmania* causing human disease are currently recognized and 8 species desrcibed as being only in animals [8].

It is in Brazil that the largest prevalence in the whole American continent is found, this being estimated as 65,000 new cases per year [6]. The coexistence is observed of a double epidemiological profile, expressed by the maintenance of cases coming from old foci or areas near them, and by the appearance of epidemic outbreaks associated with factors arising from the emergence of economic activities, such as mining, expansion of agricultural frontiers and extractivism, in environmental conditions that are highly favorable to the transmission of the disease [8].

A great number of the houses in recent population settlements are built very close to the edge of the forest and individuals are affected by the radius of action of these vectors that reach houses and are also attracted by several factors such as lighting, the presence of sinantropic animals such as Didelphis marsupialis, domestic animals and man himself [1]. Some species of rodents, marsupials, edentates and wild canids have already been recorded as hosts and possible natural reservoirs. The reservoir-parasite intersection is considered a complex system, insofar as it is multifactorial, unpredictable and dynamic, and forms a biological unit which can be in constant change as a result of the changes in the environment [8].

The disease occurs, more habitually, in the form of epidemic outbreaks. Thus, the degree of exposure of the individuals affected is related directly to agricultural population settlements which were planned or more often arise from occupation processes on the outskirts of a city, most of which are disorganized [1].

Initially, the reservoirs of the mosquito transmitter were in the wild or in rural areas, but the environmental transformations, provoked by the migratory process and by the increasing urbanization have been modifying this profile. The adaptation of the vectors to the new conditions enabled the disease to spread in the domiciliary and peri- domiciliary settings [5].

In several regions of the country, such as in the South and Southeast, intense environmental changes occurred due to anthropic action and agricultural and pastoral activities, which led to the near disappearance of cutaneous Leishmaniasis in the late 40s. However, from the 70s and 80s Leishmaniasis has reappeared in these regions, with a significant increase in the number of new cases arising from endemic areas [1]. Transmission classically was due to the bite of an insect, the so-called insect vector. This insect, also called a sandfly, belongs in the Old World to the genus Phlebotomus, and in the New World, to the genus Lutzomyia [4].

The first cases of ATL in America date from 1885 and in Brazil, the first report was in 1909. In the period 1985-1999, there were 388,155 auctothon cases in Brazil of ALT; from 1999 to 2003, 33,872 cases of ATL a year were registered [1]. In the period from 2000 to 2009, an average of 24,684 confirmed cases of Leishmaniasis was registered in Brazil the Information System for Notifiable Diseases (SINAN) [14]. In 2003, the regions with the highest prevalence of LTA were the North (14,200 cases) and the Northeast (8,005 cases) [5].

In Brazil, 23,399 confirmed cases of ATL were notified in 2009, of which 94.1% were new cases and 4.6% relapses. With respect to clinical manifestations, 93.7% of patients had the cutaneous clinical form and 6.2%, clinical mucosa. Of all patients, in 2009, only 73.5% [17, 23] were cured, 16 patients died due to ATL, and 122 died from other causes, noting that 21.2% there was no information on the evolution of 21.2% of the cases [14].

It is estimated that every year there are new cases in Brazil and the growth of this number is due in part to the emergence and growth of AIDS and deforestation areas [2]. It mostly affects young and adult males [16]. The greater number of cases of American Tegumentary Leishmaniasis among men and adults suggests extra-domiciliary transmission in the economically active population, while this occurrence among women, children and people with non-agricultural occupations suggests intra- and or peridomiciliary transmission.

The transmission of ATL in the Amazon presents a clear seasonal variation, it being more intense in the rainy season, when the temperature, solar radiation and evaporation are lower and humidity higher, thus favoring an increase in the density of the phlebotominae, including the species involved in the cycle of the disease [1]. In endemic areas, there may be significant percentages of children with the disease [16].

3. Etiological agents and vectors

In the Americas, 11 dermotropic species of *Leishmania* which cause the disease in humans are currently recognized and 8 species have been described as affecting only animals. However, in Brazil, 7 species, there being 6 of the subgenus *Viannia* and 1 of the subgenus *Leishmania,* have been identified. The three main species are: *Leishmania (Leishmania) amazonensis* - distributed throughout the primary and secondary forests of the Amazon (Amazonas, Pará, Rondônia, Tocantins and the southwest of Maranhão southwest), particularly in *igapó* and forest areas of the "swamp-forest" type. Its presence extends to the regions of the Northeast (Bahia), Southeast (Minas Gerais and São Paulo) and Midwest

(Goiás); *Leishmania (Viannia) guyanensi* - apparently limited to the north of the Amazon Basin (Amapá, Roraima, Amazonas and Pará) and extending to the Guianas. It is found mainly in *terra firme* forests in areas that do not flood during the rainy season; *Leishmania (Viannia) braziliensis* – is widely distributed, from the South of Pará to the Northeast, also reaching the center-south of the country and some areas of the Eastern Amazon East. In the Amazon, the infection is usually found in dry land areas.

As the subgenus *Viannia*, there are other species of *Leishmania* that have been recently described: *L. (V) lainsoni, L. (V) naiffi* with a few human cases in Pará; *L. (V) shawi*, with human cases found in Pará and Maranhão. More recently, the species *L. (V.) lainsoni, L. (V.) naiffi, L. (V.) lindenberg and L. (V.) shawi* were identified in states of the North and Northeast regions [8]. In areas of transmission of *L. braziliensis* concomitantly or after resolution of the cutaneous disease, about 3% of patients with cutaneous *Leishmania*sis will develop the mucosal form of the disease [3].

Mucosal Leishmaniasis (ML) is a form of tegumentary Leishmaniasis associated with *L. braziliensis, L. panamensis* and less frequently with *L. amazonensis* [11]. The vectors of ATL are insects known as phlebotominae, belonging to the order *Diptera, Psychodidae* family, sub-family *Phlebotominae*, genus *Lutzomyia*, popularly known, depending on the geographical location, as straw-mosquito straw, *tatuquira, birigui*, among others [8]. Generally not exceeding 0.5 cm in length, with long and spindly legs and a dense body follicles. A characteristic of theirs is a hopping flight and keeping their wings erect, unlike other dipteral [9]. The vectors are *Lutzomya anduzei, Lutzomyia whitmani* and *Lutzomyia umbratilis*, which is the main vector, which usually lands during the day on tree trunks and attacks people in large numbers, when disturbed [16]. It is usually brownish ("straw-mosquito"), only the females being adapted with the respective mouth part to prick the skin of vertebrates and suck blood.

The genus *Lutzomyia* is responsible for the transmission of Leishmaniasis in the Americas, and there are 350 species catalogued, which are distributed from the South of Canada to the North of Argentina. Of these, at least 200 occur in the Amazon basin. Very little is known of their breeding grounds, with immature forms being found in debris of rock crevices, caves, roots of the soil and of dead and damp leaves, and also in the forks of trees in animal burrows - ie in moist but not wet soil, and in debris rich in decaying organic matter [9].

4. Clinical state

Tegumentary Leishmaniasis is more common than the visceral disease and is characterized in its classical form by the presence of a well-bounded ulcer with raised edges. [17] ATL is an initial infection of the skin (its site of preferential location) from which it can undergo propagation or a secondary process which goes on to manifest itself in the mucosae of the upper airways [5]. The incubation period of the disease in humans is, on average, 2 months, it being possible for there to be shorter (two-week) periods and longer periods (of up to 2 years) [16].

The disease breaks out, in general, during the first five years that follow the appearance of the skin lesion, but may do so even a few decades after the primary cutaneous lesion, the scar from which can still be seen. However, in some patients the disease appears primarily in the mucosa membrane, without leaving traces on the skin. [2]. The most common manifestation is leishmaniotic ulcer: a single skin ulcer or only in small numbers, with raised edges, framed and the absence of local pain. Other morphological features can also be identified, such as: infiltrated plaque, tubercule, nodule and verrucous vegetating lesion. When the mucosa is injured, it can present an infiltrated erythema, granular or ulcerated aspect. In order of frequency, mucosal lesions are manifested mainly in the nose, hard palate, pharynx and larynx, which they can present themselves with an erythematous-infiltrated, granular, ulcerated or polypoid aspect with a roughly rounded surface [5].

Basically, it is possible to do the staging of the lesions that have occurred in the ATL by taking into consideration the time of onset, extent and spread of the lesion, and grouping them into: 1). Primary infections: which characterizes the primary accident (initial injury) or leishmaniotic cancer, found at the site of the bite, and after the incubation period (two weeks to one year), erythematous papules appear that progress to forming ulcers with serosanguinous crusts. 2) The onset of secondary Leishmaniasis ranges from one to three months after the primary infection, involving the skin, lymph nodes, lymphatic organs and mucosa and by contiguity, the mucous membranes of the nose, lips, eyelids and genitals are affected when the primary or secondary lesions settle near these regions. 3) Tertiary Leishmaniasis requires a longer period to appear, generally, five to ten years after the initial lesion and is characterized by the presence mainly of naso-oro-pharyngeal, laryngeal and ocular lesions, and it is in this period tertiary that the primary infection has already disappeared and the secondary one, in general, is still present [5]. The clinical presentation exhibits polymorphism and the spectrum of severity of the signs and symptoms is also variable, although there is a certain correspondence between the different clinical presentations and the different species of the parasite [7].

Mucosal Leishmaniasis appears under the following clinical forms: 1) Late –this is the most common form. Classically, it is associated with multiple or long-lasting skin lesions, spontaneous cures or insufficient CL treatments; 2) Of undetermined origin - when the ML is clinically isolated, it not being possible to detect any other evidence of prior CL; 3) Concomitant - when the mucosal lesion occurs at a distance, but at the same time as the active skin lesion (not contiguous to the natural orifices); 4) Contiguous – this occurs by direct propagation of the skin lesion, located next to natural orifices, to the mucosa of the aerodigestive tracts. The skin lesion may be in activity or healed at the time of diagnosis; 5) Primary – this occurs, possibly, by the bite of the vector in the mucosa or semimucosa of lips and genitals [7.8].

It is believed that untreated mucosal lesions are progressive, there being few reports of spontaneous cicatrizations of these lesions which, even if treated, may leave permanent sequelae [22]. There are several hypotheses that attempt to explain the predilection of the nasal mucosa: direct contact of the hand with the skin lesions and scratching one´s nose afterwards, the epithelium of the anterior part of the nasal cavities offer conditions to the location of Leishmanias and the lower temperature in the anterior area of the nasal septum, due to the presence of a current of inspiratory air. The transition zone between the squamous epithelia and the pseudostratified vibrating, in the anterior part of the nasal septum and the lower turbinate head, is the "*locus minoris resistentia*" to the Leishmaniasis process. However, the most consistent hypothesis says that *Leishmania* requires lower temperatures for its growth. Thus, since the anterior area of the nasal septum is cooler due to the inspiratory airflow, there would be a predilection for proliferation of the parasites [13]. The association of low temperature with Leishmaniasis may, in part, be explained by the documentation *in vitro* that macrophages grown at 29°C are less able to destroy *Leishmania* than macrophages cultured at 33°C [3].

It occurs more often in males and at age bands usually higher than CL, which is probably due to its character of secondary complication [8]. The involvement of the nasal and/or mucosa is usually more severe and thus may cause sequelae and death [20].

The initial lesion is characterized by a whitish nodulation without ulceration which is usually observed in the cartaliginous septum (Kiesselbach's area), the floor and side wall, specifically on the head of the inferior turbinate. This impairment classified as stage I of the disease, represents a very early stage of inflammation and does not resemble, from the clinical standpoint, any other nasal disease. Subsequently, a fine granular lesion appears, character- ized by superficial ulceration, documented at the anterior septum, inferior turbinates and floor of the nasal cavity (Stage II) [17]. At first, there is hyperemia and edema of the mucosa of the anterior septum, with the establishment of nodulations [3].

In Stage III, or the stage of deep ulceration, tissue reaction is more intense, with aberrant granulation tissue and infiltration of the mucosa, thus widening the nasal septum. There is sometimes edematous infiltration of the nasal pyramid itself. In this phase, hematic crusts can be observed on the septum, the inferior turbinates and the floor of the nasal cavities. These lesions are characterized by excessive fragility, as they bleed very easily when the mucosa is touched.

Clinically, the patient may complain of soreness at the level of the nasal pyramid, sanguinolent rhinorrhea and emission of hematic crusts. Nasal obstruction is a frequent symptom in this phase of the disease. From the external point of view, due to the inflammatory process that involves the cartilages and subcutaneous cell tissue and the very skin of the base of the nasal pyramid, the nose takes on the aspect known as tapir-nose.

Stage IV of the disease is characterized by the cartilaginous involvement of the anterior septum with necrosis and, sometimes, impairment of the columella. It is at this stage that perforation of the cartilaginous septum is established, also with marked infiltration of the posterior septum. In more advanced forms (Stage V), total destruction of the columella may occur and may drop, thus transforming the nasal cavity into a similar cloaca and some- times there is perforation of the dorsum of the nasal pyramid [17]. For some researchers, the specific destruction of the nasal cartilage could also indicate an autoimmune reaction that would explain why some patients undergo severe tissue destruction and others only present mucosal involvement years later [21]. In some cases there may be total destruc- tion of the anterior septum, only the entire columella remaining, with the nose being sealed. Extensive crusts of a hemorrhagic aspect or even resulting from the drying of mucous secretion caused by enlargement of the internal nasal structure can be observed as a consequence of the tissue injury, represented by the destruction of the cartilaginous septum and inferior turbinates. On this occasion, there is elimination of sanguinolent discharge and the presence of crusts is accentuated [17]. The patient's death usually occurs because of aspiration or respiratory failure [5].

The earliest signs and symptoms of mucosal Leishmaniasis are nasal obstruction, epistaxis and the establishment of granulomas in the anterior nasal septum. As the disease evolves, patients begin to present a leishmaniotic facies known as "tapir nose" due to edematous infiltration of the lining and supporting structures of the nose [3]. Lesions reach the cartilaginous nasal septum and may extend to the lateral wall and floor, the region of the palate, uvula, and less frequently, involvement of the pharynx, larynx, vocal cords and upper lip occur with varying degrees of infiltration, granulation and ulceration [17]. The infiltration of the soft palate reaches the proportions of a real tumor. The whole palate is changed: the uvula is reduced to a shapeless mass, with an irregular, vegetating surface. In the palatal vault, lobed prominences are formed, separating themselves by sinuous furrows and ulcerated erosions.

More rarely it can involve the gum and dental interstices, where voluminous and prominent granulations develop, and reach the upper lip. The tongue is usually spared [5]. The manifestations of the mucosal diseases include involvement of pillars and uvula with an increase in volume, hyperemia, roughness and superficial ulcers [12]. The pharynx is the second site of involvement when mucosal lesions caused by *L. braziliensis* set in. As in the nose, the lesion initially observed at the level of the mucosa of the pharynx takes on a lumpy aspect; however, here, there is a much more intense edematous infiltration, especially of the uvula and secondarily of the tonsillar pillars, extending also to the mucosa of the posterior pharyngeal wall.

The appearance can be observed at this stage of granulation tissue that is a little redundant intermingled with the lumpy aspect of the mucosa. The next stage is characterized by the appearance of abundant granulation tissue, which causes important tissue destruction, also involving the lymphoid tissue of Waldeyer's lymphatic ring at the level of tonsils. Areas with a tenuous fibrin layer mix in with the granulation tissue of a vegetating aspect.

Because of the intense tissue aggression, in the specific post-treatment healing process, the presence of abundant fibrous tissue, with the formation of true whitish cords can be documented. These completely deform the configuration of the anatomical structures of the velum of the palate and the posterior wall of the pharynx, leading to full stenosis in the communication of the oropharynx with the nasopharynx [3]. In the mouth, the hard palate is often involved, with dissemination of the process to the soft palate, uvula and pharynx. The proliferating infiltrative process can cause fusion of the uvula, pillars, lateral cords and posterior wall, causing obliteration of the nasopharynx. Deformity and narrowing of the lumen of the oropharynx may occur due to fibrosis of the tonsils [5].

Laryngeal mucosa is the 3rd site of election when mucosal Leishmaniasis sets in. As in the pharynx, the mucosal lesions present the same characteristics of finely granular tissue. There may be in situations of greater inflammation, the presence of granulation tissue with a vegetating aspect, covered at times with a tenuous fibrin layer, involving the mucosa that covers the cartilage of the epiglottis, extending to the mucosa of the structures of the laryngeal vestibule and vocal folds. At this stage, dysphonia characterized by a muffled voice is always present, which draws attention to the impairment of the organ [3]. Pharyngolaryngeal involvement can be intense, to the point of causing dysphagia, dyspnea, dysphonia, odyno-phagia, and coughing [15]. The hypopharynx, larynx, epiglottis, arytenoid cartilages and the posterior commissure of the vocal cords are covered by a lesion with a vegetating aspect, which sometimes come to join up. These granulations often regress and eventually disappear, making the surface affected by a smooth and slightly whitish coloration.

There is generalized laryngeal inflammation particularly in the piriform sinuses. The vocal folds appear to be moving well, but phonation is weak and the muscular control of tension can be harmed by granulomatous formation and subsequent fibrosis. Even after successful treatment, the voice rarely returns to normal and the lumen of the larynx may be reduced [5]. Painful dysphagia in degrees of greater or lesser intensity prevents the normal feeding of the individual, with consequent impairment of general condition and, in very advanced cases, becoming cachexia. In post-treatment healing, the deformities that these cartilages present are very evident, such as fibrous tissue which is also whitish, thereby completely modifying the anatomy of the organ, except for a residual permanent dysphonia [3].

Complications include pneumonia due to aspiration, bacterial infections, secondary myiasis, cachexia due to difficulties in swallowing, laryngeal edema and asphyxiation, which may be lead on to the patient's death mainly due to respiratory failure and sepsis [5]. The presentation of the clinical form with lesions exclusive of mucosa of the larynx and trachea is relatively uncommon [2]. The ear is not usually affected in mucosal Leishmaniasis. However, the involvement of the mucosa of the nasopharynx leads to impairment of the pharyngeal orifice of the Eustachian tube, situated on its sidewall. A process of otitis media with effusion (secretory otitis media chronic) can be established in these cases.

The sensation of blocked ear, tinnitus and hearing loss are complaints in these cases [3]. Morbidity of the skin and ear cartilage occurs because it is a place of lower temperature, apt for the growth of *Leishmania*, besides being an area exposed to the inoculation of the vectors. The external ear commonly presents an increase in volume, ulcers with raised edges, some-times covered with crusts, and may appear as an infiltrated plate, tubercule, vegetating warty nodule and lesion, on course in the end to mutilating the ear [5].

Mucosal Leishmaniasis can compromise the labial mucosa and gingival margin. This is a rarer manifestation of the disease [3]. The lesion in some individuals heals early, sometimes without seeking medical attention. Others remain for months with the lesion in activity and the healing process is slow. This phenomenon can be explained by the rapid or late establishment of a specific immune response which is effective in eliminating the parasite.

The cure of Leishmaniasis is not sterile. It has been possible to isolate viable parasites of ALT scars in individuals who have been cured for several years, a fact confirmed in experimental studies using an animal model. This phenomenon could thus explain the appearance of late relapses as well as the onset of the disease in immunocompromised patients, such as AIDS (Acquired Immunodeficiency Syndrome) [7].

5. Diagnosis

It is very hard to detect Leishmaniasis in the initial stage [15]. The long interval between the onset of symptoms and etiological diagnosis of the mucosal form of ATL may reflect the limitation of the training of most physicians in the proper approach to mucosal Leishmaniasis [2]. A laryngoscopy exam usually demonstrates an extensive inflammatory component, with erythema and edemas evident. The granulomatous aspect associated with the presence of ulcers is common, and may present purulent exudate. In the advanced disease, tissue destruction can be striking. As a protocol of etiological investigation on suspicion of granulomatous bodies that are difficult to access such as the larynx, laboratory tests and imaging should be requested, and should a diagnostic uncertainty be maintained, a biopsy of the lesions is recommended for histological study. If the appearance of the lesion suggests malignant neoplasm, research using noninvasive and invasive tests should occur simultaneously so as not to delay diagnosis [15].

The ENT examination associated with the Montenegro test remains the most important element for diagnosis, although it is usually of a presumptive character [20]. The encounter of *Leishmania* is the gold standard for the diagnosis of ATL [21]. The diagnosis can be confirmed by various tests: 1) Direct investigation of the parasite, which can be done by scraping the ulcerated surface or by compression of the slide on the wounded area of the lesion. The material is stained with Giemsa or Wright [2]. The direct parasitological examination is the procedure of first choice because it is faster, less expensive and easy to perform [16]. It gives good results in initial lesions, without associated bacterial infection [2], 2) Montenegro intradermoreaction: This translates the response of cell delayed hypersensitivity [16]. It consists of intradermal injection of 0.1 ml of antigen prepared from *Leishmania* promastigotes, with a reading after 48 hours. The test is considered positive that produces an induration of 5 mm or more. However, the positivity of the test indicates that the person has already been sensitized but is not necessarily a carrier of the disease [2]; 3) Histopathological examination of the tegumentary lesion [2]. The Biopsy can be performed with a "punch" of 4 mm in diameter, or a wedge, with the use of a scalpel. In ulcerated lesions, the whole edge of the whole lesion should be preferred, This, in general, shows a tumified and hyperemic aspect [16]; 4) Serology (indirect immunofluorescence or ELISA); they have good sensitivity but can give a reaction crossed with Chagas disease and visceral Leishmaniasis, this being the cause of false-positive results, thus reducing its specificity [2].

The most commonly used techniques for antibodies are: indirect immunofluorescence (IIF), counterimmunoelectrophoresis (CIE), ELISA and Western blot. The Western blot technique has a superior sensitivity to the other serologic techniques [70.6%), a sensibility of 70.3% and a precision of 72.7%. In the immunocompetents, the specificity and sensitivity are 100% [4]; 5) Immunohistochemical techniques (immunostaining with anti *Leishmania* antibodies); they permit evidence of the parasite in histological sections; 6) Method of culture: culture takes place in Novy-MacNeal-Nicolle medium from the biopsy or aspirate [4]. They are not practical for diagnosis, especially of *Leishmania brasiliensis*, since it does not grow easily in culture media; in addition, bacterial or fungal contamination often complicate this procedure [2]. Research can be done into *Leishmania* in other affected organs such as the spleen, liver and lymph node, and whenever there is a suspected diagnosis, into the pleural fluid, bronchoalveolar lavage, intestinal biopsy, skin, etc. Hepatic and spleen biopsies are used as a last resort due to the increased risk of potentially serious complications such as hemorrhaging [4].

Cases are confirmed according to the following criteria: 1) Residence, arrival in or moving away from the area with confirmation of transmission and presence of the parasite in direct and/or indirect parasitological exams; 2) Residence, arrival in or moving away from the area with confirmation of transmission and intradermoreaction of Montenegro (MRI) positive, 3) Residence, arrival in or moving away from the area with confirmation of transmission with other methods of positive diagnosis [19].

6. Differential diagnosis

The finding of symptoms and head and neck moles in patients with Leishmaniasis, paracoccidioidomycosis and leprosy underscore the need that they all undergo an ENT evaluation. In addition to these diseases, it would be an appropriate conduct to perform complete ENT examination in all patients with some form of granulomatous disease [11]. The differential diagnosis of laryngeal ATL is made with granulomatous lesions such as tuberculosis and paracoccidioidomycosis which have a predilection for the posterior portion of the larynx [2]. The diagnosis of paracoccidioidomycosis is characterized by erosion or exulceration in the oral mucosa, with a granulous base and the presence of stippled hemorrhage (Aguiar Puo's moriform stomatitis), regional lymph node and lung involvement [8]. Syphilitic laryngitis, which fortunately nowadays is rare and appears in the tertiary stage of syphilis may present diffuse infiltrate, which subsequently undergoes ulceration [2]. Tertiary syphilis can be confirmed by histopathological exam, and shows vascular lesions and plasma cell wealth, and VDRL may be positive [8].

Neoplastic lesions of the larynx are more localized and almost always there is a report of smoking and alcoholism in the medical history [2]. Epidermoid and basal cell carcinomas usually present themselves as hardened to palpation, and are confirmed by histopathological examination [8]. Histoplasmosis in its chronic disseminated form involves mucosa in 90%, and the upper airways are affected; the larynx is very adversely affected with infiltration and edema of the laryngeal vestibule, pink nodules on an infiltrated base and granulomatous ulcerations of a granulomatous depth partially covered by yellowish-white secretions that may lead to obstructive dyspnea, requiring a tracheostomy. Generally, in this form of presentation of histoplasmosis there will be alterations in the chest X-ray associated with pulmonary symptoms, which differentiates it from Leishmaniasis. Coccidioidomycosis of the larynx is very rare in our environment. Tracheobronchial amyloidosis with involvement of the larynx is very rare; however, it may present itself with pseudotumoral, bleeding, warty lesions, with a visual appearance similar to the case presented, which can lead to obstruction of the airways [2]. The differential diagnosis is made with rhinophyma, rhinosporidiosis, entomophthoromycosis, traumatic septal perforation or because of drug use, allergic rhinitis, sinusitis, sarcoidosis, Wegner's granulomatosis and other rarer diseases.

As for lymphomas, histopathological and immunohistochemical exams will help to conclude the diagnosis. In the case of rhinophyma, there is usually a history of rosacea (acne-like lesions and telangiectasias, of long evolution). In the differential diagnosis with rhinosporidiosis what are important are: the origin (Piauí, Maranhão), the history of possible exposure to the fungus in stagnant water and dams, the presence of polyps in the nasal and ocular mucous membranes, and upper respiratory tracts. Histopathological examination shows the microorganism (sporangia of 6 to 300μm). Lesions of entomophthoromycosis present a hardened or woody consistency to palpation and histopathological and mycological exams demonstrate the presence of hyphae and isolation of the fungus in cultur medium. In the differential diagnosis with leprosy, skin sensibility tests, testing of skin bacilli in the lymph of the pinna or lesions and histopathological examination will help confirm the diagnosis. The clinical history is essential when seeking information on personal or family atopy (allergic rhinitis, bronchitis, migraine), on traumatic perforation and use of drugs. Wegner's granulomatosis and sarcoidosis are rarer diseases, and sometimes difficult to confirm. Diagnosis may be aided by observation of the involvement of other organs such as the lungs and kidneys, it being stressed that the histopathology will contribute to the diagnosis [8].

7. Co-infection *Leishmania* and HIV

ATL can modify the progression of the disease due to HIV and immunosuppression caused by this virus facilitating progression of ATL [8]. Acquired immunodeficiency syndrome is caused by a retrovirus of the *Lentiviridae* family, HIV-1 and HIV-2. Those infected with the human immunodeficiency virus (HIV) progress to severe dysfunction of the immune system, as the CD4 + T lymphocytes, one of the major target cells of the virus, are being destroyed [19]. On destroying the immune system, the so-called "opportunistic infections" are manifested as this unfolds in which infections are included, namely infections by protozoa [4]. The assessment of the set of clinical manifestations of ATL in patients with HIV indicates that there is no definition of a clinical profile that may unarguably be associated with co-infection [8]. The exponential increase in the number of cases of co-infection of *Leishmania*/ HIV, especially in the late 1990s, has undergone modifications [4]. Unusual findings can be observed in co-infected patients, suchas, for example, finding *Leishmania spp* in intact skin, and overlying a Kaposi's sarcoma lesion, or *Herpes simplex* and *Herpes zoster* lesions. There may also be involvement of the gastrointestinal tract and the respiratory tract for the coinfection of ATL/AIDS [8]. The population of drug users who inject endovenously is the main group at risk of the co-infection of *Leishmania*/HIV in Southeast Europe, and form 72% of co-infected patients [4].

8. Prevention

Several thorough trials have been carried out on the production of anti- *Leishmania* vaccines: 1) "Leishmanization" has been used empirically since the distant past by people living in endemic areas. This consists of scarification covered with virulent promastigotes of virulent to avoid the appearance of disfiguring lesions in exposed areas. 2) The association of BCG with dead *Leishmania* promastigotes. 3) Vaccines produced by molecular technology from DNA, probably the future of prophylaxis in infectious diseases in immunosuppressed patients [4].

9. Treatment

ENT activity is of primary importance [5]. The drug of first choice is the pentavalent antimonial one. With a view to standardizing the therapeutic regimen, WHO recommends that the dose of this antimonial be calculated in mg /SbV/ Kg day./ (SbV meaning a pentavalent antimonial).

There are two types of pentavalent antimonial that can be used, N-methylglucamine antimonate and sodium stibogluconate [10,16]. In all forms of mucosal involvement, the recommended dose is 20mg Sb+5/kg/day, for thirty consecutive days, preferably in a hospital environment. If healing is not complete within three months (twelve weeks) after treatment ends, the scheme should be repeated only once. Should there be no response, use one of the second choice drugs [16].

If there is no satisfactory response to the treatment with pentavalent antimony, the second choice drugs are amphotericin B and pentamidine isethionate. The injections must be made parenterally, intramuscularly (IM) or intravenously (IV), with rest after application. The IM may have the drawback of local pain. It is suggested, therefore, locations be alternated, the gluteal region being preferred.

In cases of malnourished patients with low muscle mass, and those with thrombocytopenia, the intravenous route should be given preference. This is the best route because it allows the application of large volumes without the inconvenience of local pain. The application should be slow (a minimum of 5 minutes), with a fine needle (gauge 25x7 or 25x8) and without needing to be diluted. To make it possible for rest after administration, it is generally advisable to apply the medication at the end of the day. It is worth noting that there is no difference between the IV and IM routes, with respect to the efficacy and safety of the drug [8].

The use of topical products such as paromomycin and imiquimod, associated or not with parenteral medication, have also presented preliminary satisfactory results, with cure rates ranging between 74% and 85% for the former drug, and 90% for the latter [9]. The imidazo-quinoline, approved for the treatment of genital warts, [17] stimulates the Th1 response by increasing the production of TNF-α, IFN-γ and IL-12. *In vitro*, presents anti Leishmanial activity because it also stimulates the production of nitric oxide by macrophages, thus decreasing the number of parasites. Paromomycin is an antibiotic that inhibits the mitochondrial activity of *Leishmania*. rhGM-CSF is a glycoprotein that induces the growth of colonies of granulocytes and/or macrophages, by stimulating their phagocytic and metabolic functions. For this reason, it plays an important role in the immune response against intracellular pathogens. It has been used experimentally in the treatment of some inflammatory diseases as it has an inhibitory effect on TNF-α [18].

Local treatment of small lesions may not be necessary. Larger lesions may be treated with surgical excision, curettage or cryotherapy [13]. Secondary infection may occur in 54.2% of patients and the germ most frequently found is *Staphylococcus aureus* [21], which is why local care should be prescribed such as local cleansing with soap and water and if possible compresses with KMnO (potassium permanganate in a dilution of 1/5000ml) [8, 16].

The cure criterion is defined by the regression of all signs and confirmed by ENT examination, up to 6 months after completion of the treatment regimen. In the absence of the specialist, the clinician must be trained to perform, at least, anterior rhinoscopy and oroscopy. Where there is no clinician, the patient should be referred to the service that evaluates healing. The patient should return monthly for a consultation for 3 consecutive months after the end of the treatment regimen so that the clinical cure can be evaluated.

Once cured, the patient should be monitored every 2 months, until 12 months after completing treatment [8]. The control of ATL should be tackled in a comprehensive way, in five respects: epidemiological surveillance, measures of performance in the transmission chain, educational measures, administrative measures and vaccine [9]. To reduce the lethality of these diseases, what is above all necessary is early diagnosis and the timely treatment of cases [14].

The current challenges for ATL are: a) to increase investments in seeking drugs with better efficacy, safety, low cost, ease of administration and sustainability; b) to continue to be vigilant about the adverse effects of medication; c) to expand the health network for early diagnosis and adequate treatment of cases; d) to investigate and evaluate deaths; e) to implement surveillance actions in territorial units; f) to expand the activities of epidemiological surveillance [19].

Acknowledgements

Our thanks to the Teacher Roddy Kay for his dedication in translation of this chapter.

Author details

Luiz Alberto Alves Mota[1,2]* and Roberta Correia Ribeiro Ferreira de Miranda[3]

*Address all correspondence to: luizmota10@gmail.com

1 Faculty of Medical Sciences, Universidade de Pernambuco, Brasil

2 ENT service, Hospital Universitário Oswaldo Cruz, Brasil

3 Faculty of Medical Sciences, Universidade de Pernambuco, Brasil

References

[1] Guerra JAO, Barbosa MGV, Loureiro ACSP, Coelho CP, Rosa GG, Coelho LIACR. Leishmaniose tegumentar americana em crianças: aspectos epidemiológicos de casos atendidos em Manaus, Amazonas, Brasil. Cad. Saúde Pública, Rio de Janeiro. 2007, 23(9):2215-2223.

[2] Melo SMD, Todt Neto JC, Andrade LCF. Pseudo-hemoptise por leishmaniose. Jornal de Pneumologia. 1999, 25(6):347- 350.

[3] Lessa MM, Lessa HA, Castro TWN, Oliveira A, Scherifer A, Machado P, Carvalho EM. Leishmaniose mucosa: aspectos clínicos e epidemiológicos. Rev Bras Otorrinolaringol. 2007, 73(6):843-847.

[4] Catorze MGB. Leishmaniose e SIDA. Med. Cutan. Iber. Lat. Amer. 2005, 6:237-250.

[5] Neto FXP, Rodrigues AC, Silva LL, Palheta ACP, Rodrigues LG, Silva FA. Manifestações Otorrinolaringológicas Relacionadas à Leishmaniose Tegumentar Americana: Revisão de Literatura. Arq Int Otorrinolaringol./Intl Arch Otorhinolaryngol. 2008, 12(4):531-537.

[6] Silva L, Costa HO, Duprat AC, Bairão F, Della Nina M. Granulomatose laríngea. Avaliação e métodos diagnósticos e terapêuticos em 24 casos. ACTA ORL/ Técnicas em Otorrinolaringologia. 2007, 25(1):16-23.

[7] Ministério da Saúde do Brasil. Manual de Vigilância da Leishmaniose Tegumentar Americana. 2ª ed. Brasília; 2007, 1-30.

[8] Ministério da Saúde. Secretaria de Vigilância em Saúde. Leishmaniose Tegumentar Americana. Guia de Vigilância Epidemiológica; Caderno 11.

[9] Basano SA, Camargo LMA. Leishmaniose tegumentar americana: histórico, epidemiologia e perspectivas de controle. Rev Bras Epidemiol. 2004, 7(3):328-337.

[10] Secretaria Municipal de Saúde. Recomendações para o Manejo Clínico da Leishmaniose Tegumentar e Visceral. Belo Horizonte; 2007.

[11] Fornazieri MA, Yamaguti HY, Moreira JH, Takemoto LE, Navarro PL, Heshiki RE. Manifestações Otorrinolaringológicas Mais Comuns das Doenças Granulomatosas. Arq Int Otorrinolaringol./Intl Arch Otorhinolaryngol. 2008,12(3):362-365.

[12] Focaccia R, Veronesi R. Tratado de Infectologia. 3ª edição v.2 Atheneu, São Paulo, 1997.

[13] Gomes ACA, Dias EOS, Pita Neto IC, Bezerra TP. Leishmaniose muco-cutânea: relato de caso clínico Rev.Cirurgia e Traumatologia Buco-Maxilo-Facial. 2004, 4(4):223-228.

[14] Tratamento da Leishmaniose Visceral e Leishmaniose Tegumentar Americana no Brasil Epidemiol. Serv. Saúde, Brasília, 20(1):107-110, jan – mar 2011.

[15] Leishmaniose Laríngea. Arquivos Internacionais de Otorrinolaringologia. São Paulo - Brasil, v.16, n.4, p. 523-526, out – dez 2012.

[16] Ministério da Saúde. Gerência Técnica de Doenças Transmitidas por Vetores e Antropozoonoses. Coordenação de Vigilância Epidemiológica Centro Nacional de Epidemiologia. Manual de Controle da Leishmaniose Tegumentar Americana. Fundação Nacional de Saúde Brasília, 2000.

[17] Luiz Henrique Guimarães, et al. Aspectos clínicos da Leishmaniose tegumentar. Gaz. méd. Bahia 2005;75:1(Jan-Jun):66-74.

[18] Almeida OLS, Santos JB. Avanços no tratamento da leishmaniose tegumentar do novo mundo nos últimos dez anos: uma revisão sistemática da literatura. An Bras Dermatol. 2011;86(3):497-506.

[19] Penna GO, Domingues CMAS, Siqueira JB Jr, Elkhoury ANSM, Cechinel MP, Grossi MAF, et al. Doenças dermatológicas de notificação compulsória no Brasil. An Bras Dermatol. 2011;86(5):865-77.

[20] Diniz JLCP, Costa MOR, Gonçalves DU. Mucocutaneous Leishmaniasis: clinical markers in presumptive diagnosis. Brazilian Journal of Otorhinolaryngology 77 (3) Maio/Junho 2011;77(3):380-4.

[21] Silva MS, Sousa RT, Silva EB, Guerra JAO, Gomes NM, Santana RF, Mubarac RS. Primary lesion of Mucocutaneous Leishmaniasis simulating external otitis.

[22] Nunes CS, Yoshizawa JK, Oliveira RZ, Lima AP, Oliveira LZ, Lima MVN Leishmaniose mucosa: considerações epidemiológicas e de tratamento. Rev bras med fam comunidade. Florianópolis, 2011 Jan-Mar; 6(18): 52-56.

3

The Geospatial Approach on Eco-Epidemiological Studies of Leishmaniasis

João Carlos Araujo Carreira,

Mônica de Avelar Figueiredo Mafra Magalhães and

Alba Valéria Machado da Silva

1. Introduction

1.1. Leishmaniasis

Leishmaniasis is a vector-borne disease transmitted by numerous sand fly species caused by obligate intracellular parasitic protozoa of the genus Leishmania. It can infect besides the man, a wide range of sylvatic and domestic mammal hosts producing either tegumentar or visceral lesions.

The life of *Leishmania* get going, when phlebotomine sand flies, mostly *Lutzomyia* in the New Word and *Phlebotomus* in the Old Wold, become infected during the blood meal, by ingesting infected mononuclear phagocytic cells. The amastigotes in the gut of sand flies, differentiates into promastigotes and multiply. In the *Viannia* subgenus the parasites develop in the hindgut of the vectors while in the *Leishmania* subgenus, the growth occurs in the midgut. In the insect's gut several promastigotes differentiate into metacyclic forms and migrate to the proboscis.

The parasites are transmitted by the bite of infected female of phlebotomine sand flies during the blood meal when the insects inject from their proboscis, the metacyclic promastigotes. Those forms are capable to survive inside the phagolysosomes of macrophages and other types of mononuclear phagocytic cells. Once inside of the cells, promastigotes differentiate into amastigotes, a stage that is associated mammal tissues. The amastigotes multiply by simple division and continue to infect other mononuclear phagocytic cells (Figure 1).

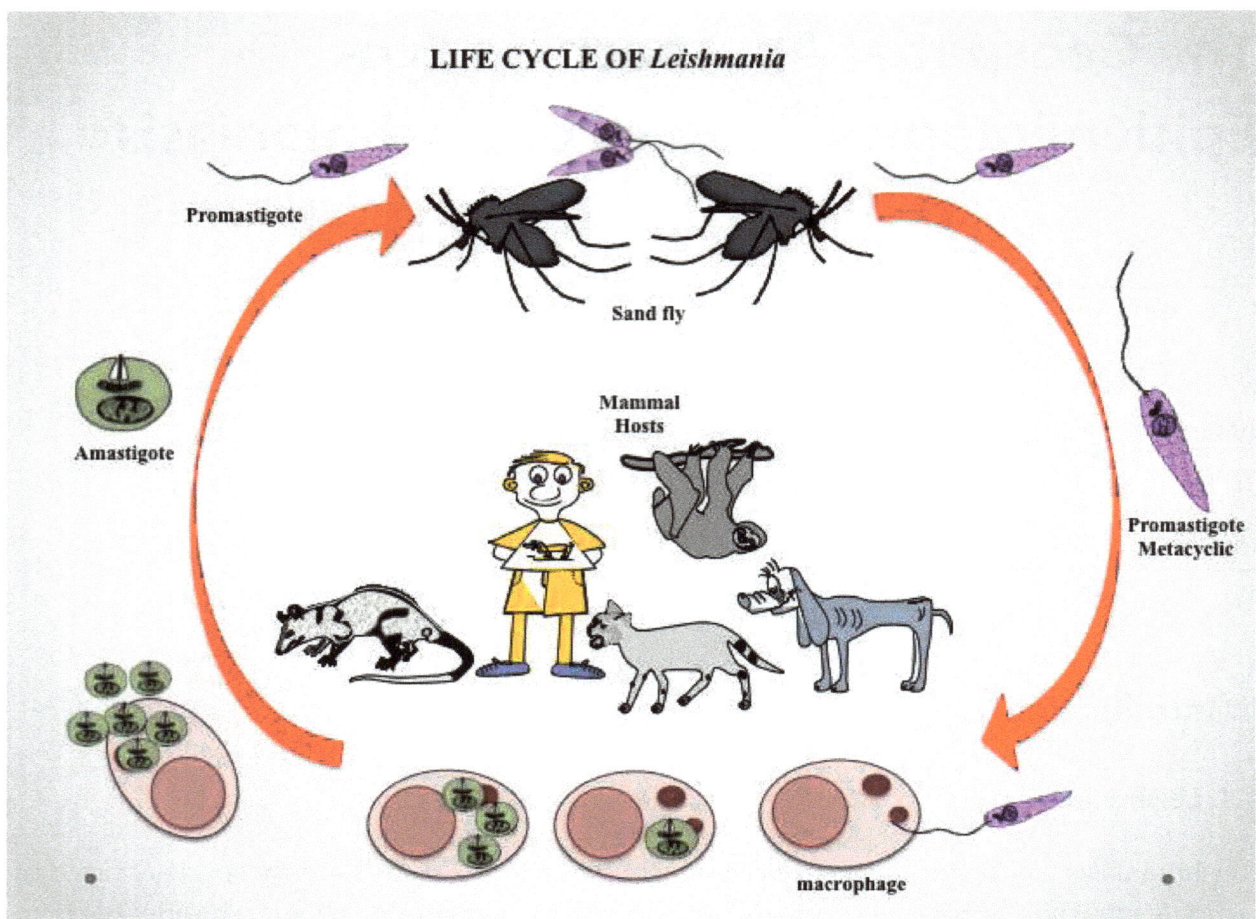

Figure 1. Life cycle of *Leishmania*.

Depending on the parasite and host species in addition to numerous factors related to the hosts' genetic background, the progress of the infection might be influenced, determining if the patient will become symptomatic or sick, eventually resulting in cutaneous or visceral leishmaniasis.

The geographical distribution of leishmaniasis includes 88 countries and almost 350 million of peoples live in these areas where the disease has been considered one of the most severe problem of public health. The majority of the countries affected are in the tropics and sub-tropics, consequently leishmaniasis covers a wide range from rain forests in Central and South America to deserts in West Asia [1,2] (Table 1 and 2).

Depending on the eco-epidemiological conditions, the leishmaniasis can present sylvatic or domestic transmission cycles (Figure 2). Among the most important factors composing those conditions, we could mention the environmental characteristics (biotic and abiotic factors) as well as the parasite, vector and host species involved.

The sylvatic cycles are quite ancient; they have been molded for millions of years before the emergence of man, through co evolutionary relationships among the parasite, vectors and

SPECIES	CLINICAL FORMS	REGION	VECTOR	HOST
Leishmania major	Cutaneous	Asia, Africa	*Phlebotomus papatasi*	Human, rodents
Leishmania tropica	Cutaneous	Europe, Asia, Africa	*P.sergenti*	Human, dogs, rock-hyraxes
Leishmania aethiopica	Cutaneous, mucocutaneous	Africa	*P. longipes, P. pedifer*	Human, hyracoids
Leishmania infantum	Visceral	Europe, Asia, Africa	*P. perniciosus, P. ariasi*	Human, dogs, sylvatic canids
Leishmania donovani	Visceral, PKDL	Asia, Africa	*P. argentipes, P. orientalis*	Human
Leishmania siamensis	Visceral	Europe, Asia, and North America	?	Human, horse, cows

Table 1. The main species of *Leishmania* from the Old World: with the correspondent clinical forms, regions of occurrence, vectors and mammal hosts. (? - Not known).

SPECIES	CLINICAL FORMS	REGION	VECTOR	HOST
L (V) braziliensis	Cutaneous, mucocutaneous	South and Central America	*Nyssomyia intermedia, N. whitmani, Migonemyia migonei*	Human, terrestrial rodents, marsupials, equines, dogs, cats
L (V) peruviana	Cutaneous	South America	*Lutzomyia peruensis, L. verrucarum*	Human, dogs, rodents* opossums*
L (V) guyanensis	Cutaneous	South America	*L. umbratilis*	Human, sloth, anteater, rodents, opossums
L (V) panamensis	Cutaneous	South and Central America	*L. panamensis, L. trapidoi*	Human, sloth, arboreal animals, monkeys, rodents, hunting dogs
L (L) mexicana	Cutaneous, diffuse cutaneous	South, Central and North America	*L. olmeca*	Human, forest rodents
L (L) amazonensis	Cutaneous, diffuse cutaneous	South America	*L. flaviscutellata, L. panamensis*	Human, forest rodents, marsupials, fox
L (L) pifanoi	Cutaneous, diffuse cutaneous	South America (Venezuela)	*L. flaviscutellata* *	Human, Rodents?
L (L) venezuelensis	Cutaneous	South America (Venezuela)	*L. olmeca* *	Human, domestic cats, rodents?
L (L) infantum	Visceral	South, Central and North America	*L. longipalpis, L. cruzi, L. evansi*	Human, sylvatic canids and felids, opossums, dogs

Table 2. The main species of *Leishmania* from the New World: with the correspondent clinical forms, regions of occurrence, vectors and mammal hosts. (*- Putative).

mammal hosts. Mammal reservoirs and insect vectors have been continuously maintaining the parasites in equilibrium without human involvement.

In our time sylvatic cycles are restricted to wild places where disease outbreaks can eventually occur when people make incursions or settlements in those areas.

Concerning to domestic cycle an intra-domiciliary type (figure 2) of transmission is characteristic and the principal components for the disease establishment and maintenance, are the occurrence of vectors with the capacity of domiciliary human landing/biting, besides humans and domestic animals as mammal hosts [2].

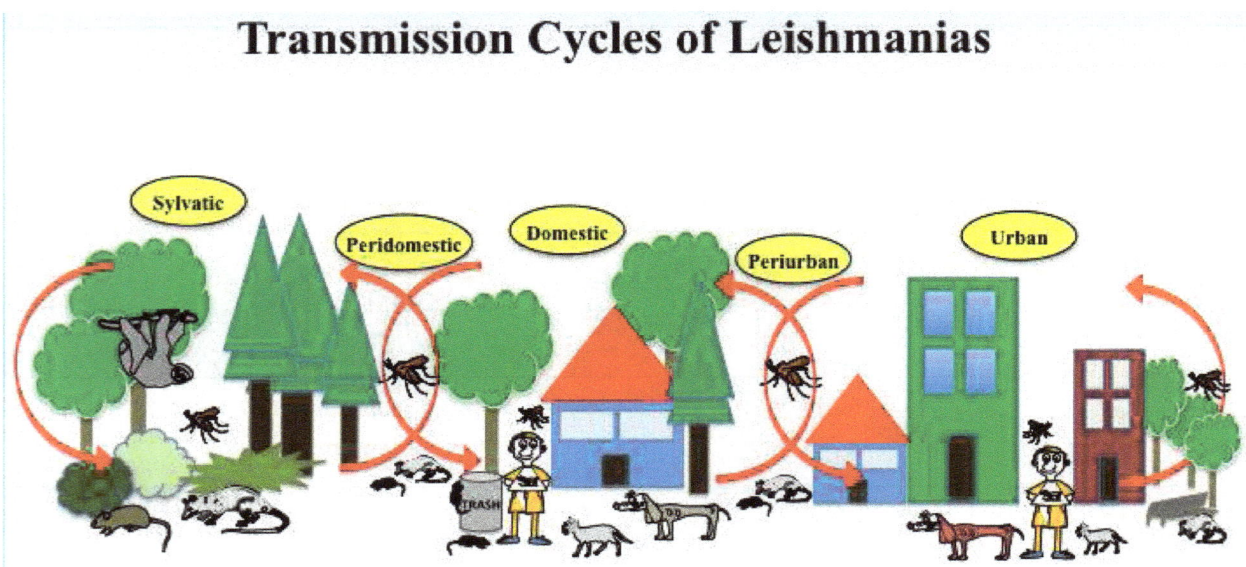

Figure 2. Schematic drawing: eco-epidemiological picture of transmission cycles of Leishmanias.

The earliest steps for the origin of domestic cycles of leishmaniasis probably started around 12.000 years ago, when the ancient human populations began to practice sedentary agriculture and also have introduced domestic animals and livestock causing drastic alterations on the natural habitats.

As a result of such environmental modifications, a large avoidance of the sylvatic animals occurred from the surroundings of human habitations; that together with the insertion of new potential mammal hosts gave rise to a progressive adaptation process in some populations of sylvatic vectors toward a domiciliary behavior. Then little by little certain sand flies populations adopted some introduced species as their new feeding sources [2-4].

In our time, after thousands of years of interaction with domestic mammals as hosts, some vectors hosts species that originally were totally sylvatic, have evolved to exist even in great urban areas, permitting the transmission of the parasite and its maintenance practically restricted to the participation of domestic and/or synanthropic hosts, sand fly and the man [5-7].

So, actually the eco-epidemiological picture of leishmaniasis could be represented as a complex puzzle where each piece is formed by the interaction of a parasite species with their correlated hosts and vectors, in a determined habitat. Nevertheless, it should not be considered as a static process because the occurrence of other parasite species, besides the action of the temporal component they can play a very important role, by influencing the whole process making it possible the occurrence of a variety of transmission patterns that sometimes may result in disease.

Considering the several difficulties to elaborate Leismaniasis control plans, probably the most significant is the high complexity of eco-epidemiological features of the disease. They are greatly influenced by the wide distribution of the parasites, the existence of a large variety of vector species in addition to the pressure of local environmental factors affecting the populations of human hosts, vectors and reservoirs [3-4,8].

The leishmaniasis control measures in use, including spraying to eliminate the adult forms of the vector, diagnosis and treatment of human patients and elimination of seropositive dogs, have failed in preventing new epidemics [9,10].

Therefore, a spatial and temporal approach to analyze endemic foci of the disease could be very a useful method to understand the dynamic of transmission [11,12].

1.2. Methods

Geographic information systems (GIS) and remote sensing (RS) are important tools that comprise computational systems, which permit to map and analyze environmental factors related to the spatial and temporal distribution environmental components that affect the distribution of diseases [12]. The availability of climatic, geological and phytographic digital data and the accessibility of GIS software also have permitted the implementation of several epidemiological studies in relation to ecological factors and disease prediction, as well as have been providing evidences that its use is indispensable before the elaboration of control plans [5, 11,12].

As examples of GIS software we could mention: ArcGis, TerraView, TerraHidro, Gvsig, etc.

The Remote Sensing is also an important data resource for presentation of vegetation, land cover and land use as well as the categorization of the habitats and population density of insect vectors, parasite and reservoir hosts [12,13].

An important feature available in GIS methodology consists of Kernel's method. It is considered a new class of pattern analysis algorithms also utilized in GIS, which can operate on a wide-ranging types of data and relationships. Correlation, factor, cluster and discriminant analysis are just some of the types of pattern analysis tasks that can be performed on data as diverse as sequences, text, images, graphs and of course vectors. The method provides also a natural way to merge and integrate different types of data [5,14].

Kernel density estimators belong to a class of estimators called *non-parametric* density estimators. In comparison to parametric estimators where the estimator has a fixed functional form (structure) and the parameters of this function are the only information we need to store, Non-parametric estimators have no fixed structure and depend upon all the data points to reach an estimate [15].

Differently from conventional histograms where it is necessary to sub-divide the whole data in equal intervals and also to determine the end point of each interval, producing a not smooth representation. On the kernel method those problems can be minimized by the production of a kind of smooth histogram [15] (Figure 3).

HISTOGRAM METHOD   KERNEL METHOD

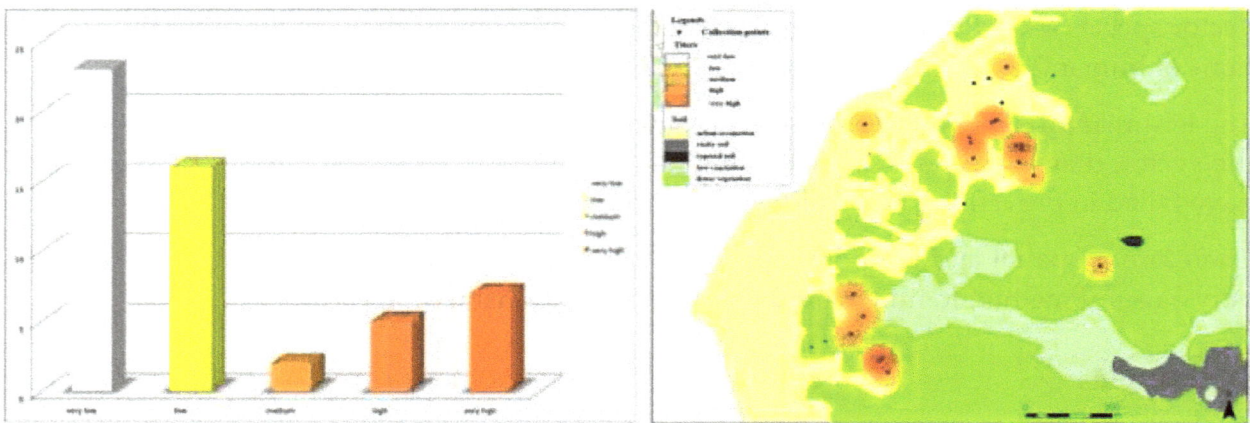

Figure 3. Depiction of doghouses geo-referenced and canine leishmaniasis cases in function of serological titers, represented by histograms and Kernel method (ArcGis).

Other attributes of GIS methodology very useful to the study epidemiology of leishmaniasis is the possibility to create digital maps after performing cluster analysis on the populations of vectors and mammal hosts, including the man; and also to represent circumscribed areas in the same maps, indicating potential regions of vector flight or putative hosts' home ranges [11,14,16] (Figure 4 and 5).

Clustering is a method also applied in GIS, and comprises a common technique for statistical data analysis used in many fields, including machine learning, data mining, pattern recognition image analysis and bioinformatics.

So, the use of new technologies based on eco-epidemiological indicators is essential on the identification of circumstances that impair the spread and maintenance of the disease and certainly could be used to set priorities for implementing disease control measures, thus reducing operational costs and increasing their effectiveness.

In conclusion, the notorious difficulty in controlling the transmission of leishmaniasis, a disease caused by a parasitic protozoa described at 1903 and that still persists currently showing a re-emerging pattern in some places, indicates that such parasites have been developing a great number of evolutionary advantages and despite all the efforts of scientists an effective control was not achieved yet. It is important to remember that those organisms

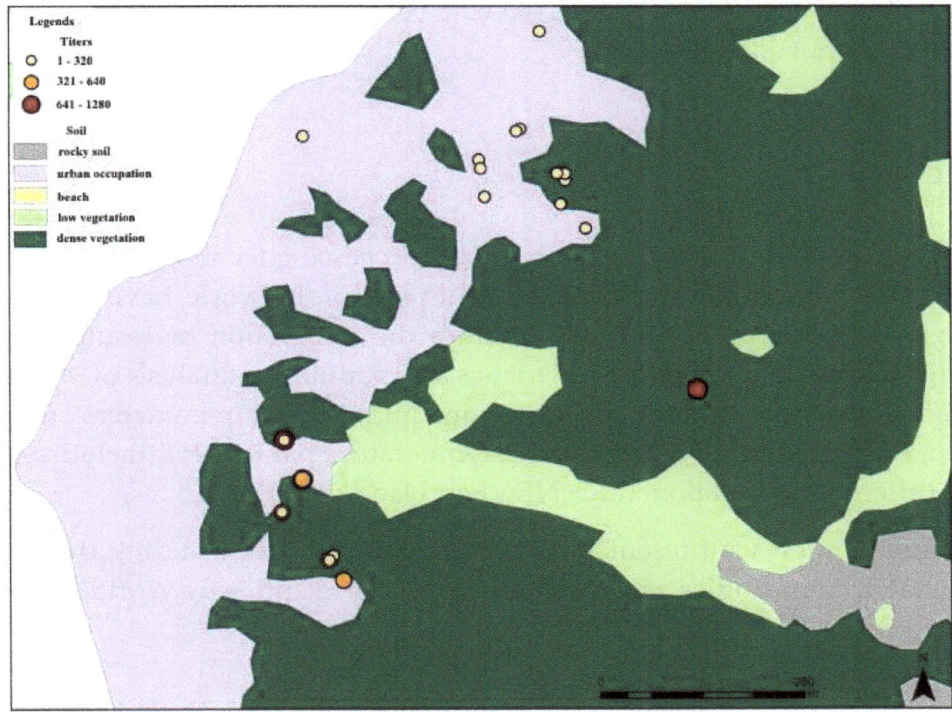

Figure 4. Vegetation, land cover and land use patterns and general distribution of canine leishmaniasis cases, with the respective serological titers, from an endemic focus in Brazil (ArcGis).

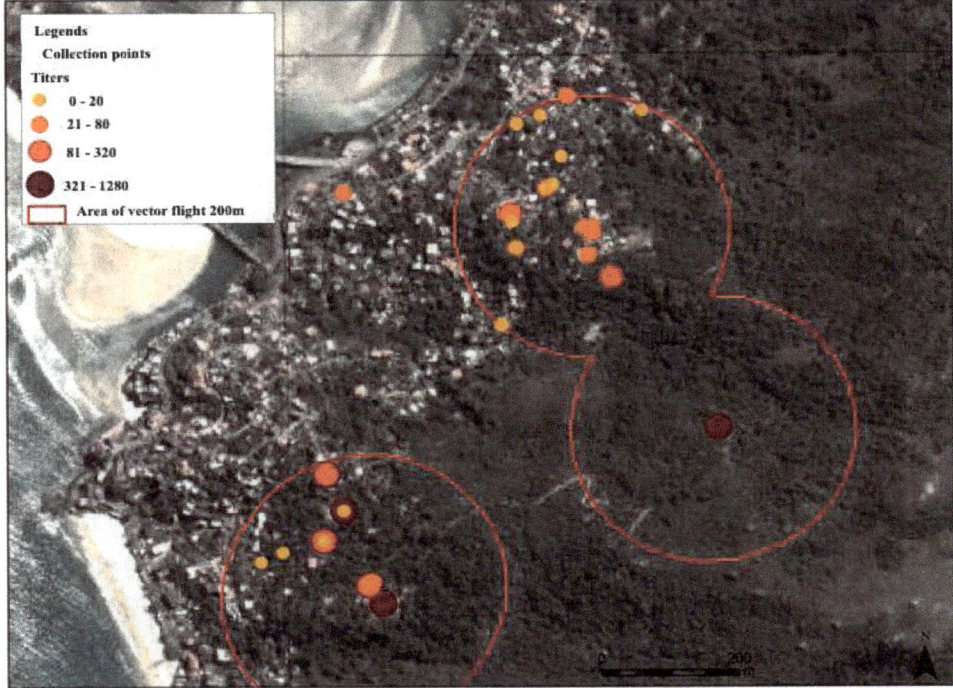

Figure 5. Visual interpretation of an aerial mosaic of photographs from an endemic focus in Brazil, showing the area of influence of the vector flight and the general distribution of canine *Leishmania* infections in addition to the serological titers (source: website of the Pereira Passos Institute http://www.armazemdedados.rio.rj.gov.br/).

have been dwelling on earth for millions of years before of us and it certainly represents that they have skills we not elucidated yet.

2. Overview

The first studies on leishmaniasis utilizing the geoprocessing technology were carried out in the 90s. After that, several groups from different parts of the world have studied important epidemiological aspects of this disease through the integration of results obtained from serological techniques, biological characteristics and population analysis of vectors and hosts with environmental factors such as: elevation, temperature parameters, mean monthly precipitation, relative humidity, land surface temperature parameters (including amplitude), normalized-difference vegetation index NDVI and land cover.

In the following section we presented a chronological review including the more relevant papers, originated from studies achieved in the Old World and New World, using the above-mentioned approach.

3. Leishmaniasis in the Old World

Elnaiem 1998 [17] in Sudan, investigating the importance of the effect of environmental data (obtained from digital records collected by satellites), such as: rainfall, minimum and maximum temperatures, soil class, vegetation and land-surface-temperature indices, on a population of *Phlebotomus orientalis*, observed a significant association of this sand fly with the presence of the tree species *Acacia seyal* and *Balanites aegyptiaca* and with the black cotton (vertisolic) soils of eastern Sudan. The authors also showed that positive sites were found to have significantly higher annual mean maximum and minimum daily temperatures and the annual mean maximum normalized-difference vegetation index (NDVI) value was also found to be significantly higher in these in comparison with those places where no *P. orientalis* were found.

Bern et al 2005 [18] studied the spatial patterns and risk factors for anthroponotic visceral leishmaniasis in Bangladesh. Integrating the GIS approach with data related to history, active case detection, and serologic screening, from residents had kala-azar, they observed that the risk was highest for persons 3–45 years of age, and no significant difference by sex. Considering the age-adjusted multivariable models, 3 factors were identified: proximity to a previous kala-azar patient, bed net use in summer and cattle per 1,000 m2. The authors observed no difference by income, education, or occupation; land ownership or other assets; housing materials and condition; or keeping goats or chickens inside bedrooms. The results confirmed a strong clustering occurrence and suggested that insecticide-treated nets could be effective in preventing kala-azar.

In this study, the households were mapped by a GPS and the data were processed into ArcGis. Through the GIS data, distances were determined from the household to the closest kala-azar cases in the previous year. Kernel density estimation was used to estimate cattle per 1,000 m^2 in order to calculate the effect of cows, oxen or calves on the kala-azar risk for nearby residents.

Ryan et al 2006 [19], studying visceral leishmaniasis in Kenya, used *Leishmania*-specific antibodies to estimate the seroprevalence and GIS and spatial clustering techniques to study the presence of spatial clusters in two villages. In only one of the villages, significant associations among seropositivity and house construction, age, and proximity to domestic animal enclosures were found. In the same place, a significant spatial cluster of VL was found and the spatial distribution of cases in the two villages was different with respect to risk factors, such as presence of domestic animals. The authors suggested that disease control efforts could be focused on elimination of sand fly habitat, placement of domestic animal enclosures, and targeted use of insecticides.

Sudhakar et al., 2006 [20] in a study carried out in India, analyzed in Silicon graphic image processing system, using ERDAS software, some data obtained from a remote sensing satellite.

The GIS functions were applied to quantify the remotely sensed landscape proportions of 5 km^2 buffer in determined places of high occurrence of sand flies in endemic and nonendemic areas. Through the combination of remote sensing (RS) and geographical information system (GIS) they developed landscape predictors of sand fly abundance an indicator of human vector contact and as a measure of risk prone areas.

It was indicated, that the environmental factors such as type and density of settlements, proximity to these with that of water bodies, marshy areas with succulent weed cover and also crops of high succulent in nature like sugarcane, bananas coupled with local prevailing conditions had definitely interactive influencing effect of vector density and also incidents of vector borne diseases.

Rossi et al 2007 [21] in Southern Italy, applied GIS and SR to analyze the distribution of the *Leishmania infantum-Phlebotomus perniciosus* parasite-vector system in relation to environmental features of two opposite sides (coastal and Apennine) of an area of intense transmission of human and canine leishmaniasis.

The cumulative density, a term determined by the authors as the number of specimens/m2 of sticky trap/two nights, of this vector species was related as significantly more abundant in the coastal side. The authors suggested that the predominance of green vegetated environments in the coastal side, in contrast with the predominance of urban environment in the Apennine side, could be responsible for the different *P. perniciosus* densities between the areas.

Ready 2010 [22] reported that climate change could affect leishmaniasis distribution, by the effect of temperature on parasite development in insect vector, or because of the effect of environmental variation on the range and seasonal abundances of the sand fly species.

He also suggested that bio-climate zones and their vegetation indicators vary regionally, and continuing climate change could alter the patterns of land cover and land use. Thus, the GIS-based spatial modeling of the Emerging Diseases in a changing European Environment was providing analysis of alterations in climate and land cover and their effects on sand flies.

Bhunia et al 2010 [23] in India, through satellite imagery complemented with a GIS database, estimated parameters such as altitude, temperature, humidity, rainfall and the normalized difference vegetation index (NDVI) for correlation with the distribution of Kala-azar. They observed that the highest prevalence was below 150 m of altitude with very few cases located above the 300 m level and a low NDVI value ranges correlated with a high occurrence of the disease. They also showed, that most of the cases occurred in non-vegetative areas or low density vegetation zones highlighting that the low density vegetation zones were significant for the *P. argentipes* vector distribution in the disturbed areas.

Khanal et al 2010 [24] in Nepal, merged results from a serological test made in humans and domestic animals with GIS technology to evaluate the exposure to *L. donovani* on two populations in a recent focus of visceral leishmaniasis (VL). They used a Poisson regression model to evaluate the risk of infection in humans associated with seropositive animals in the proximities of the household. It was also demonstrated that seropositive animals and humans were spatially clustered and the presence of positive goats, past VL cases and the proximity to a forest island increased the risk of occurrence of seropositivity in humans. The authors also suggested that goats might play some role in the distribution of *L. donovani*, in the VL focus studied.

Bhattarai et al 2010 [25] also in Nepal, with the purpose of determining possible reasons for persistence of VL during inter-epidemic periods, they mapped cases *Leishmania* infections among apparently healthy persons and animals in an area of active VL transmission. The results of a bivariate K-function analysis showed the occurrence of spatial clustering of *Leishmania* spp.–positive persons and domestic animals, addition the investigation through classification tree, determined that the proximity of *Leishmania* spp.–positive goats ranked as the first risk factor for *Leishmania* infection among persons.

Salahi-Moghaddam et al 2010 [26] in Iran performed a serological study on a population of dogs from an endemic area.

No significant correlation between topographic conditions and the prevalence of positive cases was observed after regression analysis. Nevertheless, positive correlations were found in relation to the amount of rainfall, between infected dogs with high titers (≥1/640) and the number of days with temperatures below 0 °C during one year. The same correlation was observed when they were considered past meteorological records, conversely the humidity showed an inversely correlated with the *Leishmania* infections.

The authors suggested that in mapped areas the prevailing low temperatures could represent an important factor influencing the distribution of leishmaniasis.

More recently, Bhunia et al 2013 [27] in India, assumed that the utilization of GIS and RS technologies on the control of VL dates back to the late 2000s and those control programs have mostly focused on mapping prevalence and association of *Phlebotomus argentipes* habitats, predicting transmission risk in relation to ecological transformation.

Besides, the authors proposed that the multiplicity of satellite and sensors technics offer relevant data to assembly spatial, spectral and temporal scales. They also argued about the advantages of remotely sensed imagery technology in studies in sand fly ecology and vector-borne diseases, by the generation of a proper household breeding documentation at higher spatial resolution.

4. Leishmaniasis in the New World

One of the first works, carried out in the New World that have exploited SR- satellite imagery technology on an epidemiological survey with American Cutaneous Leishmaniasis, was presented by Miranda et al 1996 [28] in Brazil. In that study, the data were plotted on a TM-LANDSAT image a color composition of bands 3, 4 and 5 (see supplementary information on table 3,4 and 5) that were considered useful to identify the relevant vegetation (shrubs and trees) within the boundaries of the studied areas and in their neighborhood about 250 meters from the perimeter of each area. It was suggested, the use of means qualified as presenting a larger view of a geographical area, composed the advantages of remote satellite sensing to study this endemic foci.

Lima et al 2002 [29] also in Brazil, studied the geographical distribution of notified human TL cases and correlated with the occurrence of the remaining vegetation and water streams, through satellite monitoring (LANDSAT level 4).

They observed that the geographical distribution of cases displayed a higher concentration in the northern and western regions of the studied area and a close relationship between TL and modified native forest areas, gallery forest areas or the remnants of both.

Landsat 4-5 Thematic Mapper (TM) and Landsat 7 Enhanced Thematic Mapper Plus (ETM+)		
Band	Wavelength	Attributes
Band 1 - blue	0.45-0.52	Bathymetric mapping, differentiating soil from vegetation and deciduous from coniferous vegetation
Band 2 - green	0.52-0.60	Highlights peak vegetation, useful for assessing plant vigor
Band 3 - red	0.63-0.69	Distinguish vegetation slopes
Band 4 - Near Infrared	0.77-0.90	Accentuates biomass content and coastlines
Band 5 - Short-wave Infrared	1.55-1.75	Categorizes wetness matter of soil and vegetation; permeates thin clouds
Band 6 - Thermal Infrared	10.40-12.50	Thermal mapping and predictable soil wetness
Band 7 - Short-wave Infrared	2.09-2.35	Hydrothermally transformed rocks related to mineral deposits
Band 8 - Panchromatic (Landsat 7 only)	.52-.90	15 meter resolution, sharper image definition

Table 3. Parameters utilized on Landsat 4-5 Thematic Mapper (TM) and Landsat 7 Enhanced Thematic Mapper Plus (ETM+) methodologies (based on the data obtained from the website http://landsat.usgs.gov).

Landsat 8 Operational Land Imager (OLI) and Thermal Infrared Sensor (TIRS)		
Band	Wavelength	Attributes
Band 1 – coastal aerosol	0.43-0.45	coastal and aerosol analyzes
Band 2 – blue	0.45-0.51	Bathymetric mapping, characterizing soil from vegetation and deciduous from coniferous vegetation
Band 3 - green	0.53-0.59	Highlights peak vegetation, which is functional for plant vigor assessing
Band 4 - red	0.64-0.67	Distinguishes vegetation slopes
Band 5 - Near Infrared (NIR)	085.-0.88	Highlights biomass and coastlines
Band 6 - Short-wave Infrared (SWIR) 1	1.57-1.65	Distinguishes wetness content of soil and vegetation; infiltrates thin clouds
Band 7 - Short-wave Infrared (SWIR) 2	2.11-2.29	Enriched wetness content of soil and vegetation and thin cloud infiltration
Band 8 - Panchromatic	.50-.68	15 meter resolution, intense image definition
Band 9 – Cirrus	1.36 -1.38	Increased detection of cirrus cloud pollution
Band 10 – TIRS 1	10.60 – 11.19	100 meter resolution, thermal mapping and predictable soil wetness
Band 11 – TIRS 2	11.5-12.51	100 meter resolution, enhanced thermal mapping and predictable soil wetness

Table 4. Parameters utilized on Landsat 8 Operational Land Imager (OLI) and Thermal Infrared Sensor (TIRS) methodologies (based on the data obtained from the website http://landsat.usgs.gov).

Landsat Multi Spectral Scanner (MSS)			
Landsat MSS 1, 2,3 Spectral Bands	Landsat MSS 4,5 Spectral Bands	Wavelength	Attributes
Band 4 - green	Band 1 - green	0.5-0.6	Sediment-laden water, delimits areas of shallow water
Band 5 - red	Band 2 - red	0.6-0.7	Cultural features
Band 6 - Near Infrared	Band 3 - Near Infrared	0.7-0.8	Vegetation boundary between land and water, and natural features of landscape
Band 7 - Near Infrared	Band 4 - Near Infrared	0.8-1.1	Infiltrates atmospheric cloud over best, highlights vegetation, boundary between land and water, and natural features of landscape

Table 5. Parameters utilized on Landsat Multi Spectral Scanner (MSS) method (based on the data obtained from the website http://landsat.usgs.gov).

Peterson et al 2004 [30] investigates the potential of ecological niche modeling techniques for interpolating into unsampled areas in order to understand the geographic distributions of vector species. They used multiple subsamples from accessible distributional points to analyze the question of how much sampling is needed to assemble a suitable distributional interpretation for vector species.

The Genetic algorithm for rule-set prediction (GARP) was utilized for modeling the ecological niches. The authors inferred that GARP associates ecological characteristics of known occurrence points to those randomly sampled from the rest of the study region, pursuing the development of a series of decision rules that can best summarize those factors related with the presence of species.

They also demonstrated that moderate sampling densities at sample sizes that possibly could characterize many epidemiological studies, including the distributions of vector or reservoir were sufficient to produce excellent briefs of the geographic distributions of species permits development of geographic predictions for poorly known species to promote the knowledge about geographic aspects of disease systems.

Carneiro et al 2004 [31] in Brazil, used geo-technologies including satellite images, as normalized difference vegetation index (NDVI), in the collection and analysis of epidemiological data from an LV endemic area. It was observed that, the power of specific variable such as: demographic density, age, occurrence of sand flies, contaminated dogs, and human living in specific area, as well as the practical value of using NDVI values to identify risk areas.

Salomón et al 2006 [32] in Argentine, utilized the RS to study the spatial distribution of Phlebotominae associated with a focus of tegumentary leishmaniasis. Satellite images were used to estimate the influence of the maximal and minimal flow of a river present on the area of study, on the transmission of the disease. The probable correlation with the gallery forest was also rated.

The images were obtained from LANDSAT 5 TM and 7 ETM, they were georreferenced using satellite ephemeris and the nearest-neighbor method. The Band 5 was also used to discriminate areas covered by the river, and the neighboring the land uncovered of vegetation trough visual identification.

The authors concluded that the fishing spots were significantly overflowed during the transmission peak because the spatial restricted flood could concentrate vectors, reservoirs, and humans in high places.

They also suggested through both spatial distribution of vectors and remote sensing data the higher transmission risk in the area it is still related with the gallery forest, despite of the urban influence.

Margonari et al 2006 [5] in Brazil, applied the GIS methodology integrated with demographic, socio-economic and environmental data to study some aspects of the epidemiology of a visceral leishmaniasis focus.

It was observed that among biogeographic parameters such as: altitude, area of vegetation influence, hydrographic, and areas of poverty, only altitude showed to influence emergence of leishmaniasis because most canine and human cases of leishmaniasis cases were localized between 780 and 880 m above the sea level and at these same altitudes, a large number of phlebotomine sand flies were collected.

Nieto et al 2006 [33] also in Brazil, used models developed within a GIS employing Genetic Algorithm Rule-Set Prediction (GARP) and the growing degree day (GDD)-water budget (WB) concept to predict the distribution and potential risk of visceral leishmaniasis (VL).

It was described a high and moderate prevalence sites for VL were significantly related to areas of high and moderate risk prediction. Indeed the area expected by the GARP model, hinged on the number of pixels that overlapped among eleven annual model years and the quantity of potential generations per year that could be completed by the *Lu. longipalpis-L. chagasi* system by GDD-WB analysis.

In both the GARP and the GDD-WB prediction models suggested that the highest VL risk was characterized by a semi-arid and hot climate (Caatinga), but the risk in the interior forest and the Cerrado was lower and the coastal forest was predicted as a low-risk area due to the unsuitable conditions for the vector and VL transmission.

Neto et al 2009 [34] in Brazil, applied GIS and SR to examine factors associated with the incidence of urban VL. They observed that the annual incidence rates were related to socioeconomic and demographic indicators as well as the vegetation index.

The highest incidence occurred in the peripheral areas of the city and areas with high population growth and abundant vegetation. On the other hand the percentage of households with piped water was inversely associated with the disease incidence.

The authors conclude that spatial distribution of the disease in the area was heterogeneous, and the incidence was associated with the peripheral neighborhoods fullest vegetation cover, considered subject to anthropic action.

Shimabukuro et al 2010 [35] in Brazil, utilized GIS and SR to study the geographical distribution of American cutaneous leishmaniasis and its phlebotomine vectors and generate risk maps. They observed that generally, the sand fly vector species evaluated have presented unique and heterogeneous distributions, although often overlapped. Numerous sand fly species were highly localized, while the others were much more largely spread.

The authors emphasized the complexity and geographical pattern of ACL transmission in the region.

Valderrama-Ardila et al 2010 [36] in Colombia, evaluate through spatial analysis, the environmental risk factors for CL. The applicant predictor variables were land use, elevation, and climatic (mean temperature and precipitation).

They observed that incidence of the disease was higher in townships with mean temperatures in the middle of the county's range. The frequency was independently associated with forest or shrubs and lower population density. The coverage of forest or shrub have not presented main changes over time.

The results confirmed the effect of weather and land use in leishmaniasis transmission.

Silva et al 2011 [14] in Brazil, studied a dog population from an endemic focus of LV. Through GIS and SR and applying kernel density estimator with Gaussian function and smooth kernel of 100 m radius, they observed local variations related to infection the incidence and distribution of serological titers, i.e. high titers were noted close to areas with preserved vegetation, while low titers were more frequent in areas where people kept chickens.

The authors conclude that the environment plays an important role in generating relatively protected areas within larger endemic regions, but it could also contribute to the creation of hotspots with clusters of comparatively high serological titers indicating a high level of transmission compared with neighboring areas.

Cluster analysis of the serological titers in dogs in the study area showed a non-random distribution, demonstrating that the patterns of transmission of canine VL can undergo local alterations, producing hotspots where the risk of infection was very high compared to neighboring areas.

It was suggested the possibility to predict the specific places of high-risk VL transmission within an endemic area through the mapping of canine serological titers.

Almeida et al 2011 [37] in Brazil, used spatial analysis to identify regions at highest risk of VL in an urban area. They showed from kernel ratios results, that peripheral census tracts were the most heavily affected. The spatial analysis showed that local clusters of high incidence of VL could change their locations depending on the time, suggesting that the pattern of VL is not static, and the disease may occasionally spread to other areas.

The authors also observed a spatial correlation between VL rates and all socioeconomic and demographic indicators evaluated, such as: 1) illiteracy rate; 2) children less than five years of age as a percentage of the total population; 3) mean income of heads-of-households; 4) percentage of permanent private households connected to the water supply; 5) percentage of households with regular garbage collection; and 6) percentage of permanent private households connected to the sewage system.

Foley et al 2012 [38], created a very useful tool that comprises a new map service within VectorMap (www.vectormap.org). Using the words of the authors, "It allows free public online access to global sand fly, tick and mosquito collection records and habitat suitability models, given the short home range of sand flies, combining remote sensing and collection point data, offering a powerful insight into the environmental determinants of sand fly distribution.

Sand fly Map uses Microsoft Silverlight and ESRI's ArcGIS Server 10 software platform to present disease vector data and relevant remote sensing layers in an online geographical information system format. Users can view the locations of past vector collections and the results of models that predict the geographic extent of individual species. Collection records are searchable and downloadable, and Excel collection forms with drop down lists, and Excel charts to country, are available for data contributors to map and quality control their data.

Sand fly Map makes accessible, and adds value to, the results of past sand fly collecting efforts. It is detailed the workflow for entering occurrence data from the literature to Sand fly Map, using an example for sand flies from South America.

The proper use of a global positioning system (GPS) device and a detailed text description of the locality are encouraged to minimize this uncertainty [39]. The calculation of spatial uncertainty, for example for Martins et al [40], allows data to be matched to appropriate resolution remote sensing data, for modeling or other spatial analyses".

Saraiva et al 2012 [41] in Brazil, utilizing GIS methodology associated with serological tests, studied a VL focus. They described the occurrence of serologically positive dogs was spread out throughout all geographical area. The places of concentration of serologically positive dogs appeared both in risk areas and outside them.

Overlaying the map of the human and canines cases with factors traditionally related to VL as vegetation, hydrography, and areas of poverty, it was not possible identify a spatial correlation between them, which demonstrates that in urban areas there are still unknown parameters.

Souza et al 2012 [42] in Brazil, carried out a space-time analysis of AVL cases in humans. They conclude by the time series analysis, a positive tendency over the period analyzed, completing that the disease was clustered in the Southwest side of area of study, suggesting it could require special attention with regard to control and prevention measures.

Finally, González et al 2013 [43] in Colombia, have surveyed the spatial distribution of two vector species of *L. infantum*, after predicting its future dispersal into climate change situations to establish the potential dissemination of the disease. They used ecological niche models through the Maxent software and 13 Worldclim bioclimatic coverages. Through predictions for the pessimistic CSIRO A2 scenario, was calculated the higher increase in temperature in function of non-emission reduction, and by the optimistic Hadley B2 Scenario, was predicted the minimum increase in temperature.

Concerning the climate change projections, they observed an overall reduction in the spatial distribution of the two vector species, progressing a shift in the vertical distribution for one species and restricting the other to certain regions at the sea level.

The authors predicted an outcome for VL vectors in Colombia and suggested that Changes in spatial distribution patterns could be affecting local abundances due to climatic pressures on vector populations thus reducing the incidence of human cases.

4. Conclusion

In conclusion, the employment of a geospatial approach to interpret eco-epidemiological phenomena related to vector borne diseases have been used for some groups in significant studies. The possibilities of use of that very effective tool, considering the advances on computational knowledge and the possibilities of accessing information at a global level, make this technology indispensable to make a broad analysis objecting the optimizing of planning control campaigns.

Author details

João Carlos Araujo Carreira[1*], Mônica de Avelar Figueiredo Mafra Magalhães[2] and Alba Valéria Machado da Silva[3]

*Address all correspondence to: carreira@ioc.fiocruz.br; jcacarreira@gmail.com

1 Núcleo IOC- Jacarepaguá/Fundação Oswaldo Cruz, Rio de Janeiro, Brazil

2 Laboratório de Geoprocessamento, Fundação Oswaldo Cruz, Rio de Janeiro, Brazil

3 Laboratório de Bioquímica de Proteínas e Peptídeos, Fundação Oswaldo Cruz, Rio de Janeiro, Brazil

References

[1] TDR for research on diseases of poverty. http://www.who.int/tdr/research/ntd/leishmaniasis (accessed 04/03/2013).

[2] Lainson R, Rangel E. *Lutzomyia longipalpis* and the ecoepidemiology of American visceral leishmaniasis, with particular reference to Brazil – A review. Memórias do Instituto Oswaldo Cruz 2005; 100: 811-827.

[3] Ashford RW. The Leishmaniasis as emerging and reemerging zoonoses. International Journal for Parasitology 2000; 30: 1269-1281.

[4] Maia-Elkhoury ANS, Alves WA, Sousa-Gomes ML, Sena JM, Luna EA. Visceral leishmaniasis in Brazil: trends and challenges. Cad Saúde Pública 2008; 24: 2941-2947.

[5] Margonari C, Freitas CR, Ribeiro RC, Moura ACM, Timbó M, Gripp AH, Pessanha JE, Dias ES. Epidemiology of visceral leishmaniasis through spatial analysis, in Belo Horizonte municipality, state of Minas Gerais, Brazil. Memórias do Instituto Oswaldo Cruz 2006; 101: 31-38.

[6] Silva, AVM, Paula AA, Pereira DP, Brazil RP, Carreira JCA. Canine Leishmaniasis in Brazil: Serological Follow-Up of a Dog Population in an Endemic Area of American Visceral Leishmaniasis. Journal Parasitology Research 2009; 2009: 1-6.

[7] Carreira JCA, Silva AVM, Pereira DP, Brazil RP. Natural infection of *Didelphis aurita* (Mammalia: Marsupialia) with *Leishmania infantum* in Brazil. Parasites & Vectors 2012; 5:111 - 116.

[8] Cabrera MAA, De Paula AA, Camacho LAB, Marzochi CA, Aguiar GM, Xavier SC, Da Silva AVM, Jansen AM. Canine Visceral Leishmaniasis in Barra de Guaratiba, Rio de Janeiro, Brazil: assessment of some risk factors. Revista do Instituto de Medicina Tropical de São Paulo 2003; 45: 79-83.

[9]   Ministério da Saúde. Brasil: Editora MS. Manual de Vigilância e Controle da Leish-
       maniose Visceral; 2003.

[10]   Palatnik-de-Souza CB, Dos Santos WR, França-Silva JC, Da Costa RT, Reis AB, Palat-
       nik M, Mayrink W, Genaro O. Impact of canine control on the epidemiology of ca-
       nine and human visceral leishmaniasis in Brazil. American Journal of Tropical
       Medicine and Hygiene 2001; 65: 510-517.

[11]   Bavia ME, Carneiro DDMT, Costa Gurgel H, Madureira Filho C, Rodrigues Barbosa
       MG. Remote Sensing and Geographic Information Systems and risk of American Vis-
       ceral Leishmaniasis in Bahia, Brazil. Parassitologia 2005; 47: 165-169.

[12]   Beck LR, Lobitz BM, Wood BL. Remote sensing and human health: new sensors and
       new opportunities. Emerging Infectious Diseases 2000; 6: 217-226.

[13]   Zhou XN, Lv S, Yang GJ, Kristensen TK, Bergquist R, Utzinger J, Malone JB. Spatial
       epidemiology in zoonotic parasitic diseases: insights gainedat the 1st International
       Symposium on Geospatial Health in Lijiang, China, 2007. Parasites & Vectors 2009;
       2:10-26.

[14]   Silva AVM, Magalhães MAFM, Brazil RP, Carreira JCA. Ecological study and risk
       mapping of leishmaniasis in an endemic area of Brazil based on a geographical infor-
       mation systems approach. Geospatial Health 2011; 6 (1) 33-40.

[15]   Shawe-Taylor J, Cristianini N. Kernel Methods for Pattern Analysis. Cambridge Uni-
       versity Press; 2004.

[16]   Elnaiem DA, Schorscher J, Bendall A, Obsomer V, Osman ME, Mekkawi AM, Connor
       SJ, Ashford RW, Thomson CM. Risk mapping of visceral leishmaniasis: the role of lo-
       cal variation in rainfall and altitude on the presence and incidence of kala-azar in
       Eastern Sudan. American Journal of Tropical Medicine and Hygiene 2003; 68: 10-17.

[17]   Elnaiem DA, Connor SJ, Thomson MC, Hassan MM, Hassan HK, Aboud MA, Ash-
       ford RW. Environmental determinants of the distribution of Phlebotomus orientalis in
       Sudan. Annals of Tropical Medicine and Parasitology 1998; 92(8) 877-887.

[18]   Bern C, Hightower AW, Chowdhury R, Ali M, Amann J, Wagatsuma Y, Haque R,
       Kurkjian K, Vaz LE, Begum M, Akter T, Cetre-Sossah CB, Ahluwalia IB, Dotson E,
       Secor WE, Breiman RF, Maguire JH. Risk Factors for Kala-Azar in Bangladesh.
       Emerging Infectious Diseases 2005; 11 (5) 655- 662.

[19]   Ryan JR, Mbui J, Rashid JR, Wasunna MK, Kirigi G, Magiri C, Kinoti D, Ngumbi PM,
       Martin SK, Odera SO, Hochberg LP, Bautista CT, Chan AS. Spatial clustering and ep-
       idemiological aspects of Visceral Leishmaniasis in two endemic villages, Baringo Dis-
       trict, Kenya. American Journal of Tropical Medicine and Hygiene 2006; 74(2) 308-
       317.

[20] Sudhakar S, Srinivas T, Palit A, Kar SK, Battacharya SK. Mapping of risk prone areas of kala-azar (Visceral leishmaniasis) in parts of Bihar state, India: an RS and GIS approach. Journal of Vector Borne Diseases 2006; 43: 115-122.

[21] Rossi E, Rinaldi L, Musella V, Veneziano V, Carbone S, Gradoni L, Cringoli G, Maroli. Mapping the main Leishmania phlebotomine vector in the endemic focus of the Mt. Vesuvius in southern Italy. Geospatial Health 2007; 2: 191-198.

[22] Ready PD. Leishmaniasis emergence in Europe. EuroSurveillance 2010; 15(10) 1-11.

[23] Bhunia GS, Kesari S, Jeyaram A, Kumar V, Das P. Influence of topography on the endemicity of Kala-azar: a study based on remote sensing and geographical information system. Geospatial Health 2010; 4(2) 155-165.

[24] Khanal B, Picado A, Bhattarai NR, Auwera GVD, Das ML, Ostyn B, Davies CR, Boelaert M, Dujardin JC, Rijal S. Spatial analysis of *Leishmania donovani* exposure in humans and domestic animals in a recent kala azar focus in Nepal. Parasitology 2010; 137: 1597-1603.

[25] Bhattarai NR, Auwera GV, Rijal S, Picado A, Speybroeck N, Khanal B, Doncker S, Das ML, Ostyn B, Davies C, Coosemans M, Berkvens D, Boelaert M, Dujardin JC. Domestic animals and Epidemiology of Visceral Leishmaniasis, Nepal. Emerging Infectious Diseases 2010; 16(2) 231- 237.

[26] Salahi-Moghaddam A, Mohebali M, Moshfae A, Habibi M, Zarei Z. Ecological study and risk mapping of visceral leishmaniasis in an endemic area of Iran based on a geographical information systems approach. Geospatial Health 2010; 5(1) 71-77.

[27] Bhunia GS, Kesari S, Chatteerjee N, Kumar V, Das P. The Burden of Visceral Leishmaniasis in India: Challenges in Using Remote Sensing and GIS to Understand and Control. Infectious Diseases 2013; 2013: 1-14.

[28] Miranda C, Massa JL, Marques CCA. Analysis of the occurrence of American Cutaneous Leishmaniasis in Brazil by remote sensing satellite imagery. Revista de Saúde Pública 1996; 30 (5) 433-437.

[29] Lima AP, Minelli L, Teodoro U, Comunello E. Tegumentary leishmaniasis distribution by satellite remote sensing imagery, in Paraná State, Brazil. Anais Brasileiros de Dermatologia 2002; 77(7) 681-692.

[30] Peterson AT, Pereira RS, Neves VFC. Using epidemiological survey data to infer geographic distributions of leishmaniasis vector species. Revista da Sociedade Brasileira de Medicina Tropical 2004; 37: 10-14.

[31] Carneiro DDMT, Bavia ME, Rocha WJSF, Lobão JSB, Oliveira CMFJB, Silva CEP, Barbosa MGR, Rios RB. Identificação de áreas de risco para Leishmaniose Visceral Americana, através de estudos epidemiológicos e sensoriamento remoto orbital, em Feira de Santana, Bahia, Brasil (2000-2002). Revista Baiana de Saúde Pública 2004; 28(1) 19-32.

[32] Salomón OD, Orellano PW, Lamfri M, Scavuzzo M, Dri L, Farace MI, Quintana DO. Phlebotominae spatial distribution asssociated with a focus of tegumentary leishmaniasis in Las Lomitas, Formosa, Argentina, 2002. Memórias do Instituto Oswaldo Cruz 2006; 101(3) 295-299.

[33] Nieto P, Malone JB, Bavia ME. Ecological niche modeling for visceral leishmaniasis in the state of Bahia, Brazil, using genetic algorithm for rule-set prediction and growing degree day-water budget analysis. Geospatial Health 2006; 1:115-126.

[34] Neto JC, Werneck GL, Costa CHN. Factors associated with the incidence of urban visceral leishmaniasis: an ecological study in Teresina, Piauí State, Brazil. Cadernos de Saúde Pública 2009; 25(7) 1543-1551.

[35] Shimabukuro PHF, Silva TRR, Fonseca FOR, Baton LA, Galati EAB. Geographical distribution of American cutaneous leishmaniasis and its phlebotomine vectors (Diptera: Psychodidae) in the state of São Paulo, Brazil. Parasites & Vectors 2010; 3:121-133.

[36] Valderrama-Ardila C, Alexander N, Ferro C, Cadena H, Marin D, Holford TR, Munstermann LE, Ocampo CB. Environmental Risk Factors for the Incidence of American Cutaneous Leishmaniasis in a Sub-Andean Zone of Colombia (Chaparral, Tolima). American Journal of Tropical Medicine and Hygiene 2010; 82(2) 243-250.

[37] Almeida AS, Medronho RA, Werneck GL. Identification of Risk Areas for Visceral Leishmaniasis in Teresina, Piaui State, Brazil. American Journal of Tropical Medicine and Hygiene 2011; 84(5) 681-687.

[38] Foley DH, Wilkerson RC, Dornak LL, Pecor DB, Nyari AS, Rueda LM, Long LS, Richardson JH. Sand flyMap: leveraging spatial data on sand fly vector distribution for disease risk assessments. Geospatial Health 2012; 6(3) S25-S30.

[39] Foley DH, Wilkerson RC, Rueda LM. Importance of the "what", "when", and "where" of mosquito collection events. Journal of Medical Entomology 2009; 46: 717-722.

[40] Martins AV, Williams P, Falcao AL. American sand flies (Diptera: Psychodidae, Phlebotominae). Academia Brasileira de Ciencias, Rio de Janeiro; 1978.

[41] Saraiva L, Leite CG, Carvalho LOA, Filho JDA, Menezes FC, Fiuza VOP. Information System and Geographic Information System Tools in the Data Analyses of the Control Program for Visceral Leishmaniases from 2006 to 2010 in the Sanitary District of Venda Nova, Belo Horizonte, Minas Gerais, Brazil. Journal Tropical Medicine 2012; 2012: 1-10.

[42] Souza VAF, Cortez LRPB, Dias RA, Amaku M, Neto JSF, Kuroda RBS, Ferreira F. Space-time cluster analysis of American visceral leishmaniasis in Bauru, São Paulo State, Brazil. Cadernos de Saúde Pública 2012; 28(10) 1949-1964.

[43] González C, Paz A, Ferro C. Predicted altitudinal shifts and reduced spatial distribution of *Leishmania infantum* vector species under climate change scenarios in Colombia. Acta Tropica 2013; In Press.

4

Utilization of Composites and Nanocomposites Based on Natural Rubber and Ceramic Nanoparticles as Control Agents for *Leishmania braziliensis*

Aldo Eloizo Job, Alexandre Fioravante de Siqueira,
Caroline Silva Danna, Felipe Silva Bellucci,
Flávio Camargo Cabrera and
Leandra Ernst Kerche Silva

1. Introduction

Nanoscience and Nanothecnology are revolutionizing the world of science and technology, bringing high expectations for technological innovation and the development of areas, such as: aerospace, agribusiness, defense, energy, environment, nanodevices, nanosensors, textiles, biotechnology and health. As part of its application to the health sciences, one of the priority targets are negligible diseases such as Leishmaniasis. In this context, the main objective of this chapter is to show the potential of some classes of ceramic nanoparticles and magnetic and ferroelectric nanocomposites based on natural rubber to modulate the growth of parasite colony of *Leishmania braziliensis* (LB) and to evaluate the toxicity of these materials against mammal cells.

1.1. Nanoscience and nanotechnology applied to neglected diseases

Materials with sizes ranging between 1×10^{-9} m and 100×10^{-9} m are called nanomaterials regardless of their nature, whether ceramic, polymer, metal or composite. When a material has dimensions on the nanometric scale, its surface properties and volume are differentiated in relation to material properties at a higher dimensional scale. These differences occur because the surface/volume ratio or high aspect ratios are not linear for different dimensional scales and this is in part responsible for the differentiated properties presented by nonascale materials. These differentiated properties can be transferred to other materials by the insertion of the nanomaterials in a matrix of a different nature and nanometric scale not generating a nanocomposite material[1, 2]. In general, the choice of polymer as a matrix or continuous phase is preferable since most have appreciable thermal and mechanical properties. Other properties must also be taken into account, such as hydrophobic/hydrophilic balance, chemical stability and biocompatibility. The nanometric component, generally inorganic, known as the dispersed phase, can provide a higher mechanical, thermal stability and also biological properties [3].

Multidisciplinary researches involving nanoscience, nanotechnology, materials science and engineering, biotechnology and health sciences have gained great strength in recent decades, aiming to increase the number of tools for addressing problems [4]. Each day new materials and methodologies are tested in fighting diseases such as cancer and diseases neglected by the pharmaceutical industry, for example, malaria, leishmaniasis and Chagas' disease. As a result of this innovation, nanocomposites and composites based in natural rubber filled with ceramic particle and nanoparticles can be used in biological applications, aiming at development of devices such as intelligent bandages or agents of control and reduction of parasitic colonies [5].

1.2. *Leishmania braziliensis*

Leishmaniasis is a endemic and parasitic infection caused by the Leishmania genus protozoa. Approximately 1.5 million people were affected by cutaneous leishmaniasis, which reaches 88 countries and has compulsory notification in only 30 of them. Presents itself throughout the Americas and Brazil is the country that has the highest prevalence of cases. Leishmaniasis is a typically tropical disease from Trypanosomatidae family, affecting the skin (cutaneous leishmaniasis, caused by *Leishmania braziliensis* protozoans) or viscera (visceral leishmaniasis, caused by *Leishmania donovani* protozoans), transmitted by the bite of the vector, a phlebotomine sand fly popularly known as "straw mosquito", which utilizes both animals and humans as host [6, 7].

Protozoans of Leishmania genus are unicellular, eukaryotic, heterotrophic, with asexual reproduction by binary fission, and feed via uptake of non-self-generated food. Within the human body, Leishmania protozoans feed of proteins present intracellularly or in blood plasma, and reproduce only within macrophages or similar cells of the immune system[6, 7].

1.3. Ceramic materials

Ceramic materials (in general, oxides, carbides or nitrides) are inorganic, non-metallic substances consisting of metallic and non-metallic elements connected together by covalent and/or ionic bonds. This class of materials displays a set of distinguished physical and chemical properties such as high mechanical strength, high hardness, low tenacity, low thermal and electrical conductivity, high melting point, among others. As a result of the variety of properties that ceramic materials exhibit, these materials has various industrial applications as, for example, bricks, crockery, refractory glass mortars, magnetic materials, electronic devices, fibers, abrasives and aerospace components.

Ceramic phases preparation processes can be classified primarily in chemical and physical routes, and the appropriate processing route selection depends on several aspects associated with the desired final product characteristics, such as desired dimensional scale, final product purity degree, ceramic phase complexity, amount of obtained material, desired physical and chemical properties and cost of the final product. Among several ceramic phases currently known, investigated and used, those with magnetic and ceramic properties with ferroelectric properties can be highlighted, e.g. ferrite with inverse spinel type structure and niobate potassium strontium with tetragonal tungsten bronze structure [8, 9].

1.3.1. Inverse spinel structure and the nickel-zinc ferrite

Among the materials with inverse spinel type structure, is highlighted the Ni-Zn ferrite paramagnetic or superparamagnetic ceramic phase, with cubic symmetry and space group Fd3m unit cell displaying an occupation represented by $(Zn_x^{2+}Fe_{1-x}^{3+})[Ni_x^{2+}Fe_{1+x}^{3+}]O_4^{2-}$ [10, 11]. In this formula the transition metal ions inside the parentheses occupy the tetrahedral site D, while the metal ions inside the brackets occupy the octahedral site E.

Considering the absence of Zn^{2+} cations in the ferrite, the amount of iron in both atomic sites would be equal and their contribution to the magnetic dipole moment would be canceled, and the formation of the material magnetic dipole moment would be responsibility for Ni^{2+} cations. Doping the ferrite with Zn^{2+} cations, there is a migration of Fe^{3+} cations from tetrahedral sites to octahedral sites, unbalancing initial equality of Fe^{3+} cations. Therefore there is an abrupt increase in magnitude of the magnetic dipole moment, because Fe^{3+} and Zn^{2+} cations are contributing to the dipole moment of the material. Thus, it is possible to produce a large number of intrinsically magnetic ferrite by appropriate substitution of metallic ions. Figure 1 presents a representation of a portion of nickel-zinc ferrite with $Ni_{0.5}Zn_{0.5}Fe_2O_4$ stoichiometry and structure type inverse spinel, with octahedral sites FeO_6 or NiO_6 in blue and tetrahedral sites FeO_4 or ZnO_4 in red.

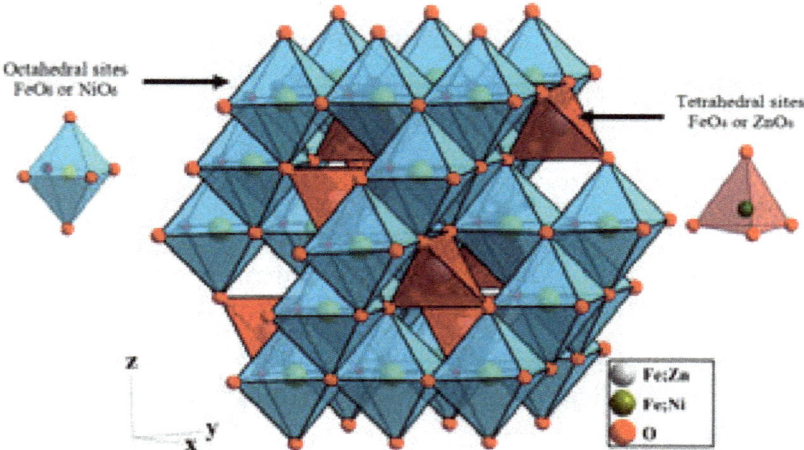

Figure 1. Oxide nickel-zinc ferrite representation, with stoichiometry $Ni_{0.5}Zn_{0.5}Fe_2O_4$ with structure type inverse spinel. Octahedral sites FeO_6 or NiO_6 are presented in blue and tetrahedral sites FeO_4 or ZnO_4 are presented in red.

Regarding magnetic ceramics, Ni-Zn ferrites stand out and attract scientific community interest, due to its high electrical resistivity, differentiated magnetic properties and several technological applications in electronics, telecommunications and biotechnology [8]. They are generally used in cores of transformers and inductors for high-frequency microwave devices, telecommunication systems and radars, high-speed read and recording magnetic heads, cellular telephony, hospital equipments, among others. In microwave-absorption devices (e.g. electromagnetic interference shielding), absorption capacity may be generated/potentiated by altering material magnetic or dielectric properties [12].

1.3.2. TTB structure and potassium-strontium niobate

Tetragonal tungsten bronze (TTB) crystalline structure is considered a structure derived from classic perovskite, where the central octahedral structure BO_6 is converted into three different types of cavities, tetrahedral and pentagonal tunnels similar to those found in perovskite structure which are favorable for substitution by cations, and trigonal tunnels are favorable for substitution by smaller cations and anions [9].

TTB structure can be described by chemical formula $A'_2B'_4C'_4Nb_{10}O_{30}$, where A', B' and C' represent different sites on the structure [13]. Depending on the number of sites available, TTB niobates are natural candidates to host structures, due to the possibility of a wide variety of cation substitutions, similar to what occurs with lead zirconate titanate ($PbZnTiO_3$). B' cavity has a cube-octahedral coordination of oxygen atoms; A' cavities have pentagonal prismatic coordinations, while C' cavities have trigonal prismatic coordinations. The size of these cavities decreases following the order A' > B' > C'. In TTB-type compounds, alkali and alkaline earth metals are located at A' and B' sites, while only cations with small atomic radius such as Li are located in C' site. TTB-type compounds with formula $A_6Nb_{10}O_{30}$, A'= Sr or Ba exhibit semiconductor characteristics which can be incremented when dopants are added.

Niobates with TTB-type structure such as $KSr_2Nb_5O_{15}$, $NaSr_2Nb_5O_{15}$, $KBa_2Nb_5O_{15}$, $NaBa_2Nb_5O_{15}$ and $K_3Li_2Nb_5O_{15}$ have created interest mainly by high anisotropy of the crystal structure. Among TTB-structure oxides, strontium potassium niobate oxide ($KSr_2Nb_5O_{15}$) stands out for being a classic ferroelectric material with Curie temperature close to 430 K[14], belonging to a class of ceramic composites which have great potential application as sensing devices, actuators, memories, transducers, filters and capacitors.

Figure 2 shows a representation of strontium potassium niobate oxide structure, with oxygen and niobium octahedra in blue and yellow dark, pentagonal sites with potassium atoms (K^{1+}), tetrahedral sites with strontium atoms (Sr^{2+}) and vacant trigonal sites. This type of structure has two niobium types, which differ from each other by crystallographic position, multiplicity and occupancy factor. Nb(I) leads to NbO_6 sites identified by their blue color, and Nb(II) leads to NbO_6 sites identified by dark yellow color. The ratio between Nb atoms is 4 Nb(I) to 1 Nb (II).

1.4. Natural rubber

Latex is extracted from rubber tree stem, more specifically, from lactiferous vessels located in the cortex, and is responsible for bringing food to the tree top. From a chemical point of view,

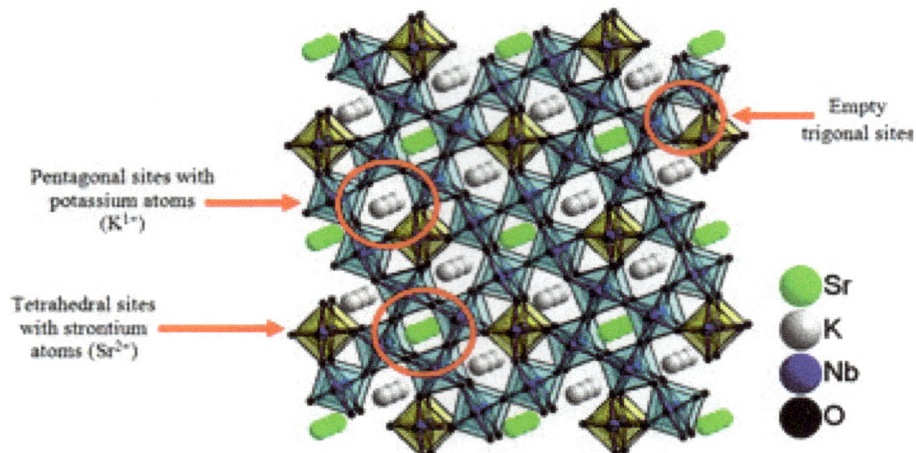

Figure 2. Representation of strontium potassium niobate oxide ($KSr_2Nb_5O_{15}$) with tetragonal tungsten bronze structure. Pentagonal sites occupied by atoms of potassium (K^{1+}), tetragonal sites occupied by atoms of strontium (Sr^{2+}) and trigonal vacant sites are highlighted.

latex is a stable colloidal dispersion of a polymer in an aqueous medium. The dispersed polymer is aggregated in the form of particles with approximately spherical geometry (natural rubber micelles), with typical diameters between 30 and 1, 000 nm [15].

The latex used in this work was collected from rubber trees of *Hevea brasiliensis* species, clone RRIM 600. This is a secondary clone developed by the Rubber Research Institute of Malaysia - RRIM, the most planted in the plateau region of São Paulo Brazilian state, due to its good performance and effect on production. This clone presents tall trees with vertical stem and fast growing when young. Its high production is highlighted, being one of the clones that has a higher dry rubber productivity.

Latex composition is, on average, 35% natural rubber (hydrocarbons), which compound is 2-methyl-1, 3-butadiene (C_5H_8), commercially known as isoprene. Recently-extracted latex is a neutral substance at room temperature with a pH between 6.0 and 7.2, depending on weather conditions, and density between 0.975 and 0.980 g/cm³. When exposed to air for 12 - 24 hours, latex pH decreases to values close to 5.0 and spontaneous coagulation process begins, separating rubber and non-rubber fractions. Rubber fraction can be represented by $(C_5H_8)_n$, where n is the number of monomers in the chain (between 2, 000 and 10, 000), presenting an average molecular weight from 600, 000 to 950.000 g/mol.

Figure 3 presents the *Hevea brasiliensis* cultivation (a), the bleeding process, in order to collect latex (b), and dry natural rubber, "Brazilian pale crepe" type (*Crepe Claro Brasileiro - CCB*) (c).

1.5. Nanocomposite materials

As commented by P. M. Ajayan and co-workers [16], the field of nanocomposites involves the study of multiphase material where at least one of the constituent phases has one dimension less than 100 nm. The promise of nanocomposites lies in their multifunctionality, the possibility of realizing unique combinations of properties unachievable with traditional materials. The

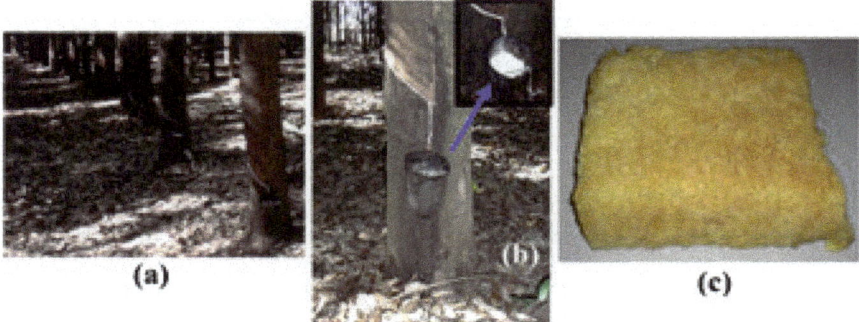

Figure 3. (a) Rubber tree plantation, *Hevea brasiliensis* species, (b) latex collection process using the bleeding method; detail: storage vessel, and (c) dry natural rubber, "Brazilian pale crepe" type.

challenges associate to this area are immense. They include control over the distribution in size and dispersion of the nanosize constituents, tailoring and understanding the role of interfaces between structurally or chemically dissimilar phases on bulk properties. Large scale and controlled processing of many nanomaterials has yet to be achieved.

An special class of composites and nanocomposites is the one formed by polymer and ceramic materials. In general, choosing a polymer as a matrix or continuous phase is interesting, since many of them have appreciable mechanical and thermal properties. Other properties are also regarded, e.g. hydrophobic/hydrophilic balance, chemical stability and bio-compatibility. The nanometric component is usually inorganic, and called dispersed phase. It can provide high mechanical and thermal stability and novel properties and functionalities that depend on component chemical nature, structure, size and crystallinity [17]. The dispersed phase provides or improves the redox properties, electronic, magnetic, density, refractive index, and others. In most cases, the main features of each of the components present in the nanocomposite is preserved or even improved and, in addition, one can obtain new properties resulting from the synergy of both components. Typical examples of polymer/ceramic nanocomposites of technological interest are formed by ceramic nanoparticles such as barium strontium titanate phase in a matrix with low dielectric loss [18] or nickel-zinc ferrite ($Ni_{0.5}Zn_{0.5}Fe_2O_4$ or NZF), dispersed in a polymeric matrix such as vulcanized natural rubber (NR) [19].

When mechanical properties of composites and nanocomposites are investigated, it is seen that the main contribution comes from the polymeric matrix. However, an appropriate nanoparticle engineering and dispersion process can act amplifying, reducing or creating new features in mechanical properties of nanocomposites. Interface and interaction between nanoparticles/matrix exert a significant influence on the mechanical properties, mainly due to the reorganization of chemical bonds and physical attractions of electrostatic nature. Therefore, properties of nanoparticles such as shape, size, surface activity, crystallinity and network microstrain become relevant. Depending on nanocomposites composition, external factors such as temperature, application of electric and magnetic fields can alter and modulate their properties, expanding application options for these materials. Thus, nanocomposites can be used in intelligent membranes, new catalysts and sensors, new generations of photovoltaic and fuel cells, intelligent micro-electronics systems, micro-optical and photonic components, and also therapeutic systems that combine marking, visualization, therapy and control of drug release [20, 21].

2. Employed methods

In the next topics, the preparation methods used in nanoparticles synthesis will be explored. The nanoparticles mentioned are magnetic (nickel-zinc ferrite, with stoichiometry $Ni_{0.5}Zn_{0.5}Fe_2O_4$ (NZF)), ferroelectric (strontium potassium niobate, stoichiometry $KSr_2Nb_5O_{15}$ (KSN)), besides magnetic and ferroelectric nanocomposites based on vulcanized natural rubber. Characterization techniques used are also covered, as well as biological testing of cell viability and against leishmaniasis.

2.1. Preparation of ceramic nanoparticles

Preparation of ceramic phases $KSr_2Nb_5O_{15}$ (KSN) and $Ni_{0.5}Zn_{0.5}Fe_2O_4$ (NZF) was performed using Modified Polyol Method [22, 23]. The main advantages of this method are high chemical homogeneity, the possibility of obtaining single phase powders and the large material portion produced in a single synthesis process (10 to 100g). Chemical formula and purity of starting reagents employed in oxides synthesis are listed in Table 1.

Component	Chemical formula	Purity
Fuel for nanoparticles synthesis		
Ethylene glicol	$C_2H_4(OH)_2$	P.A.
Nitric acid	HNO_3	65%
$KSr_2Nb_5O_{15}$ nanoparticles		
Strontium carbonate	$SrCO_3$	P.A.
Potassium carbonate	K_2CO_3	P.A.
Niobium complex salt	$NH_4H_2[NbO(C_2O_4)_3].3H_2O$	P.A.
$Ni_{0.5}Zn_{0.5}Fe_2O_4$ nanoparticles		
Nickel oxide	Ni_2O_3	P.A.
Zinc oxide	ZnO	P.A.
Iron oxide	Fe_2O_3	P.A.

Table 1. Chemical formula and purity of the materials used in the preparation of ferroelectric and paramagnetic nanoparticles (respectively, $KSr_2Nb_5O_{15}$ and $Ni_{0.5}Zn_{0.5}Fe_2O_4$).

- **Description:** in a 2 L beaker, under stirring and heating, the dissolution in nitric acid of all precursor oxides was performed in proper proportion to the desired oxide stoichiometry. 50 g of niobate oxide and ferrite were prepared for each synthesis and stoichiometric calculations were based on this mass value. Upon dissolution of all starting materials, 100 ml of ethylene glycol were added. In a chapel, the temperature was raised to 180 °C using a magnetic stirrer. With the gradual increase of temperature occurred the emanation of a yellowish-brown coloured gas, due to decomposition of NO_3 groups, similar to the process developed in synthesis via Pechini method [24]. After this initial process, the material generated in the beaker was placed in a chamber-type oven.

- **Pre-calcining:** precursors pre-calcination was carried out in two stages, under an O_2 atmosphere with a flow of 500 ml/min for the niobate phase and under a N_2 atmosphere with a flow of 300 ml/min for the ferrite phase. In the first step, the temperature was increased from room temperature at a rate of 10 °C/min to 150 °C, which was held constant for 2 hours for elimination of low molecular mass molecules such as water vapor and some organic groups. In the following, keeping the same heating rate, temperature was raised to 300 °C and maintained for 1 h, in order to remove part of non-stoichiometric elements of the phase. During pre-calcination significant elimination of organic material fraction occurs, thus obtaining a black precursor powder for KSN and reddish-brown powder for NZF.

- **Calcination:** Both precursors were calcined with a final temperature of 450 °C. For niobate phase, a ten-hour threshold (600 m) was performed at 300 °C for disposal of organic wastes, and a two-hour threshold (120 m) in the final calcination temperature. A heating rate of 5 °C/min and nitrogen flow of 150 mL/min were used during heating, for avoiding sample oxidation in second phase formation. For ferrite, a three-hour threshold (180 minutes) was performed at final calcination temperature, in order to provide sufficient time for occurring of diffusional mass processes. A heating rate of 5 °C/min and air flow equal to 7 L/min were used during heating. For both phases, the cooling process was performed at a natural rate.

Figure 4 presents a flowchart of the steps for preparing and calcining the niobate and ferrite by modified Polyol method until to characterization stage.

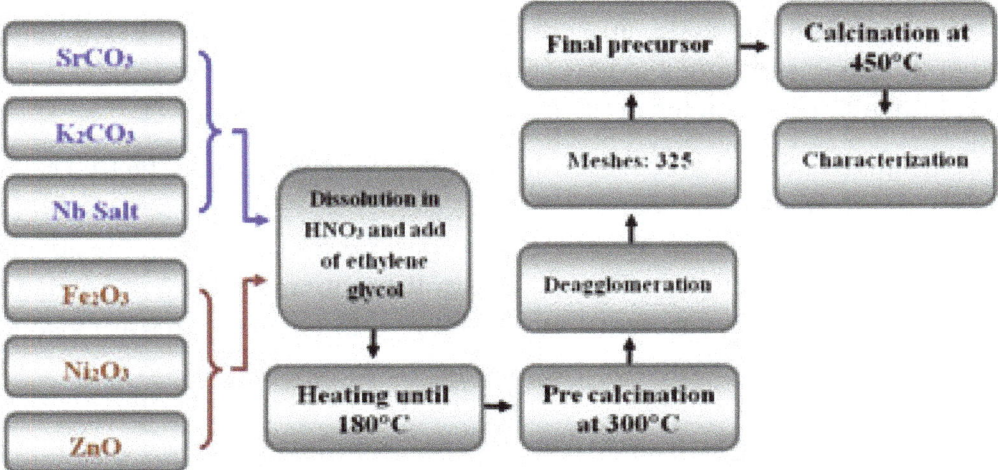

Figure 4. Flowchart of ferroelectric $KSr_2Nb_5O_{15}$ and paramagnetic $Ni_{0.5}Zn_{0.5}Fe_2O_4$ ceramic phases preparation by Modified Polyol Method. In blue, starting reactants from phase $KSr_2Nb_5O_{15}$ and in red, starting reactants from phase $Ni_{0.5}Zn_{0.5}Fe_2O_4$.

2.2. Nanocomposite magnetic and ferroelectric preparation

Magnetic and ferroelectric nanocomposites were obtained from mechanical blending of dry natural rubber, various concentrations of ceramic nanoparticles and vulcanization system. Chemical formula and purity of the starting reactants employed in preparation of vulcanized natural rubber nanocomposites are listed in Table 2.

Component	Chemical formula	Purity
Nanocomposites		
Natural Rubber	$(C_5H_8)_n$	-
Zinc oxide	ZnO	P.A.
Stearic acid	$CH_3(CH_2)_{16}COOH$	P.A.
Mercaptobenzothiazole	$S_2NC_7H_5$	P.A.
Sulfur	S_8	P.A.

n: number of monomers in the polymer chain, between 2, 000 and 10, 000.

Table 2. Names, chemical formula, and purity of materials used in preparation of functional nanocomposites based on vulcanized natural rubber.

Nanocomposites preparation was initiated with dry mechanical mixing of the activation system in a open chamber mixer for 20 minutes. The activation system consists of 4 phr of zinc oxide and 3 phr of stearic acid with various concentrations of nanoparticles and 100 phr of dry natural rubber. At this stage the samples are called "activated samples". These samples were stored at a temperature of 25 °C and without light exposure for 24 hours.

After the storage step, vulcanization (2 phr of sulfur) and acceleration (1 phr of 2-mercapto-benzothiazole) agents were added to the activated samples by using the same mixing route. At this stage the samples are termed "accelerated samples". Accelerated samples were then thermo-conformated in thicknesses equal to 200 μm, 2 mm and 6 mm in a press with a heating system at 150 °C for 8 min and 30 s, and closing uniaxial pressure equal to 2.5 MPa. Vulcanization temperature and pressure used are indicated for natural rubber [25], and the vulcanization time parameter can be determined through rheometry test [26, 27].

Two sets of vulcanized natural rubber nanocomposites were prepared. The first set (NR/KSN) with $KSr_2Nb_5O_{15}$ ferroelectric nanoparticles, and the second set (NR/NZF) with $Ni_{0.5}Zn_{0.5}Fe_2O_4$ nanoparticles, both at various concentrations (1, 2, 3, 4, 5, 10, 20 and 50 phr). Figure 5 presents NR, NR/NZF and NR/KSN films and membranes with 5 phr of nanoparticles. Images of other samples with different concentrations and temperatures are visually similar and were not included in this section.

2.3. Main characterizations of nanoparticles and nanocomposites

- **XDR:** characterization by X-ray diffraction of KSN and NZF phases was performed on a X-ray diffractometer with Cu-Kα radiation (λ = 1.54060 Å), angular range of $5° \leq 2\theta \leq 80°$, and variation rate (or step) of 0.02°. Diffraction data were refined using the software FullProf

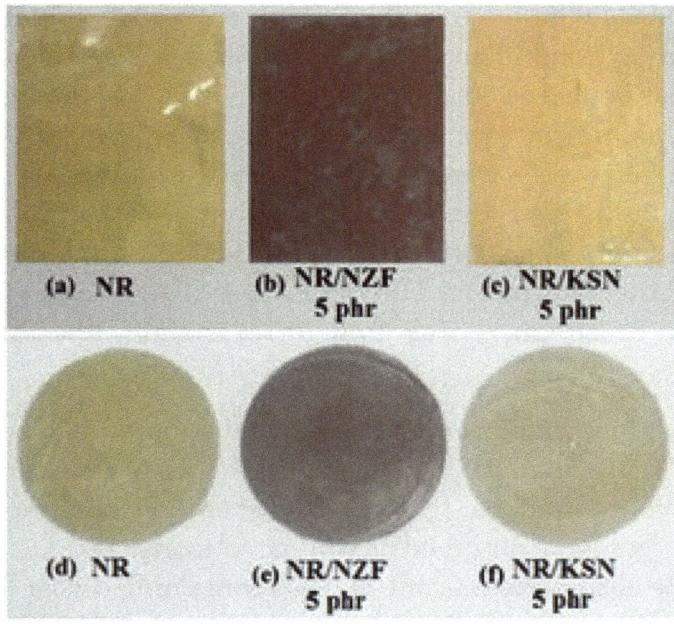

Figure 5. Thin films with a thickness of 200 μm (a, b and c) and membranes with a thickness of 2 mm (d, e and f) of NR, NR/NZF, NR/KSN and NR/KSN/NZF respectively, with 5 phr of nanoparticles.

[28]. KSN, with a bronze tungsten tetragonal structure was indexed to JCPDS-34-0108 and NZF, with a inverse spinel structure was indexed to JCPDS-08-0234 [29].

- **TEM:** images of transmission electron microscopy of KSN and NZF nanoparticles at a temperature of 25 °C were obtained from the supernatant fraction of the dispersion, nanoparticles and methanol, deposited on a polymer film. A field-emission (FEG) micro-scope with tungsten filament was used; accelerating voltage between 40 and 100 kV, CCD chamber.

- **SEM:** scanning electron microscopy images of vulcanized natural rubber and nanocomposites NR/KSN and NR/NZF were performed using a microscope with field emission (FEG) and energy dispersive analysis of x-ray analysis (EDX). Images were obtained on the sample and cryogenically fractured surfaces.

- **AFM:** atomic force microscopy AFM/STM was used in contact mode. AFM were performed to characterize nanoparticles morphology, vulcanized natural rubber and functional nanocomposites. The public domain software Gwyddion was used to generate the three-dimensional projection of the sample surface from the height mode AFM images (height).

2.4. Cell viability or toxicity assays

Assays of cell viability or the nanoparticles toxicity, vulcanized natural rubber and nanocomposites compared to mammalian cells were performed using "violet crystal method", as described by J. Moraes et al [30]. Mammalian cell lineage used in these experiments was of Vero cells ATCC CCL-81, originating from "American Type Culture Collection" (Manassas, VA, USA), a cell line from African green monkey *Cercopithecus aethiops (L.)* kidney. In the experiments, Vero cells were grown in culture plates of 96 wells containing nanoparticles at concentrations between 15.6 and 1000 µg/mL or nanocomposites based on vulcanized natural rubber at concentrations between 250 and 4000 µg/mL in DMEM (Dulbecco's Modified Eagle Medium) environment, supplemented with 10% serum at 37 °C in an CO_2 atmosphere of 5%. Anova and Kruskal-Wallis tests were used to compare multiple normal or non-normal samples, respectively. Student's t-tests and Mann-Whitney test were used to compare two normal or non-normal samples, respectively. The BioEstat 5.0 software package [ACHO QUE ERA LEGAL COLOCAR UMA NOTA DE RODAPÉ FALANDO SOBRE ONDE OBTER O PROGRAMA] (Belém, Brazil, 2007) was used for performing the statistical tests and for graphical representations.

After 24 and 48 hours, supernatants were removed and adhered cells were fixed and stained with crystal violet 0.2% in methanol 20%v. It is noted that tests were carried out with concentrations of 150 mg/ml, concentrations significantly higher than those reported in the literature and no significant changes were observed as compared to essays up to 4000 µg/mL. Toxicity was evaluated from the absorbance of control wells containing cells in DMEM environment. Throughout the incubation period, cultures were monitored daily in inverted optical microscope. All assays were performed in triplicate and the obtained average standard deviation was less than 2%.

2.4. Leishmaniasis assays

In vitro population growth kinetics: In a BHI (brain heart infusion) environment supplemented with 10%v fetal bovine serum (FBS), 2% v human urine, 100 µg/ml potassium G penicillin and 100 µg/mL of streptomycin sulfate, a sample with rectangular dimensions 10x10x2mm of vulcanized natural rubber or nanocomposites with an inoculum of five hundred thousand parasites in the promastigote form of *Leishmania braziliensis* species, ARQ-1 strains isolated from clinical cases of Santa Cruz do Rio Pardo city, São Paulo state, in 1997.

From that instant, every three hours for a week, cell counts on the supernatant portion of the colony were performed using a Neubauer chamber. With data count a curve of parasite colony development was sketched. For comparison, control colonies, i.e. without the introduction of samples or natural rubber nanocomposites were also investigated. Throughout the tests, the temperature was maintained between 27 and 32 ºC, and hydrogen potential (pH) between 6.0 and 6.9. All assays were performed in triplicate and the average standard deviation obtained was less than 1%.

3. Main results and discussions

To support discussions related to the applications of nanoparticles and magnetic and ferroelectric nanocomposites in cultures of Leishmaniasis, morphological and structural characterization of nanometric materials were performed. Thus, information is obtained mainly about the interaction of the nanoparticles and nanocomposites with the biological material, cooperating in the understanding of the results.

3.1. Structural and morphological nanoparticle essays

Figure 6 presents the diffraction pattern at room temperature for KSN and NZF nanoparticles, calcined at 450 °C for 2 hours. Lines and vertical bars represent experimental data and diffraction patterns respectively, categorized in JCPDS database: 34-0108 (KSN) and 08-0234 (NZF).

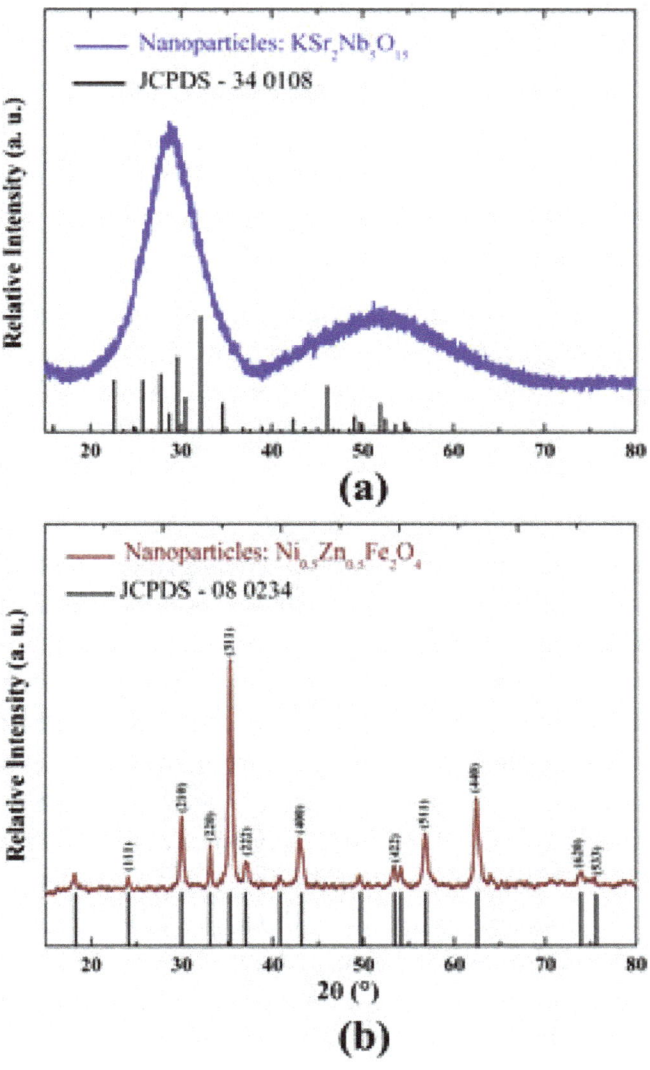

Figure 6. X-ray diffraction: (a) $KSr_2Nb_5O_{15}$ phase, calcined at 450 °C, together with experimental data, columns of the identity card JCPDS-34-0108 and (b) $Ni_{0.5}Zn_{0.5}Fe_2O_4$ phase, calcined at the temperature of 450 °C, together with experimental data, columns of the identity card JCPDS-08-0234.

As can be seen in Figure 6, and according to studies conducted previously by the authors [31], the diffraction pattern obtained for the KSN shows the typical profile of a material with short-distance ordering (amorphous), identifying only two large sets of overlapping diffraction lines indicating that the thermal energy supplied during the heat treatment was not sufficient for obtaining a crystalline material. Relative crystallinity obtained for KSN was equal to approximately 10%, compared with the same material calcined at 1150 °C.

A diffractogram obtained for NZF phase displays a set of well-resolved diffraction lines, indicating that heat treatment was suitable for the production of a material with a high crystallinity degree, relative crystallinity of 74% when compared with the same material calcined at 650 °C. For KSN phase, the formation of a tetragonal tungsten bronze structure (TTB) with P4bm spatial group (No. 100) was identified, while for phase NZF the formation of a inverse spinel structure with space group Fd3m (No. 227) was identified. Network parameters "a", "b" and "c" obtained from KSN phase and "a" for NZF phase are equal to "a" = 12.4585 Å, "b" = "c" = 3.9423 Å and "a" = 8.394 Å, respectively. The unit cell volume is equal to V = 611.90 Å^3 and V = 591.435 Å^3 to KSN and NZF.

Average crystallite size, obtained by Scherrer's equation, was equal to 2 nm for KSN and 14.7 nm for NZF. Network microstrain (γ), calculated by Williamson-Hall equation, was equal to 0.32 for KSN and 0.05 for NZF. Structural parameters obtained in this study are in agreement with values reported in previous publications [32, 33].

Figure 7 presents transmission electron microscopy (TEM) images at a temperature of 25 °C of KSN ferroelectric and NZF paramagnetic nanoparticles, both calcined at 450 °C, where (a) and (c) are 10, 000 times magnifications while (b) and (d) are 600, 000 times magnifications. The images (b) and (d) were generated from amplifications of specific regions of the images (a) and (c).

As can be seen in Figure 7 (b) and (d), for both types of primary particles, their geometry are approximately spherical due to nucleation-type particle growth mechanism, predominant in ceramic materials and also to the principle of surface energy minimizing. Average particle diameter of strontium potassium niobate is approximately 15 nm, while the average size for a primary particle of nickel-zinc ferrite is approximately 10 nm; both values are consistent with particle diameters in the scientific literature [32, 33] and agree with average-size crystallite values. As expected, KSN particle diameter for is larger than NZF particle diameter, due to the fact that tetragonal tungsten bronze structure (23 atoms/ minimal formula, pentagonal, tetragonal and trigonal sites) has greater complexity than cubic inverse spinel-type structure (7 atoms/minimal formula, octahedral and tetrahedral sites), thus the minimum cluster size to stabilize the particle tends to be higher for KSN than for NZF. Due to the difference of stage complexity, it is also expected that as both received the same heat treatment and then the same amount of thermal energy, NZF phase would be more crystalline than KSN phase, since NZF phase requires less energy to the atoms achieve their ideal atomic positions.

According to Figure 7 (a) and (c), one can identify that both ceramic phases present clusters even at nanometric scale, due to the action of secondary forces and coalescence phenomena. For KSN phase one can identify clusters with an average size of 80 nm or approximately 112 nanoparticles/cluster and for NZF phase, agglomerates with an average size of 100 nm or around 740 nanoparticles/cluster. For both estimates, clusters with spherical shape and a close-packing bundling type were considered [34]. In principle, magnetic properties displayed by NZF nanoparticles could contribute to formation of larger clusters when compared with non-magnetic phase clusters, as reported and discussed by E. M. A. Jamal et al., for nickel magnetic particles [35]. However, cluster formation is attributed essentially to preparation method used to synthesize ceramic nanoparticles; in this case, a chemical route.

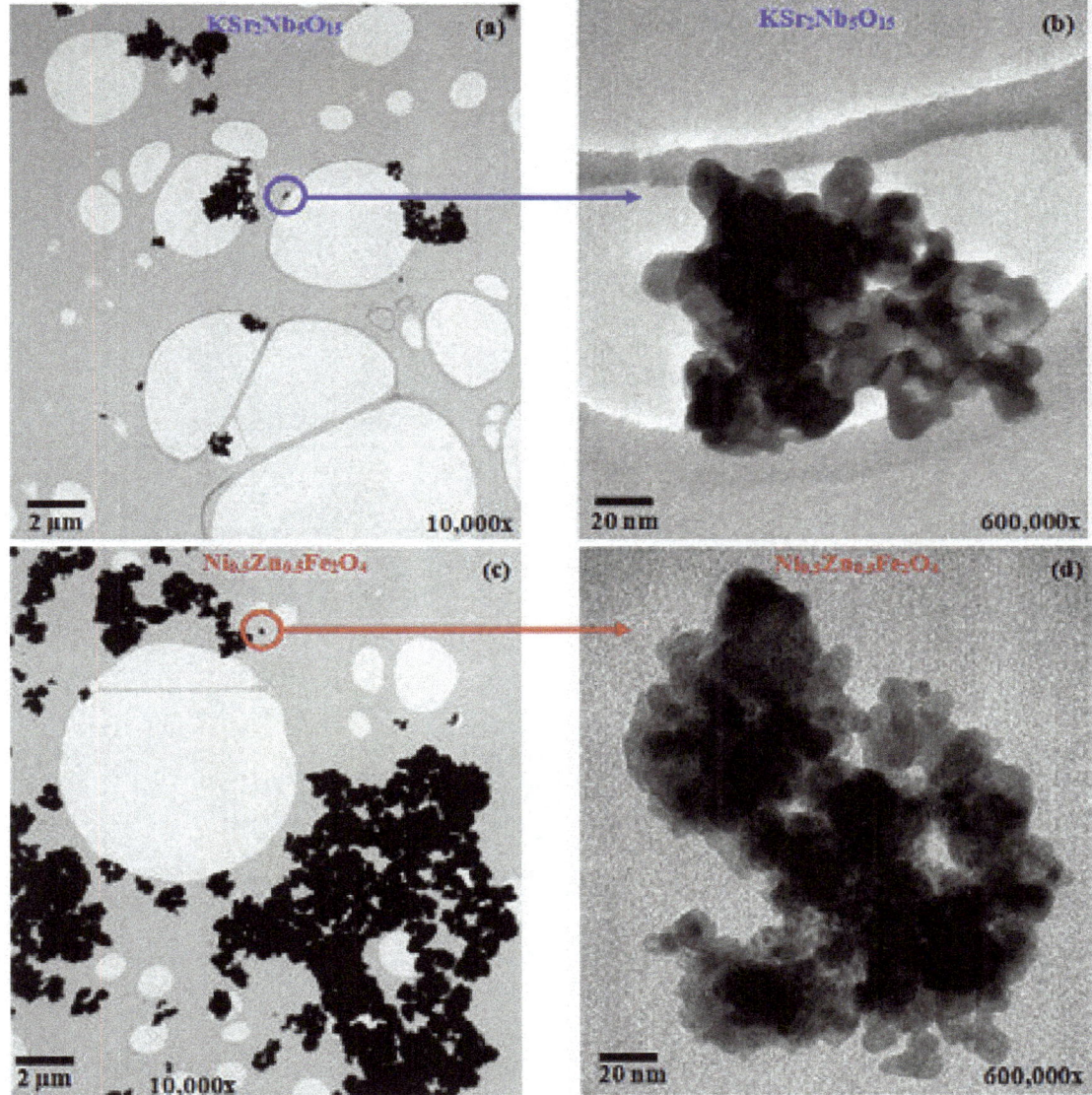

Figure 7. Transmission electron microscopy (TEM) at a temperature of 25 °C, of KSN ferroelectric [(a) and (b)] and NZF paramagnetic nanoparticles [(c) and (d)], calcined at 450 °C and at different magnifications.

Images acquired by Atomic Force Microscopy (AFM) at room temperature (25 °C) for KSN ferroelectric (a) and NZF paramagnetic nanoparticles (b) calcined at 450 °C are shown in Figure 8. Details on the grain boundary and the three-dimensional nanoparticle projection are given on the right.

According to Figure 8, structures on a nanometric scale were identified for both ceramic phases, in agreement with Figure 7. Images generated from amplitude data (main figure) provide qualitative information of nanostructure shape, while images generated from elevation data (three-dimensional projection) provide significant information about surface topography. Details on the grain boundary can be obtained from deflection data of the phase angle (image positioned in the third quadrant). For KSN ferroelectric nanoparticles, Figure 8 (a), a small

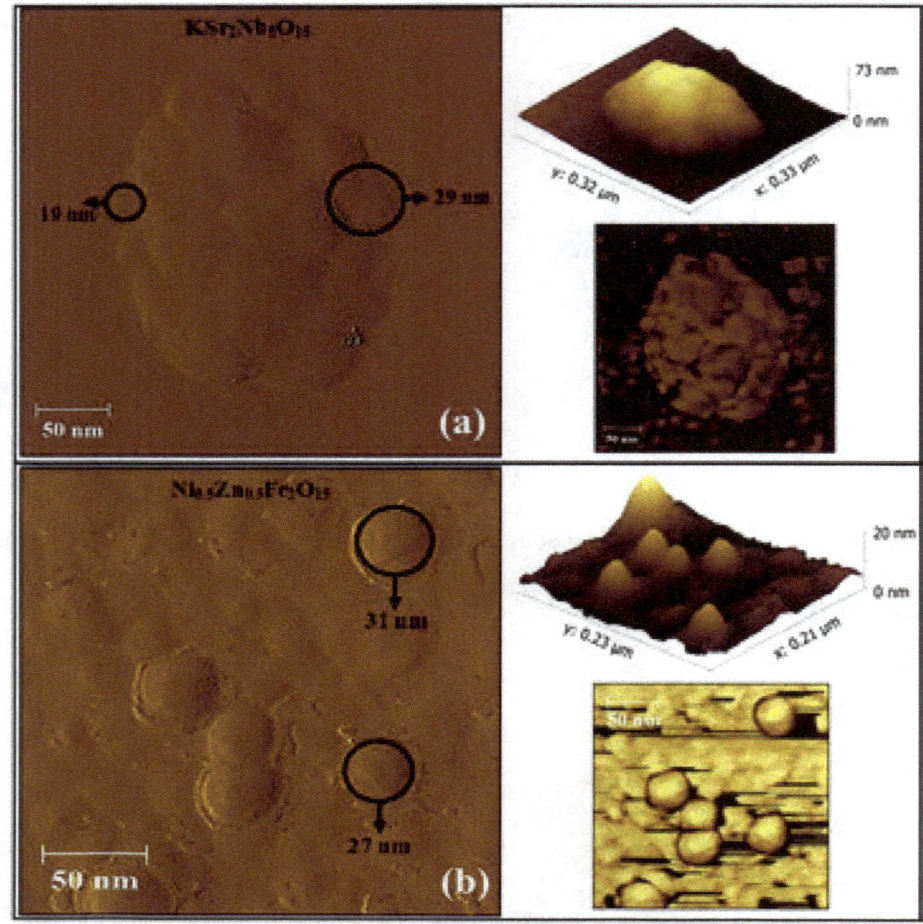

Figure 8. Atomic Force Microscopy (AFM) images generated from range, surface elevation and phase angle deflection data for KSN ferroelectric (a) and NZF paramagnetic nanoparticles (b). On the right, grain boundary details and three-dimensional nanoparticle projection.

cluster is observed in detail, with size approximately equal to 100 nm composed of nanoparticles with particle size distribution between 15 and 30 nm.

Small clusters formation is a typical feature of nanoscale materials processing using chemical routes. However, it is emphasized that the nanoparticles that compose the clusters are weakly linked together through secondary interactions of electrostatic origin. For NZF paramagnetic nanoparticles, Figure 8 (b), individual nanoparticles with approximately spherical geometry are identified, as well as the union of two or more nanoparticles by coalescence process. It is feasible to notice a particle size distribution between 25 and 40 nm for NZF phase. It should be noted that the particle size distribution for KSN and NZF is consistent with previously published work [36, 37].

3.2. Nanocomposite morphological study

Figure 9 presents scanning electron microscopy images obtained from the sample surface, a representation of the polymer chain and the EDX spectrum for the vulcanized natural rubber

NR/KSN-1phr ferroelectric and NR/NZF-1phr magnetic nanocomposites. Magnifications used were equal to 50, 000, 50, 000, and 150, 000 times.

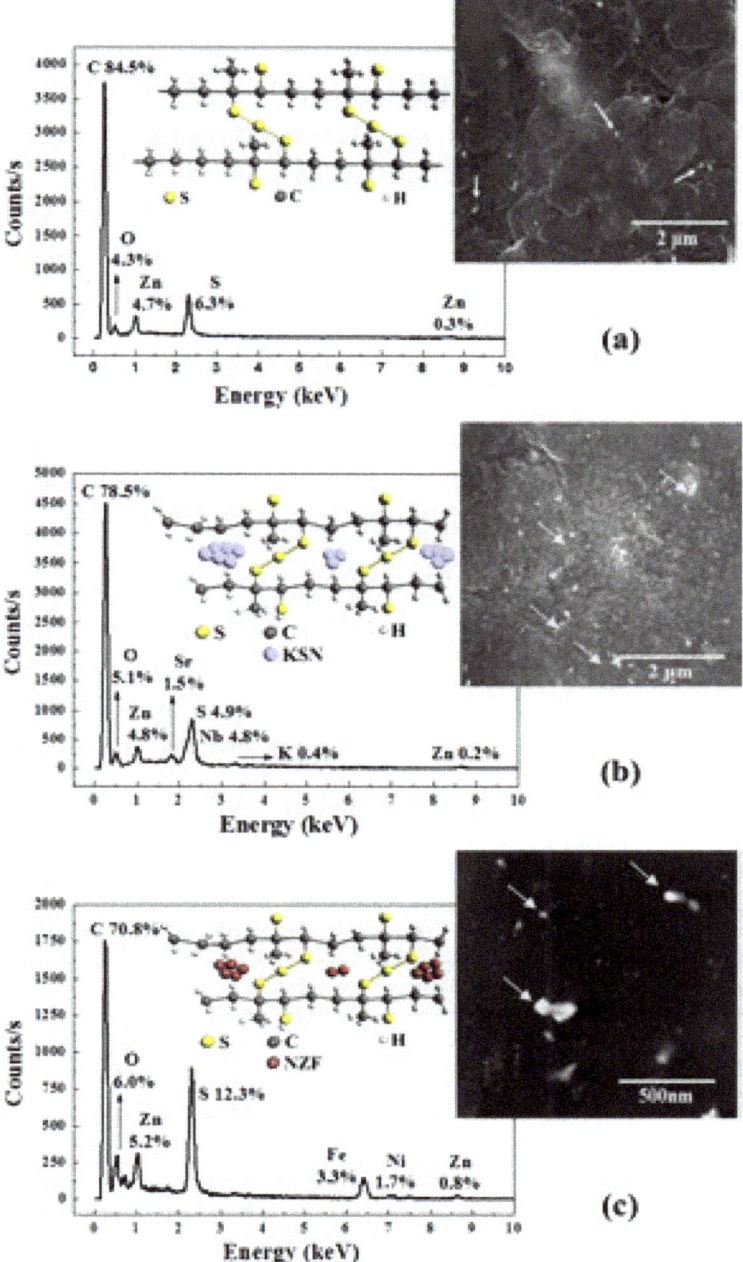

Figure 9. (a) Scanning electron microscopy images of the sample surface, polymer chain representation and EDX spectrum for vulcanized natural rubber, (b) ferroelectric nanocomposite NR/KSN-1phr and (c) magnetic nanocomposite NR/NZF-1phr.

In Figure 9 (a), a satisfactory surface homogeneity was observed, indicating that a vulcanization system in appropriate amounts and a efficient nanocomposite-preparing system was used. White spots were noticed and indicated with white arrows. Such points may be associated with the vulcanization system, in agreement with the results obtained by XRD, particularly zinc and sulfur with submicrometer dimensions (> 250 nm). According to Figure 9 (b) and (c), it is possible to identify a high dispersion of particles and small agglomerates with dimensions on the nanometer scale, between 20 nm and 80 nm, and a particle size in the submicron range.

It is suggested that the particles and small clusters are KSN and NZF nanoparticles, in accordance with the dimensional scale, dark grayish and reddish brown color in surface and inside of the nanocomposites, respectively. In EDX spectra, peaks of C, O, S and Zn were identified and are associated with the curing system and the polymer chains. EDX percentage differences observed for S and Zn among NR, NR/KSN-1phr and NR/NZF-1phr samples refer only to the position of the investigated sample and sample time exposure to X-ray.

Low percentages of K, Sr and Nb and Fe, Ni and Zn were found for samples of NR/KSN and NR/NZF and were assigned respectively to KSN and NZF nanoparticles. The values obtained are in agreement with the amount estimated by stoichiometric calculations. The difference in surface roughness observed in Figure 9 (a) and Figures 9 (b) and (c) may be associated to the mobility difference of the natural rubber polymer chain, due to the incorporation of nanoparticles, even in small mass quantities.

Images obtained by atomic force microscopy (AFM) for vulcanized natural rubber, NR/KSN-10phr ferroelectric nanocomposite and NR/NZF-10phr magnetic nanocomposite were performed directly on the surface of the samples, and their three-dimensional projections are presented in Figure 10, while Table 3 lists the values for NR surface roughness, NR/KSN ferroelectric and NR/NZF magnetic nanocomposites, depending on the nanoparticle concentration.

Sample	Superficial rugosity (nm)						
	NR	1 phr	3 phr	5 phr	10 phr	20 phr	50 phr
NR/KSN	0.45	0.68	0.83	0.70	0.55	0.50	0.58
NR/NZF	0.45	0.50	0.63	0.55	0.45	0.43	0.45

Table 3. Surface roughness values obtained from elevation mode AFM images, for vulcanized natural rubber (NR) and nanocomposites NR/KSN and NR/NZF.

According to Figure 10 and the data in Table 3, a satisfactory superficial homogeneity is noted for vulcanized natural rubber and both functional nanocomposites samples, suggesting that appropriate parameters and vulcanization system were used. Significant differences between the natural rubber nanocomposites were observed for surface roughness. At low nanoparticle concentrations, smaller than 3 phr, there is considerable roughness growth, followed by a reduction and stabilization of this parameter with increasing concentration of nanoparticles. This suggests that for low concentrations, local phenomena of elastomeric chain orientation as stress-induced crystallization [38, 39] can be significant.

Probably, differences in roughness identified between ferroelectric and magnetic nanocomposites are due to: (i) difference in interface between the nanoparticles that generate changes in polymer chains folding, (ii) different coefficients of thermal diffusion due to different ceramic phases and (iii) different anisotropies for polymer chains mobility [39].

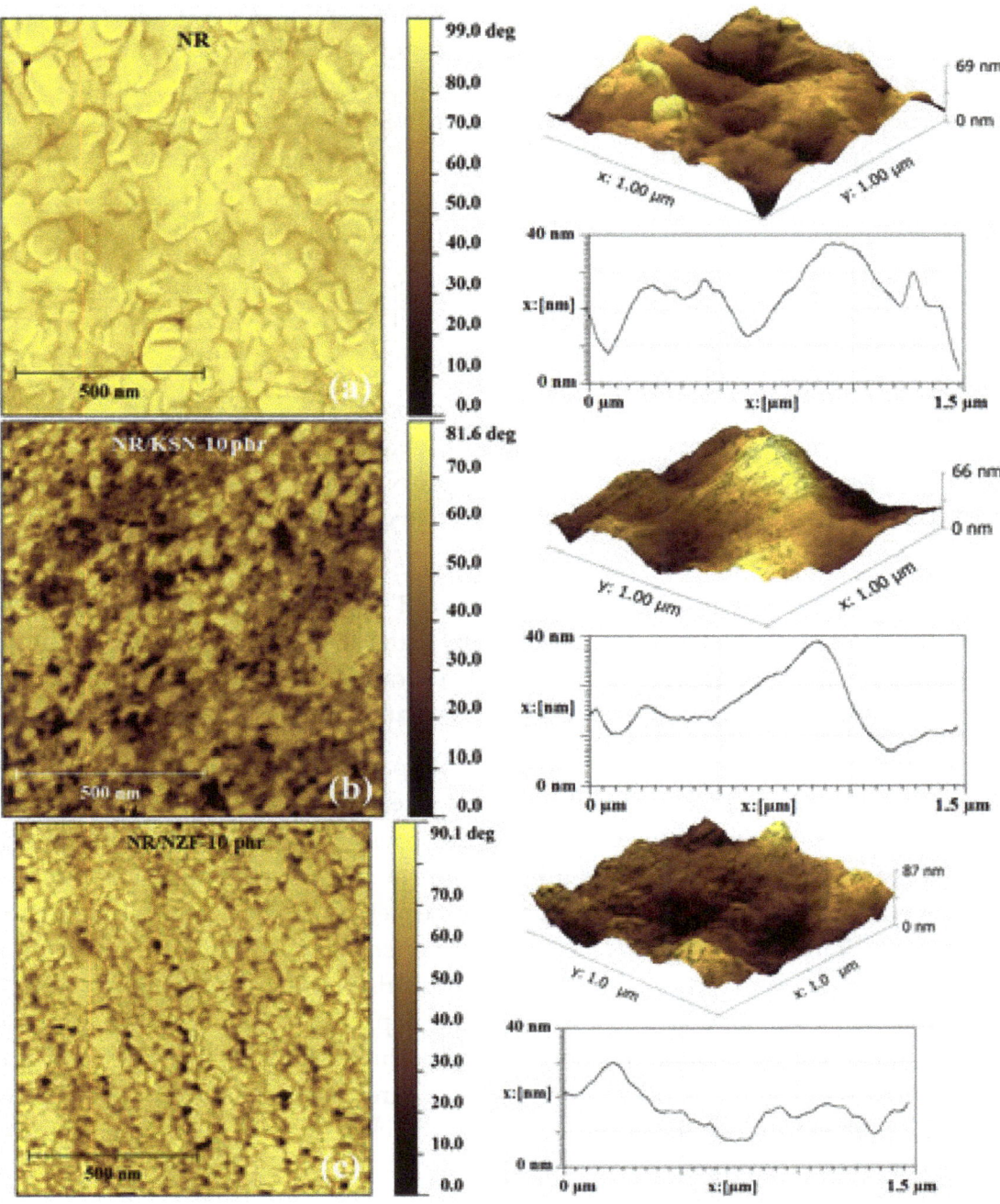

Figure 10. Images obtained using atomic force microscopy (AFM) to: (a) vulcanized natural rubber, (b) NR/KSN-10phr ferroelectric nanocomposite and (c) NR/NZF-10phr magnetic nanocomposite, performed directly on the surface of samples and their three-dimensional projections.

3.3. Polymer/ceramic composites and nanocomposites as an agent of control in Leishmaniasis colonies

Neglected diseases are illnesses that prevail not only in poverty conditions, but also contribute to the framework maintenance of economic and social inequality in the country (e.g. leishmaniasis, dengue, Chagas disease, schistosomiasis, leprosy and others [40]). As a result of this framework, multidisciplinary research involving materials science and biotechnology areas has gained significant strength, in order to develop new materials and methods to combat these diseases. For stimulating angiogenic processes [41] and due to its significant ability to disperse particulate fillers, natural rubber and its nanocomposites emerge as potential candidates for a new generation of bioactive agents with biocide character in biotechnology.

3.3.1. Biological study: toxicity evaluation

Due to great demand for innovation in biotechnology, nanoparticles and nanocomposites emerge as potential candidates for a new generation of biocides, and tests that assess the toxicity of these materials compared to mammalian cells comprises an important phase of the development process biotechnology.

Figure 11 presents the results of toxicity or viability evaluation of Vero cells after 48 h incubation in the presence of ceramic nanoparticles $KSr_2Nb_5O_{15}$ and $Ni_{0,5}Zn_{0,5}Fe_2O_4$ and their respective constituent elements, depending on particle concentration in the cellular environment [42].

According to Figure 11 for both ceramic phases and its constituent elements, except for potassium carbonate (K_2CO_3), there is no statistically significant decrease in cell viability at the end of the incubation period until the maximal concentration tested in this case (1000 µg/mL), compared to cells incubated only in the culture environment.

For cells culture in contact with potassium carbonate particles, there is clearly a statistically significant reduction ($P < 0.01$) in cell viability for concentration equal to or greater than 62.5 µg/mL. Potassium carbonate in aqueous environment tends to dissociate, originating potassium ions (K^+) that transform the extracellular environment, which should be hypotonic, in a highly hypertonic environment. Thus, cells pass for a excessive water-loss process through the cytoplasmic membrane and unbalances in key mechanisms for cell life maintenance, such as the sodium-potassium pump, mechanisms of nerve impulse conduction, protein synthesis and cell respiration. The combination of these processes is probably the responsible for the cell death observed for mammalian cells exposed to potassium carbonate particles. However, in $KSr_2Nb_5O_{15}$ ferroelectric phase, potassium ions (K^+) are isolated in the interstices of the crystallographic pentagonal structure (see Figure 4), which prevents the presence of these ions in the extracellular environment.

The results of toxicity or viability evaluation of Vero cells after 48 h incubation in the presence of vulcanized natural rubber NR/KSN ferroelectric and NR/NZF magnetic nanocomposites as a function of sample concentration in the cellular environment are shown in Figure 12. In detail, images generated by optical microscopy of cells exposed to NR/KSN-50 phr and NR/NZF-50 phr nanocomposites, and also the control sample.

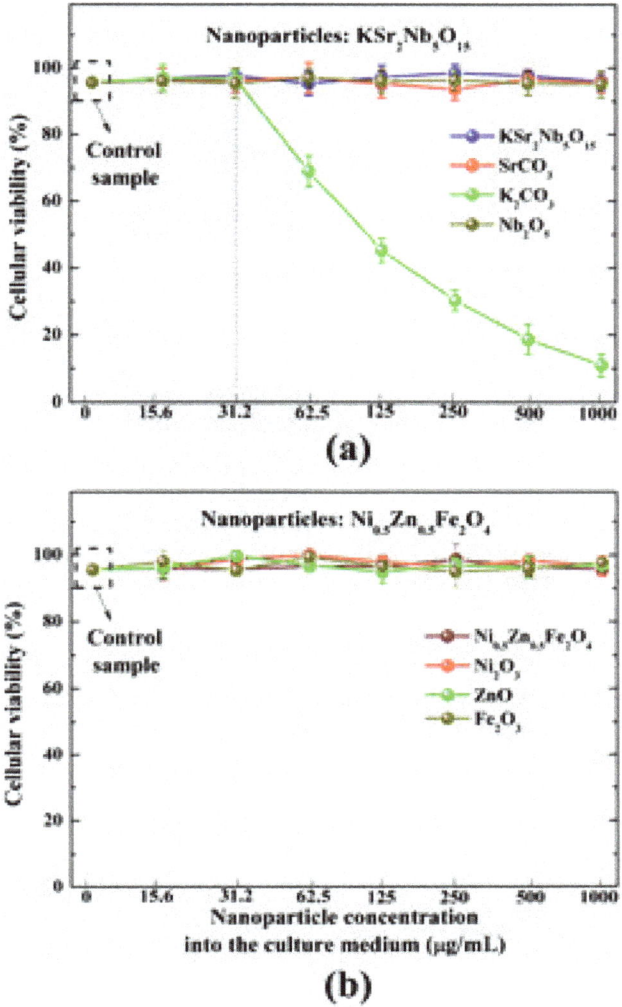

Figure 11. Cell viability in the presence of (a) ferroelectric nanoparticles, (b) magnetic nanoparticles and their respective constituents on the basis of the concentration of particles present in the culture environment. Vero-type mammalian cells cultured in particles presence were used.

As can be seen in Figure 12, for vulcanized natural rubber and both classes of nanocomposites, regardless of nanoparticles concentration, it is not possible to observe a statistically significant reduction in cell viability at the end of the incubation period until the maximal concentration tested (in this case 4000 µg/mL), compared to cells incubated only in the culture environment. In both images generated by optical microscopy, cells attached to the substrate are observed, indicating that cells remain biologically viable and comparing the cells exposed image to the two nanocomposites types with cells grown freely, it is not possible to identify significant morphological alterations, confirming that mammalian cells were not significantly affected due to nanocomposites presence. So as significant reductions were not identified in cell viability when mammalian cells were exposed to $KSr_2Nb_5O_{15}$ and $Ni_{0,5}Zn_{0,5}Fe_2O_4$ nanoparticles, vulcanized natural rubber and nanocomposites, one can consider that such systems have potential for using in biological systems composed by mammalian cells.

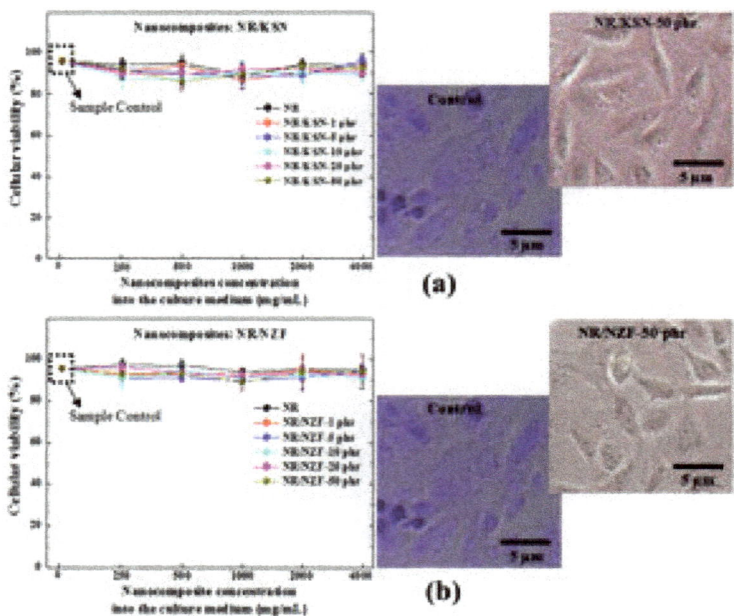

Figure 12. Cell viability in the presence of vulcanized natural rubber (a) NR/KSN ferroelectric and (b) NR/NZF magnetic nanocomposites as a function of sample concentration in the cell environment. In detail, images generated by optical microscopy of cells exposed and not exposed to nanocomposites. Vero-type mammalian cells were used, cultured in the presence of nanocomposites.

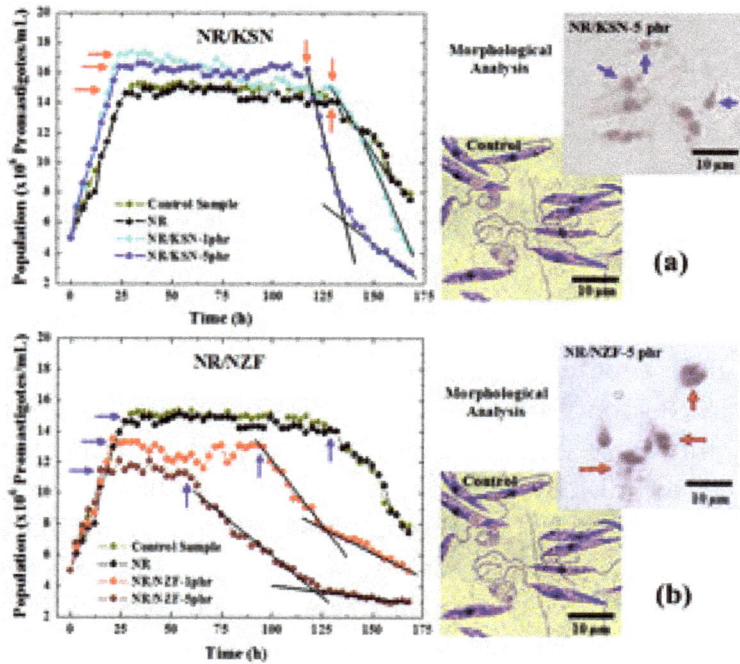

Figure 13. Population growth kinetics of Leishmania braziliensis (LB) parasite colony exposed to samples of vulcanized natural rubber, (a) NR/KSN and (b) NR/NZF nanocomposites. In detail, morphological comparison of parasites via optical microscopy.

Figure 13 presents the kinetics of colony population development of Leishmaniasis parasites exposed to vulcanized natural rubber samples, (a) NR/KSN ferroelectric and (b) NR/NZF magnetic nanocomposites in different nanoparticles concentrations. In detail, morphological comparison of the parasites after samples exposure.

Values for parameters maximum population density, phase duration, increase and decrease rates and also colony population of Leishmania braziliensis (LB) promastigotes exposed to samples of vulcanized natural rubber and nanocomposites are listed in Table 4.

Parameter	Sample							
	NR control	NR/KSN 1 phr	Δ%	NR/KSN 5 phr	Δ%	NR/NZF 1 phr	Δ%	NR/NZF 5 phr	Δ%
Generation time* (h)	14.4	9.3	-35%	9.7	-33%	13.1	-9%	12.0	-17%
Maximum population density (10^6 parasites/mL)	15.1	17.2	+14%	16.4	+9%	13.5	-11%	11.5	-24%
Length of logarithmic phase (h)	30	24	-20%	24	-20%	21	-30%	15	-50%
Average growth of logarithmic phase (10^6 cells/h mL)	0.3	0.51	+50%	0.48	+41%	0.4	+33%	0.4	+33%
Continuous phase duration (h)	102	108	+6%	93	-9%	75	-27%	42	-59%
Fall phase duration (h)	36	36	0%	51	+42%	72	+100%	111	+208%
Average rate of fall phase decrease (10^6 cells/h mL)	0.2	0.3	+50%	0.3	+50%	0.1	-50%	0.05	-75%

* Generation or double time: required time for doubling the cell population.

Table 4. Values for population development parameters of *Leishmania braziliensis* (LB) promastigotes colonies exposed to samples of natural rubber and vulcanized nanocomposites with different nanoparticle concentrations.

According to Figure 13 and data listed in Table 4, the increase curve evolution of LB promastigote population is similar for all samples studied, indicating that the presence of the samples did not change the colony global behavior. As expected, this evolution follows the standards of a colony of microorganisms grown in an artificial environment, being composed of three well-defined stages:

- **First stage:** denominated logarithmic phase, in which the pathogen has a large nutrient amount, conditions for their physiological maturation and mitotic cell division, a linear increase of promastigotes as a function of time is identified, and the average growth rate in this stage is higher for colonies exposed to samples. This suggests that the samples presence in the culture environment promotes the cell nutrition process;

- **Second stage:** denominated continuous phase, in which stabilize the processes of cell division, the parasites are mature and new members of the population do not arise; a constant number of promastigostas in function of time was identified. Oscillations in population density observed in this phase are due to cell death and reproduction, dependent on the environment nutritional availability or possible interaction between the parasite and the nanocomposite;

- **Third stage:** denominated fall phase, in which the nutritional resources of the culture environment are reduced and the process of cell death by depletion of internal micro-organism begins. A decreasing linear is identified, depending on time for control colony, and for the colonies exposed to vulcanized natural rubber samples and also linear decreasing for colonies exposed to samples of both nanocomposites and both nanoparticle concentrations, but with two different decrease rates, suggesting that there could be generations of parasites more resistant to the presence of samples in the colony, because they have already been evolved in nanocomposites presence.

Comparing the results for the control colony and the colony with a sample of vulcanized natural rubber samples, there is no statistically significant alterations in the of population growth kinetics, thus keeping unchanged the stages of cell development and maturation. However, for colonies exposed to nanocomposite samples having both nanoparticles, there are significant changes in microbial growth patterns. It should be mentioned that, regardless of the nanoparticle type associated with natural rubber, when the concentration of nanoparticles increases, the differences between the growth curves accentuate.

There is a progressive increase in the population of promastigotes in the logarithmic phase of the colonies exposed to NR/KSN nanocomposites (Figure 13 (a)), indicating that or KSN nanoparticles could come loose from nanocomposite surface, or something related to the interaction between the nanoparticles and the polymeric matrix is generating a change of or electronic nature significant structural proteins in the medium such that the parasites are able to ingest larger amounts of nutrients coming then to be reproduced more frequently. This hypothesis corroborates the reduction of over 30% in the generation time of the colonies.

The largest amount of immature parasites generated in logarithmic phase justifies the reduction in hours of the stationary phase, since the presence of large parasite quantities implies in a reduction of the amount of nutrients per parasite. It is worth mentioning that the population decrease noted in fall phase is intensified with increasing nanoparticles concentration in the nanocomposite, indicating that probably the same reason that is causing changes in culture proteins, facilitating their ingestion, is also hindering the absorption of these proteins by the parasites, accelerating nutritional starvation. Comparing the morphological characteristics of the parasites exposed to NR/KSN-5phr nanocomposites with colony control parasites [43, 44], one could clearly identify the kinetoplast and nucleus cell, but no significant morphological differences were observed, confirming the similarity of the curves in Figure 13 (a).

In the case of the colonies exposed to NR/NZF nanocomposite samples (Figure 13 (b)), one can identify a linear decrease in intensity of the logarithmic phase, depending of increasing concentration of nanoparticles, indicating that the presence of such nanoparticles difficult culture protein consumption and cell division by the parasite. However, a slight reduction (lower than 20%) can still be noticeable to the generation time of the colonies. With a smaller amount of parasites in culture and limited capacity of nutritional consumption in the environment, there is a smaller stationary phase and a fall phase greater than that of control colonies than the sample and exposed to natural rubber samples.

Comparing the morphological characteristics of the parasites exposed to NR/NZF-5phr nanocomposites with colony control parasites [43, 44], there is a clear morphological difference in cell design. Control parasites has elongated cell bodies, while for parasites in contact with NR/NZF-5phr, the cell body has approximately a circular shape.

Whereas both types of nanoparticles have nanometric sizes, the first factor to justify the identified differences is that the sum of factors such as differences in crystallinity, surface area, micro-deformations of the crystal lattice, cell volume and especially chemical composition that generate surface characteristics particular to each nanoparticle type is responsible for the differences noted in each colony. However, intrinsic interactions between cells and magnetic/ferroelectric nanoparticle properties, which would help to explain the high specificity exhibited by nanoparticles against leishmaniasis parasites and not against mammalian cells can not be discarded, although less likely.

4. Conclusions

Modified polyol method was used in the chemical synthesis of potassium strontium niobate ferroelectric oxide with stoichiometry $KSr_2Nb_5O_{15}$ and of nickel zinc ferrite paramagnetic oxide, stoichiometry $Ni_{0.5}Zn_{0.5}Fe_2O_4$. Single-phase ceramic phases with average crystallite size in nanometric scale were obtained. Using XRD and AFM essays, average crystallite size and particle surface parameters could be determined, mainly. We employed a method for the preparation of functional composites and nanocomposites based on vulcanized natural rubber, grounded in the dry mixing of the constituents using a open chamber mixing. A vulcanization system based on sulfur (S_8), suitable for natural rubber and ceramic nanoparticles was used. The development of a potential application for composites and nanocomposites based on vulcanized natural rubber was started and the preliminary results are encouraging, namely: use of paramagnetic and ferroelectric nanocomposites as modulating agents of the development of colonies of *Leishmania braziliensis* parasites.

Acknowledgements

The authors would want to acknowledge the Brazilian research agencies FAPESP, CAPES and CNPq for financial support, the graduate program of Materials Science and Technology, Carlos Gomes Barbosa-Filho and Dr. Josué de Moraes for the biological tests, Dr. José Antonio de Saja-Saéz, Prof. Dr. Miguel-Ángel Rodrigues-Pérez and Dr. Marcos Augusto de Lima Nobre for the scientific discussions and also Dr. Ricardo F. Aroca and Ariel Guerrero for the AFM measurements.

Author details

Aldo Eloizo Job*, Alexandre Fioravante de Siqueira, Caroline Silva Danna, Felipe Silva Bellucci, Flávio Camargo Cabrera and Leandra Ernst Kerche Silva

*Address all correspondence to: job@fct.unesp.br

Department of Physics, Chemistry and Biology, Univ Estadual Paulista, Presidente Prudente, Sao Paulo, Brazil

References

[1] Schneider P, Schmidt G. Nanocomposite polymer hydrogels. Colloid Polym Sci. 2009;287: 1-11.

[2] Bellucci FS et al. Preparation and structural characterization of vulcanized natural rubber nanocomposites containing nickel-zinc ferrite nanopowders. J. Nanosci. Nanotechnol. 2012; 12(3): 2691-2699.

[3] Oriakhi CO. Polymer nanocomposition approach to advanced materials. J. Chem. Educ. 2000; 77(9): 1138-1146.

[4] Moraes J et al. Schistosoma mansoni: In vitro schistosomicidal activity of piplartine. Exp. Parasitol. 2011; 127: 357-364.

[5] Joseph OH, Robert JN, Frank MC. Advantages of measuring changes in the number of viable parasites in murine models of experimental Cutaneous Leishmaniasis. Infect. Immun. 1983; 39(3): 1087-1094.

[6] Sepulveda C., editor. Leishmaniasis: Symptoms, Treatment and Potential Complications. Nova Publishers; 2013.

[7] Lindoso JAL et al. Review of the current treatments for leishmaniases. Research and Reports in Tropical Medicine. 2012;3: 69–77.

[8] Li XS et al. Synthesis and applications of functionalized magnetic materials in sample preparation. Trends Anal. Chem. 2013;45: 233-247.

[9] Lanfredi S et al. Síntese e Caracterização Estrutural do Niobato de Potássio e Estrôncio com Estrutura tipo Tetragonal Tungstênio Bronze (TTB). Cerâmica. 2005;51: 151-156.

[10] Zahi S. Synthesis, permeability and microstructure of the optimal nickel-zinc ferrites by sol-gel route. J. Electromagn. Anal. App. 2010;2: 56.

[11] Sharma S et al. Influence of Zn substitution on structural, microstructural and dielectric properties of nanocrystalline nickel ferrites. Mater. Sci. Eng., B. 2010;167: 189.

[12] Pessoa F. Síntese e caractarização de ferrita de níquel e zinco nanocristalina por combustão, para aplicação em compósito elastoméricoa absorvedores de micro-ondas. MSc dissertation. UFRJ; 2006.

[13] Lanfredi S. Structural characterization and Curie temperature determination of a sodium strontium niobate ferroelectric nanostructured powder. J. Solid State Chem. 2011;184(5): 990-1000.

[14] Das PS et al. Electrical properties of $Li_2BiV_5O_{15}$ ceramics. Physica B. 2007; 395: 98-103.

[15] Wititsuwannakul R et al. A rubber particle protein specific for Hevea latex lectin binding involved in latex coagulation. Phytochemistry. 2008;69(5): 1111-1118.

[16] Ajayan, P. M., Schadler, L. S. and Braun, P. V. Nanocomposite Science and Technology. Wiley-VCH GmbH & Co. KGaA. ISBN 3-527-30359-6, 2003.

[17] Calebrese C et. al. A review on the importance of nanocomposite processing to enhance electrical insulation. IEEE Trans. Dielectr. Electr. Insul. 2011; 18: 938.

[18] Zhou K et al. Dielectric response and tunability of a dielectric-paraelectric composite. Appl. Phys. Lett. 2008;93: 102908-102911.

[19] Ismail H et al. Properties of ferrite-filled natural rubber composites. Polym. Plast. Technol. Eng. 2007;46: 641-650.

[20] Spaldin NA. Magnetic materials: Fundamentals and device applications. Cambridge University Press; 2003.

[21] Malini KA et al. Magnetic and processability studies on rubber ferrite composite based on natural rubber and mixed ferrite. J. Mater. Sci. 2001;36: 5551.

[22] Daigle A et al. Structure, morphology and magnetic properties of $Mg_{(x)}Zn_{(1-x)}Fe_2O_4$ ferrites prepared by polyol and aqueous co-precipitation methods: a low-toxicity alternative to $Ni_{(x)}Zn_{(1-x)}Fe_2O_4$ ferrites. Nanotechnol. 2011;22(30): 305708.

[23] Feldman C. Polyol-mediated synthesis of nanoscale functional materials. Solid State Sci. 2005;7: 868-873.

[24] Nobre MAL. Varistores a Base de ZnO Obtidos a Partir das Fases $ZnSb_2O_6$ e $Zn_7Sb_2O_{12}$: Correlação entre as Fases, Microestrutura e Propriedades Elétricas. PhD thesis. Universidade Federal de São Carlos; 1999.

[25] Grison EC, Hoinacki E, Mello JB. Curso de tecnologia da borracha. Associação Brasileira de Química; 1984.

[26] Bellucci FS et al. Método de produção de nanocompósitos funcionais e produtos obtidos. Patent filing n° BR102012005278-4, 2012, international extension n° PCT/BR 2013/000063; 2013.

[27] Bellucci FS et al. Mechanical Properties of Vulcanized Natural Rubber Nanocomposites Containing Functional Ceramic Nanoparticles. Sci. Adv. Mater. 2013;5: 637.

[28] Rodriguez-Carvajal J. FullProf: A Program for Rietveld refinement and Pattern Matching Analysis. Collected Abstracts of Powder Diffraction Meeting, Toulouse, France, 1990;127.

[29] CPDS: Diffraction Data Base. Newton Square: International for Diffraction Data, CD-ROM, 1999.

[30] Moraes J et al. Schistosoma mansoni: In vitro schistosomicidal activity of piplartine. Exp. Parasitol. 2011;127: 357-364.

[31] Bellucci FS. Caracterização dielétrica de partículas nanométricas e nanoestruturadas de óxido de niobato da família tetragonal tungstênio bronze com estequiometria $KSr_2Nb_5O_{15}$. MSc dissertation. Univ Estadual Paulista; 2008.

[32] Lanfredi S, Cardoso CX, Nobre MAL. Crystallographic properties of $KSr_2Nb_5O_{15}$. Mater. Sci. Eng., B. 2004;112: 139-143.

[33] Ma R et al. Synthesis, characterization and electromagnetic studies on nanocrystalline nickel-zinc ferrite by polyacrylamide gel. J. Mater. Sci. Technol. 2008;24: 419-422.

[34] Desmond KW, Weeks ER. Random close packing of disks and spheres in confined geometries. Phys. Rev. E. 2009;80: 051305.

[35] Jamal EMA et al. On the magnetic, mechanical and rheological properties of rubber-nickel nanocomposites. Polym. Bull. 2010;64: 907.

[36] Lanfredi S. Thermistor behaviour and electricconduction analysis of Ni-doped niobate ferroelectric: the role of multiple β parameters. J. Phys. D: Appl. Phys. 2012;45: 435302.

[37] Ma R et al. Synthesis, characterization and electromagnetic studies on nanocrystalline nickel-zinc ferrite by polyacrylamide gel. J. Mater. Sci. Technol. 2008;24: 419.

[38] Trabelsi S, Albouy PA, Rault J. Stress-induced crystallization around a crack tip in natural rubber. Macromolecules. 2002;35: 10054-10061.

[39] Ozbas B et al. Strain-induced crystallization and mechanical properties of functionalized graphene sheet-filled natural rubber. J. Polym. Sci., Part B: Polym. Phys. 2012;50: 718-723.

[40] Departamento de Ciência e Tecnologia, Secretaria de Ciência, Tecnologia e Insumos Estratégicos, Ministério da Saúde. Doenças negligenciadas: Estratégias do Ministério da Saúde. Rev. Saúde Pública. 2010;44: 200.

[41] Ferreira M et al. Angiogenic properties of natural rubber latex biomembranes and the serum fraction of Hevea Brasiliensis. Braz. J. Phys. 2009;39(3): 564-569.

[42] Bellucci FS. Preparação e caracterização de nanocompósitos multifuncionais obtidos com nanopartículas ferroelétricas e paramagnéticas em filmes de borracha natural. PhD thesis. Univ Estadual Paulista and Universidad de Valladolid; 2013.

[43] Devorak G, Rovid-Spickler A, Roth JA. Handbook for zoonotic diseases of companion animals Interaction effects on the coercivity and fluctuation field in granular powder magnetic systems. Bayer Healthcare Animal Health; 2008.

[44] Barboza-Filho CG et al. The influence of natural rubber/Au nanoparticle membranes on the physiology of Leishmania brasiliensis. Exp. Parasitol. 2012;130: 152-158.

5

Environmental Changes and the Geographic Spreading of American Cutaneous Leishmaniasis in Brazil

Elizabeth F. Rangel, Simone M. da Costa and
Bruno M. Carvalho

1. Introduction

Global human population is facing the impacts of centuries of constant changes in natural environments. Impacts in the dynamics of infectious diseases are not only expected, but can already be noticed. Vector-borne diseases are particularly susceptible to environmental changes, since their occurrence depends on the ecological balance between different species in complex transmission cycles [1-3]. Leishmaniases are among the vector-borne diseases most affected by this *ecological chaos* driven by human actions [4], and one of the expected impacts is the expansion of its geographical distribution [5-7].

Leishmaniases are among the world's six most neglected diseases, affecting indistinctively men, women and children. Usually they occur among the poorest of the poor, mainly in developing countries, contributing to establishment and maintenance of social inequities [7]. They can be divided in two main clinical forms: visceral leishmaniasis (VL) and cutaneous leishmaniasis (CL). Despite this simple classification, a wide clinical spectrum is observed, mostly because of the high diversity of parasites (Trypanosomatidae of *Leishmania* genus), vectors (Phlebotominae sand flies) and reservoir hosts (mammals of several orders) involved in its transmission cycles [7, 8].

The geographical distribution of leishmaniases includes 98 countries in American, European, Asiatic, African and Australian continents. The World Health Organization estimates the yearly occurrence of about 200,000 to 400,000 VL human cases and 700,000 to 1.2 million CL human cases. More than 90% of global VL cases are recorded in six countries: India, Bangladesh, Sudan, South Sudan, Ethiopia and Brazil. Cutaneous leishmaniasis is more widely distributed, with about one-third of cases occurring in tropical regions of the Americas, the

Mediterranean basin, western and central Asia. In the American continent, Brazil is the country with the highest estimated incidences of both visceral and cutaneous leishmaniases [9].

The distribution of leishmaniases in the world can be partially explained by its widely distributed vectors. The sand flies are small insects (adults of about 3-5 mm) from order Diptera, family Psychodidae, subfamily Phlebotominae. Although occurring mainly in the tropical, hottest areas of the world (Latin America, South Europe, Africa, South Asia and Australia), their distribution stretches north and south to latitudes of over 40°, such as in Germany [10] and Argentinean Patagonia [11]. Sand flies have primarily crepuscular and nocturnal habits, but adults were captured during the day in dense forests [12], caves [13] and dark, humid animal shelters [14]. Only females are haematophagous and thus are related with *Leishmania* transmission. Their broad feeding habits contribute to the transmission of pathogens between hosts in sylvatic and peridomestic areas [15, 16]. Of approximately 900 described sand fly species, no more than 70 have been implicated in leishmaniases transmission [17]. All New World vector species belong to *Lutzomyia* genus, while the Old World vectors are grouped in *Phlebotomus* genus [15, 18].

In Brazil, the concept of leishmaniases as a sylvatic zoonosis is restricted to the Amazon Forest, Atlantic Forest fragments and parts of Cerrado. A new transmission profile has emerged, driven mostly by human-made environmental changes. In past decades, human migration of different origins and purposes resulted in major deforestation and unplanned settlements. These changes favor the dispersion of sylvatic animals (some *Leishmania* reservoir hosts) and sand flies (especially those species with eclectic feeding habits) to peridomestic areas, where new transmission cycles may establish close to human dwellings [19-21].

This new transmission profile is especially evident for American Cutaneous Leishmaniasis (ACL), which is caused by a variety of *Leishmania* parasites. Although some clinical manifestations are more frequently associated with a particular *Leishmania* species or subgenus (*Viannia* or *Leishmania*), none is unique to a species. In addition, a substantial but variable proportion of infections are asymptomatic. Human cases have been occurring with different clinical forms, including localized, disseminated, diffuse and atypical cutaneous and mucosal lesions. Different species of sand flies and reservoirs interact in complex transmission cycles, with particular ecoepidemiological features on each disease focus [22, 23].

According to Brazilian Ministry of Health [23], ACL can be categorized in three epidemiological patterns:

1. Sylvatic: In this case, transmission occurs in primary vegetation areas, where the disease is characterized as a strictly sylvatic zoonosis. Humans get infected occasionally when entering these areas, where the enzootic cycle is maintained;

2. Sylvatic/occupational and impacted areas: This pattern is associated with exploitation of natural environments and deforestation, originated mostly from constructions of roads, hydroelectric power plants, human settlements, wood extraction, agricultural activities, military training and ecotourism. In this case, humans are more intensively exposed to vector contact;

3.   Rural/periurban (colonization areas): ACL occurrence is related to human migration, occupation of slopes and aggregation in periurban areas associated with secondary and residual vegetation. Synanthropic and domestic animals such as dogs, horses and rodents are suggested reservoir hosts.

Brazil is currently facing an increasing geographical expansion of ACL, with a shift from the classical predominant epidemiological pattern 1 to frequent observations of pattern 2. All of its states have records of the disease, with a growing number of municipalities affected each year (Figure 1).

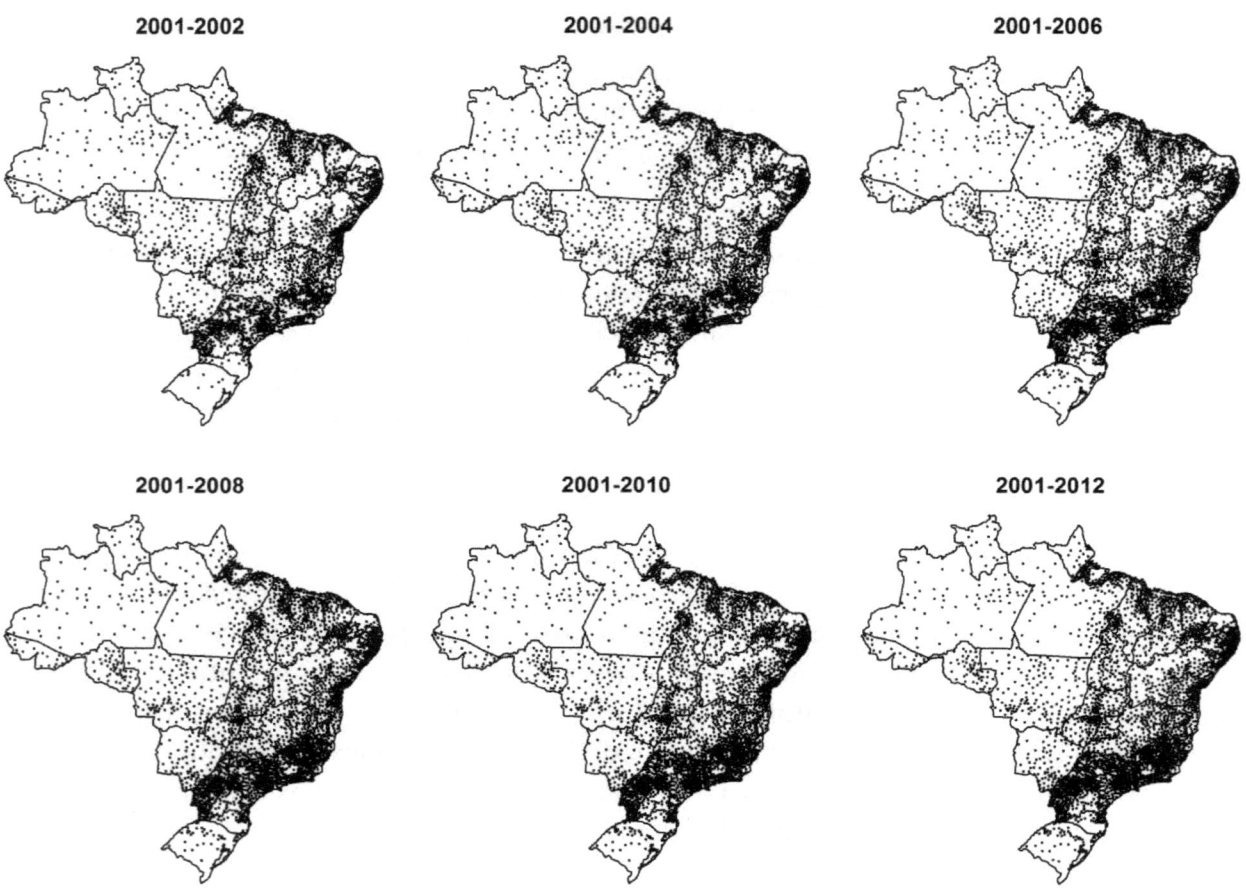

Figure 1. Brazilian municipalities with records of American Cutaneous Leishmaniasis, 2001 to 2012. Each point on the map represents one municipality with ACL human case records

This expansion can probably be explained by the growing environmental changes, which in turn affect vector behavior. Some ACL vector species have been showing evidences of adaptation to man-modified environments, establishing in peridomestic areas, even in outskirts of large cities [22, 23]. In this case, two sand fly species are particularly good examples, in different ecoepidemiological situations: *Lutzomyia (Nyssomyia) whitmani* and *Lutzomyia (Nyssomyia) flaviscutellata*. On the following sections the geographical distribution in Brazil and relation with ACL transmission of these species are presented.

2. *Lutzomyia* (*Nyssomyia*) *whitmani* (Antunes & Coutinho 1939)

Lutzomyia (N.) whitmani was described by Antunes & Coutinho in 1939 [24] as *Flebotomus whitmani* in honor of Dr. Whitman, from Rockefeller Foundation, an institute that collaborated with the Brazilian government at the time in the Yellow Fever Service. The new species was described based on male and female specimens captured in Ilhéus municipality, Bahia state. This species can be observed in all five regions of Brazil and, in the American continent it is also present in Argentina, French Guiana, Paraguay and Peru [7, 18].

The role of *L. (N.) whitmani* as ACL vector is evident throughout the Brazilian territory. The first observation of its importance in ACL transmission cycle was made in São Paulo state, where females were caught naturally infected by flagellates, possibly *Leishmania* [25]. In the same state, the biology of some sand fly species was studied, and *L. (N.) whitmani* was frequently found in deforested areas [26]. According to Pessoa & Coutinho [25], this species is considered highly anthropophilic, constantly invading houses for biting humans.

Between decades of 1930 and 1940, during the human colonization of South and Southeast Brazilian regions, ACL transmission was related with *L. (N.) whitmani*, with its occurrence mainly in sylvatic areas [27]. At this time, this sand fly species used to inhabit mainly forests. Man and domestic animals were bitten when they entered these areas or when houses were built near or inside forests [26]. Other studies on the ecology of *L. (N.) whitmani* showed aspects of its natural breeding places, monthly variation, high density and adaptation to domestic areas [28].

In Brazil, *L. (N.) whitmani* was already detected in 634 of its 5566 municipalities, occurring in all 27 federative units (Figure 2). The states with the higher spatial aggregation of municipalities with the vector occurrence are Pernambuco, Minas Gerais, São Paulo and Paraná, which are also areas of high concentration of ACL human cases [29] (see Figure 1).

Lutzomya (N.) whitmani is widely distributed across Brazilian biomes. Its presence was recorded in Amazon, Cerrado, Caatinga, Atlantic Forest and Pantanal (Figure 3), occurring mainly in Cerrado and Atlantic Forest [30]. When observing its occurrence in different Brazilian vegetation types, the vector occurs in municipalities with predominance of dense ombrophilous forest, deciduous ombrophilous forest, semideciduous ombrophilous forest, savannah and steppe (Figure 4). The species was not observed in municipalities predominantly covered by marshes and sandbanks [29].

In São Paulo state, *L. (N.) intermedia* and *L. (N.) whitmani* were the predominant species during deforestation of primary forests [28]. However, as deforestation continued to expand, *L. (N.) whitmani* showed lower abundances, suggesting that this species would be more dependent of primary forest than *L. (N.) intermedia*. On the other hand, *L. (N.) whitmani* was found frequently inside houses built near the forest. In Southeast Region, this species can be found during all months of the year [22, 26]. In São Roque municipality, São Paulo state, *L. (N.) whitmani* was the predominant sand fly species among *Leishmania (V.) braziliensis* transmission areas [31], showing higher abundances in the hotter months of the year [32].

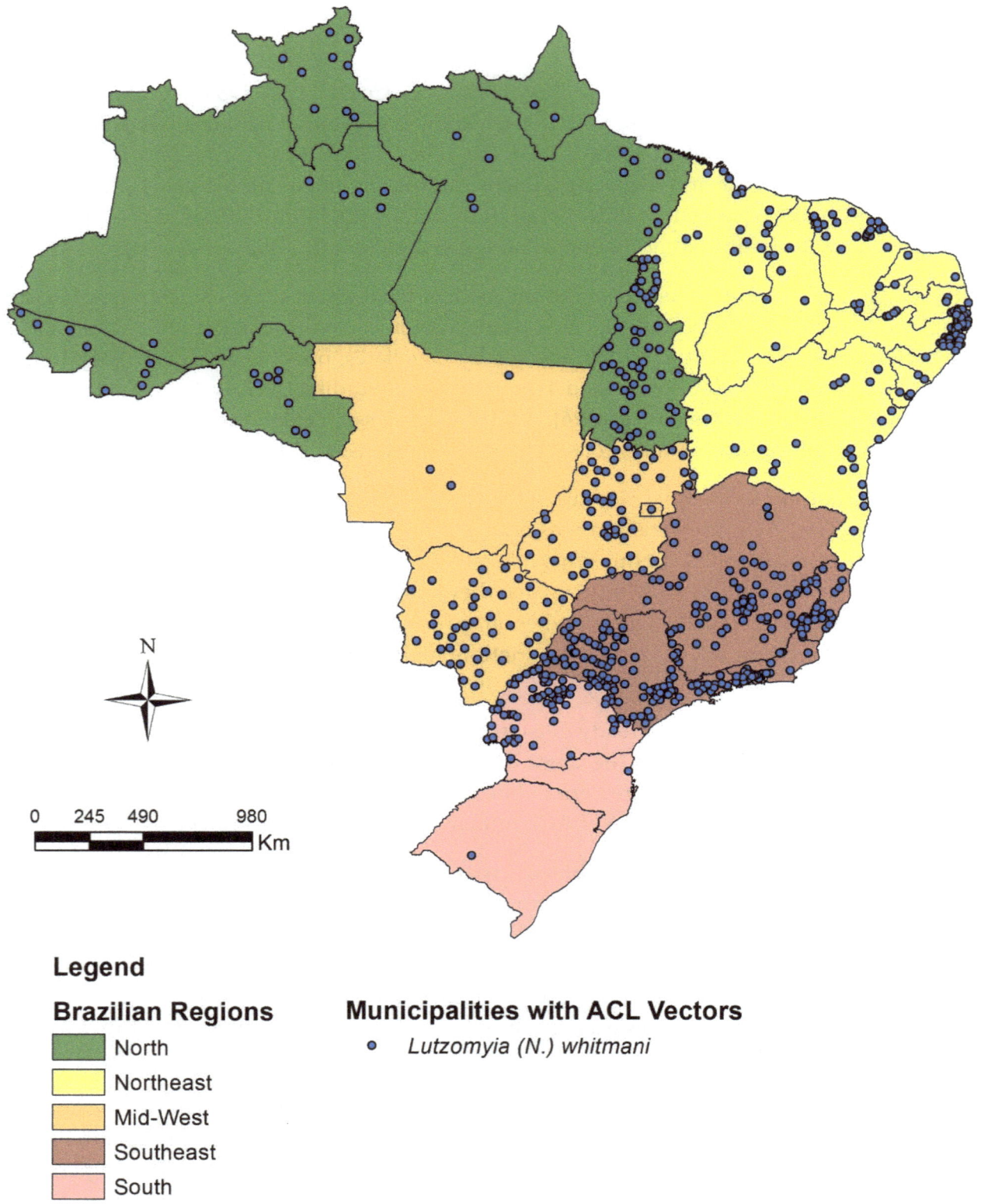

Legend

Brazilian Regions

- North
- Northeast
- Mid-West
- Southeast
- South

Municipalities with ACL Vectors

- *Lutzomyia (N.) whitmani*

Figure 2. Brazilian municipalities with *Lutzomyia (Nyssomyia) whitmani* occurrence

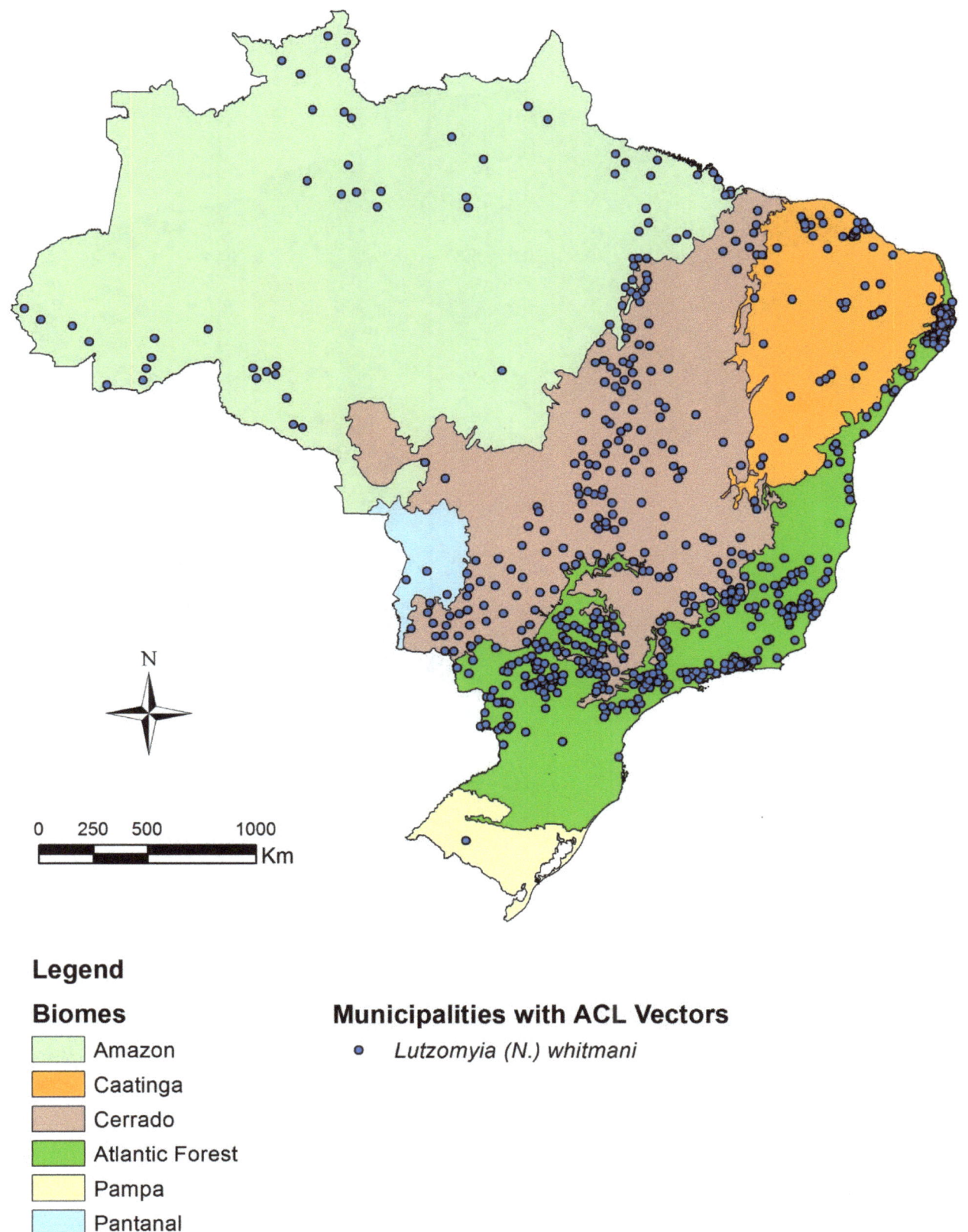

Figure 3. Brazilian municipalities with *Lutzomyia (Nyssomyia) whitmani* occurrence and biomes

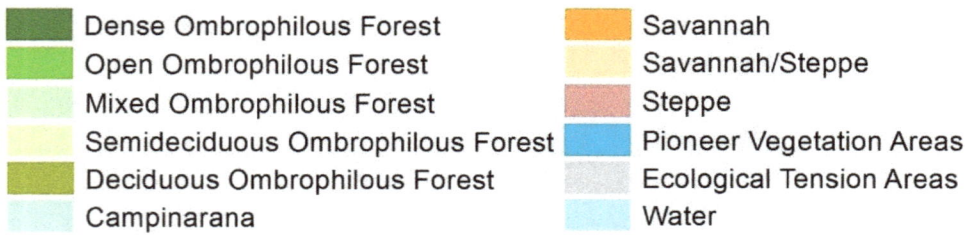

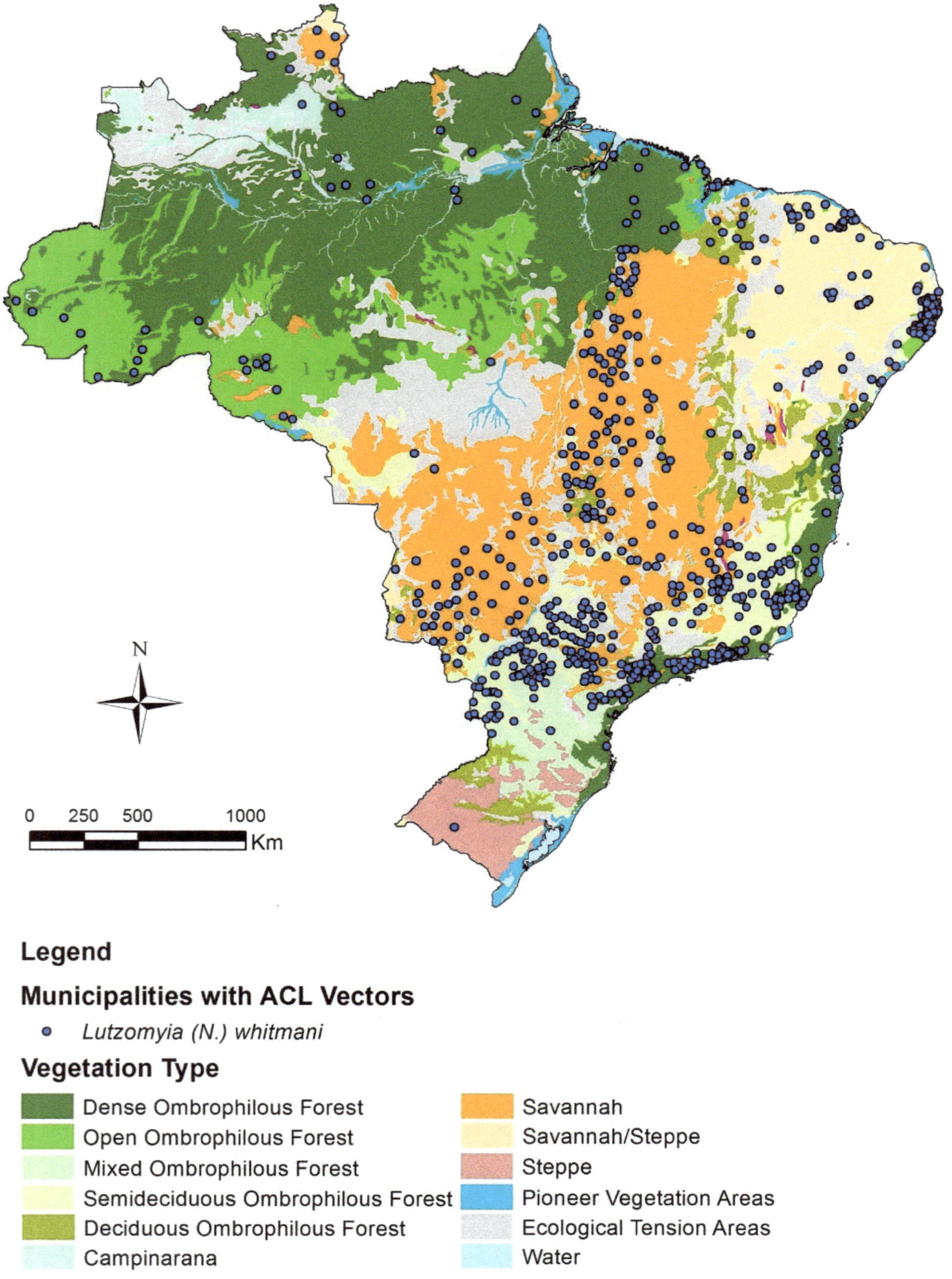
N
0 250 500 1000
Km
Legend
Municipalities with ACL Vectors
Lutzomyia (N.) whitmani
Vegetation Type
Dense Ombrophilous Forest
Open Ombrophilous Forest
Mixed Ombrophilous Forest
Semideciduous Ombrophilous Forest
Deciduous Ombrophilous Forest
Campinarana
Savannah
Savannah/Steppe
Steppe
Pioneer Vegetation Areas
Ecological Tension Areas
Water

Figure 4. Brazilian municipalities with *Lutzomyia (Nyssomyia) whitmani* occurrence and vegetation types

This species was also observed in Atlantic Forest protected areas and inside houses near the forest in Rio de Janeiro state [33]. In the same state, studies performed in rural areas of ACL transmission showed the co-occurrence of *L. (N.) intermedia* and *L. (N.) whitmani* biting humans. In peridomestic areas, *L. (N.) intermedia* was predominant, while *L. (N.) whitmani* was more frequent in the nearest forest. With this spatial separation, the authors suggested that both species would be sharing *Leishmania (V.) braziliensis* transmission on the same focus, throughout the year. *Lutzomyia (N.) whitmani* was captured during all year, but was more frequent in months with lower temperatures [34].

Also in Southeast region, besides São Paulo and Rio de Janeiro states, *L. (N.) whitmani* was associated with *Leishmania (Viannia) braziliensis* transmission in Caratinga (Minas Gerais state) and in a mountainous region of Afonso Cláudio (Espírito Santo state) [35, 36].

In South Brazil, *L. (N.) whitmani* is probably associated to ACL transmission in Paraná state. Studies performed in the north of this state detected it as predominant sand fly species and naturally infected by *Leishmania (V.) braziliensis* parasites [37].

Leishmania (V.) braziliensis in Northeast region is also probably transmitted by *L. (N.) whitmani*. In Bahia and Ceará states this vector shows similar habits to the Southeast region populations: high anthropophily and presence in domestic areas [38-40]. In Ceará state, *L. (N.) whitmani* was found naturally infected by *Leishmania* of *Viannia* subgenus [41]. Afterwards, new infections were detected and the parasite characterization confirmed to be *Leishmania (V.) braziliensis* [42]. Other evidences of this vector's role in ACL transmission in the region were its high abundance and anthropophily [40, 42].

In Bahia state, *L. (N.) whitmani* was found naturally infected by *Leishmania (V.) braziliensis* in Três Braços [43]. This finding, associated with the high frequency of this sand fly in peridomestic and domestic areas allowed the hypothesis of occurrence of a domestic transmission cycle in this area [44]. In Ilhéus municipality, *L. (N.) whitmani* was suggested as ACL vector, considering its almost absolute predominance over other sand fly species (99.7%), its high anthropophily and its occurrence on every sand fly capture point, most of them coincident with areas of ACL human cases [40].

In the Mid-West Region, in Corguinho municipality (Mato Grosso do Sul state), *Leishmania (V.) braziliensis* was isolated from every tested ACL patient by monoclonal antibodies. *Lutzomyia (N.) whitmani* was suggested as vector because it was observed in high abundances and anthropophilic [45]. Furthermore, its predominance over other sand flies was observed in eight of ten ecotopes studied in the locality. *Lutzomyia (N.) whitmani* was present both in ground level and in the forest canopy, suggesting its eclectic feeding habits on mammals and birds. Although in this locality the species is not very common in peridomestic areas, its high abundance and anthropophily are strong evidences of its role in ACL transmission [46].

The behavior of *L. (N.) whitmani* in North region seems to be different from other regions. In these areas, the species was considered mainly sylvatic, being captured on tree trunks and canopies, besides showing low attractiveness for humans [47]. Afterwards, novel studies confirmed such observations and suggested that, if the species were to be anthropophilic, it would be only in some situations [48, 49]. In 1989, in Pará state, a parasite was isolated from

L. (N.) whitmani, and after its characterization as *Leishmania (V.) shawi,* the sand fly species was suggested as its vector [50].

3. *Lutzomyia (Nyssomyia) flaviscutellata* (Mangabeira 1942)

Lutzomyia (N.) flaviscutellata was described by Mangabeira [51] as *Flebotomus flaviscutellatus,* based on two male specimens captured in Belém (Pará state). Later, Sherlock & Carneiro [52] described a female collected in Salvador (Bahia state), although its identification has been questioned by several authors [18, 27, 53]. At the same time, the species *Phlebotomus apicalis* was described by Floch & Abonnenc [54] in French Guiana. Three years later, after a review of the specimens, *P. apicalis* was considered synonym of *L. (N.) flaviscutellata* [55].

In the following years, descriptions of *L. (N.) olmeca* [56], *L. (N.) olmeca bicolor* [53] and *L. (N.) olmeca nociva* [57], all of them morphologically similar to *L. (N.) flaviscutellata,* led some authors to consider these four species as the "*L. flaviscutellata* complex" [58]. However, they are all currently considered valid species, with more recent taxonomic reviews supporting their status [18, 59].

Lutzomyia (N.) flaviscutellata is currently widely distributed across Latin America, occurring in Bolivia, Brazil, Colombia, Ecuador, French Guiana, Peru, Suriname, Trinidad and Venezuela [7, 18].

This sand fly species is associated with *Leishmania (Leishmania) amazonensis* transmission in Brazil. This parasite, when infecting humans, can cause localized cutaneous lesions and eventually develop a more severe clinical form, diffuse cutaneous leishmaniasis (DCL). This clinical form is rare, with chronic development, where the immunodepressed patient shows frequent relapses and insufficient responses to available therapies [60].

The first observation of this sand fly's role in ACL transmission cycle was from a study in the Utinga forest, an Amazon area in Belém municipality (Pará state) [61]. In this area, wild rodents of *Proechimys* and *Oryzomys* genus were captured with cutaneous lesions on tails and feet, from where *Leishmania* parasites were isolated. These rodents were then used as baits and 98% of captured sand flies were *L. (N.) flaviscutellata.* Captured sand flies were dissected and flagellates were isolated from eight females.

Studies of the feeding habits of *L. (N.) flaviscutellata* showed higher preference for small sylvatic rodents (*Proechimys* sp., *Oryzomys* sp.), agoutis (*Dasyprocta* sp.) and porcupines (*Coendou* sp.), having the species also fed on opossums (*Philander* sp.), monkeys (*Saimiri* sp.) and chickens (*Gallus gallus*). Few females fed on humans, so the authors considered the species as having low anthropophily [62]. This preference for biting small rodents indicates that captures of this species tend to be more efficient when using animal baited traps, such as the Disney trap [63].

Despite its strong zoophilic habits and low anthropophily, *Lutzomyia (N.) flaviscutellata* has recently been captured in peridomestic areas, suggesting its dispersion to human dwellings [64-67]. This hypothesis is plausible, since the species also occurs in secondary forests in the

Amazon. In a study performed in the late 1980s in Pará state, *L. (N.) flaviscutellata* was the predominant sand fly species in an area where the primary forest was replaced with exotic trees (*Pinus* and *Gmelina*), with occasional captures in peridomestic areas of houses near the forest [68]. In a review of the Amazonian ACL transmission cycles, *L. (N.) flaviscutellata* was considered one of the few vector species that could adapt to deforestation and become peridomestic [69].

In Brazil, *L. (N.) flaviscutellata* was detected in 131 municipalities, mostly in North and Mid-West regions, with occurrences also in Southwest and Northeast regions (Figure 5).

Lutzomya (N.) flaviscutellata is considered mainly an Amazonian species, although it can also be found in Cerrado and some few occurrences were recorded in Atlantic Forest, Caatinga and Pantanal (Figure 6).

In the Amazon, *L. (N.) flaviscutellata* is more commonly found in seasonally flooded areas of "igapó forests", when compared with non-flooded areas of "terra-firme forests" [70]. Its vertical distribution was also studied in the Amazon. The species has a very low flight, with 26 times more specimens captured 0.2 meters above ground than at 1.2 meters. This observation reinforces its association with small rodents and the fact that human cutaneous lesions caused by *Leishmania (L.) amazonensis* are mainly located in the lowest parts of the body [71].

The species was also captured in peridomestic areas of Manaus (Amazonas state) [72], Ilha de Marajó (Pará state) [73] and Santarém (Pará state) [74]. Other examples of surveyed Amazon forest areas of the North region with records of *L. (N.) flaviscutellata* include the states: Acre [75, 76], Amazonas [13, 76-79], Amapá [80], Pará [61, 62, 68, 70, 81], Rondônia [82, 83] and Roraima [84, 85].

Also in the North region, Tocantins state has most of its area covered by Cerrado. It was in this biome that *L. (N.) flaviscutellata* was captured during a four-year sand fly fauna monitoring in the ACL endemic areas of Porto Nacional and Guaraí municipalities. This vector species was found in peridomestic captures in rural settlements and periurban areas [66, 67] and was suggested as *Leishmania (L.) amazonensis* vector in Porto Nacional [66]. In municipalities of the south of the same state, *L. (N.) flaviscutellata* was captured near houses in areas directly and indirectly impacted by a hydroelectric power plant construction in Tocantins River [86].

In Bela Vista municipality (Mato Grosso do Sul State, Mid-West region), an ACL outbreak associated with *Leishmania (L.) amazonensis* in a military training unit led to a sand fly fauna monitoring during years 2004 to 2006. Using light traps, few specimens of *L. (N.) flaviscutella-ta* were caught [87]. When a modified Disney trap baited with hamsters (*Mesocricetus auratus*) was used, *L. (N.) flaviscutellata* was the species with the highest female abundance [88]. Despite its capture with these methodologies, some females were also captured in white and black Shannon traps [89], suggesting that the species can also feed on humans, and therefore be a possible *Leishmania (L.) amazonensis* vector in this locality [87].

The sand fly fauna of an ecotourism area in Bonito (Mato Grosso do Sul state) was studied. In Cerrado areas, *L. (N.) flaviscutellata* was caught with light traps mainly inside the forest, but it was also found in yards and kennels of houses [64].

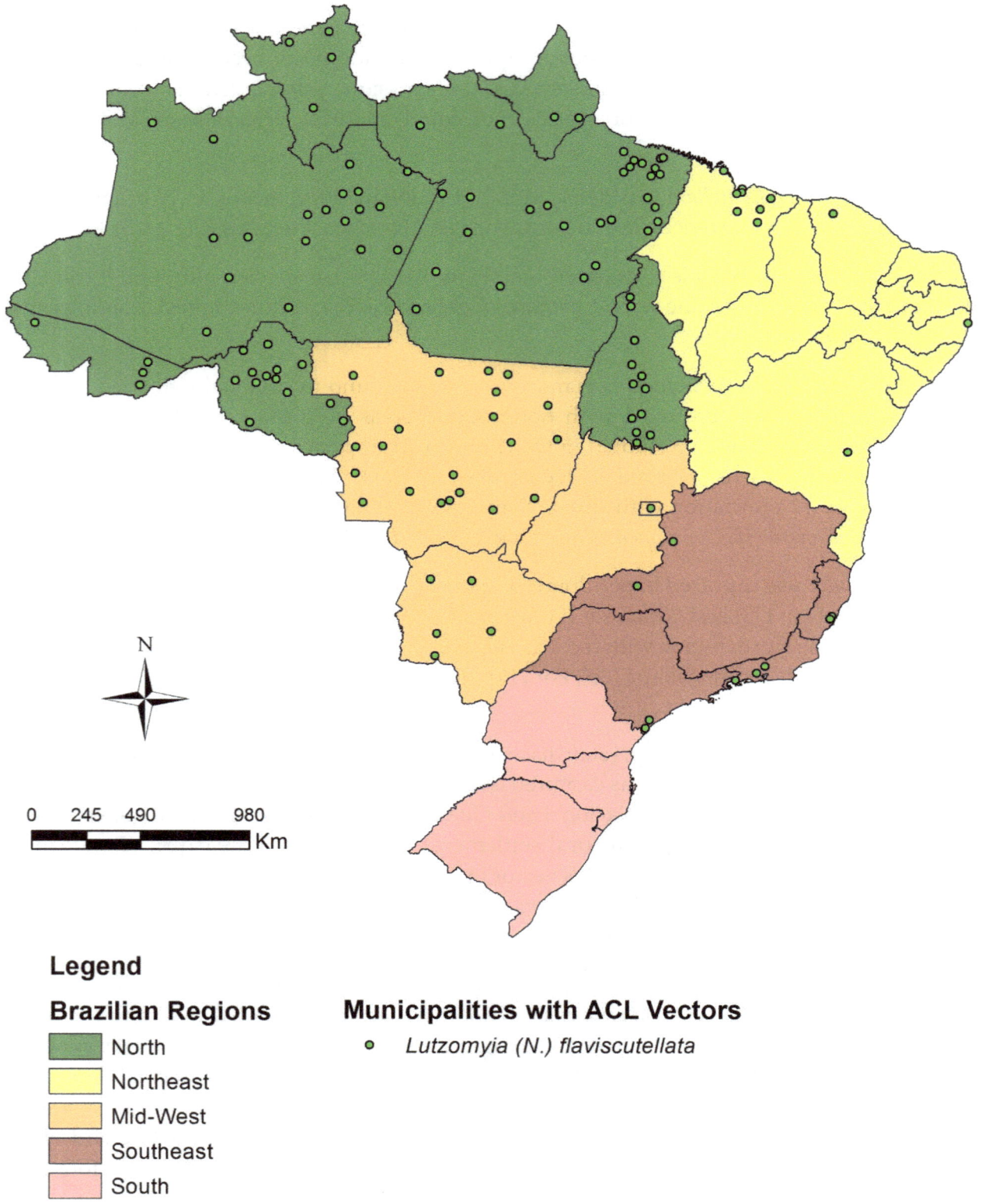

Figure 5. Brazilian municipalities with *Lutzomyia (Nyssomyia) flaviscutellata* occurrence

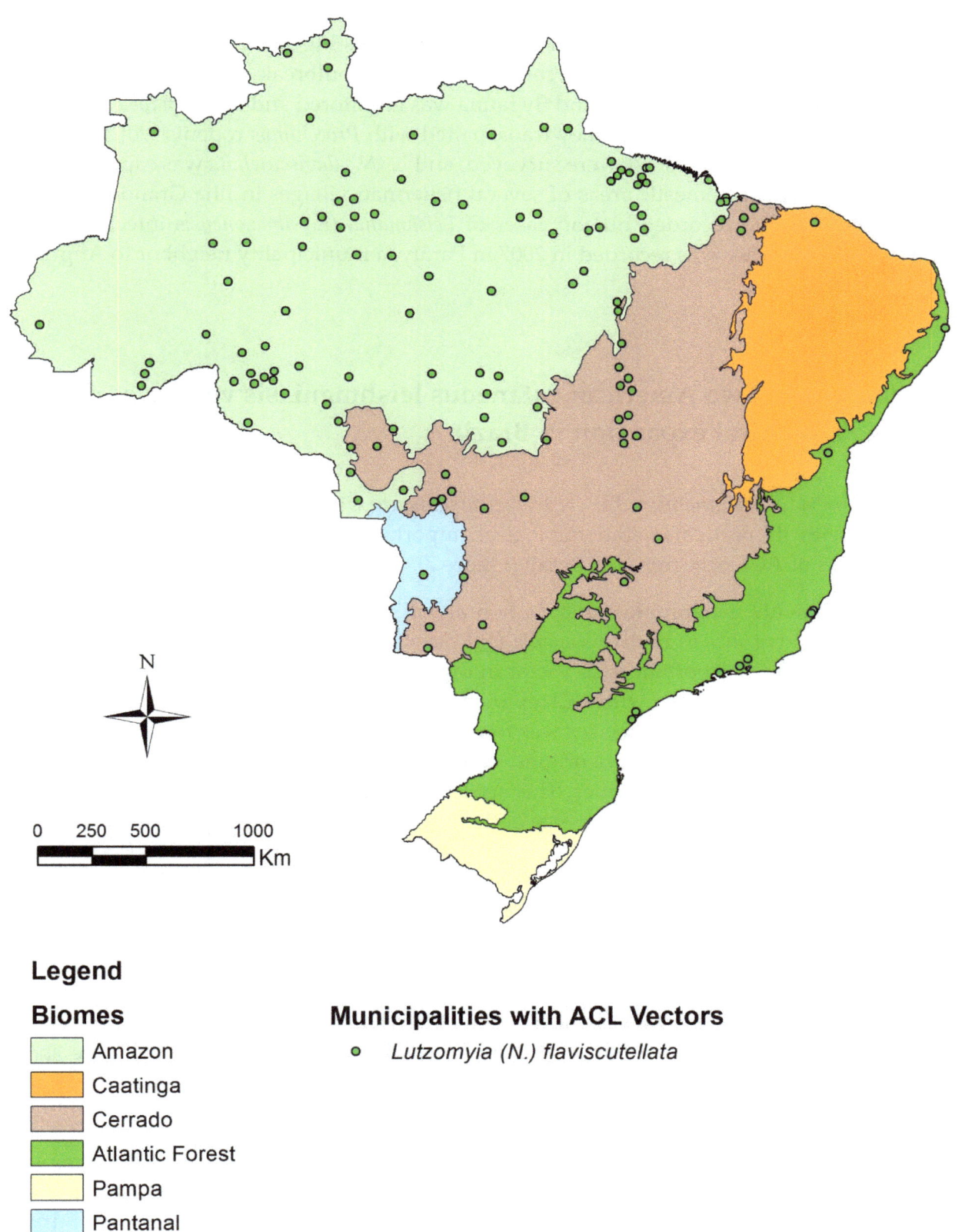

Legend

Biomes

☐ Amazon
☐ Caatinga
☐ Cerrado
☐ Atlantic Forest
☐ Pampa
☐ Pantanal

Municipalities with ACL Vectors

○ *Lutzomyia (N.) flaviscutellata*

Figure 6. Brazilian municipalities with *Lutzomyia (Nyssomyia) flaviscutellata* occurrence and biomes

In Southeast region, another ecotourism area was surveyed, in Rio de Janeiro state, Atlantic Forest biome. In Angra dos Reis municipality, the state's biggest continental island - Ilha Grande - has records of sporadic ACL cases since the first outbreak in the decade of 1970. At the time of the ACL outbreak, the sand fly fauna was monitored and *L. (N.) flaviscutellata* was captured inside the forest with Disney traps, baited with *Proechimys* rodents [90]. Over three decades later, the same localities were surveyed, and *L. (N.) flaviscutellata* was captured inside the forest and in peridomestic areas of several fisherman villages in Ilha Grande [65]. Even though there are no recorded human cases of *Leishmania (L.) amazonensis* infection in Ilha Grande, one DCL case was recorded in 2007 in Paraty, a municipality neighbor to Angra dos Reis [91].

4. Conclusion: Two American cutaneous leishmaniasis vectors as drivers of its geographical expansion in Brazil

Both *Lutzomyia (N.) whitmani* and *L. (N.) flaviscutellata* are widely spread in Brazilian territory. Each one with its particular epidemiological importance, their geographical distributions overlap areas of ACL occurrence in Brazil (Figure 7).

Since it has a wide geographical distribution and it is associated with two ACL parasites (*Leishmania (V.) braziliensis* and *Leishmania (V.) shawi*), currently, *Lutzomyia (N.) whitmani* is considered the most important ACL vector in Brazil. Its importance is due mainly to its role in transmission cycles related with ACL epidemiological pattern 2 (sylvatic/occupational and impacted areas). This sand fly species was found in several localities associated with areas of environmental changes of different origins, such as deforestation, road constructions, human settlements and agricultural activities. This epidemiological pattern is frequently observed in Brazil, and constitutes the main evidence of the disease's geographical spreading.

Lutzomyia (N.) flaviscutellata, with evidences of dispersion to peridomestic areas especially in the Cerrado biome, confirms the ruralization process of the previously considered strictly sylvatic cycle of *Leishmania (L.) amazonensis*. The possibility of this enzootic cycle to be maintained in secondary forests and even become peridomestic was previously discussed [69]. This could be happening, in part, because of the adaptation process of the vector to man-modified environments. At first, it would be logical to think that a strictly sylvatic cycle would disappear with deforestation of primary forests [92], but the *Leishmania (L.) amazonensis* cycle shows evidences of occurrence in secondary forests and peridomestic areas, where the vector could be dispersing to domestic animal shelters [22].

Considering the great challenge that is controlling ACL, a disease with complex epidemiology directly associated with environmental changes, studies that aim to characterize and monitor its spatial and temporal trends can support the Epidemiological and Entomological Surveillance actions of Health Departments. These studies can help to identify receptive areas for new ACL outbreaks and population groups at higher risk of infection, so that control actions can be better planned and more effective.

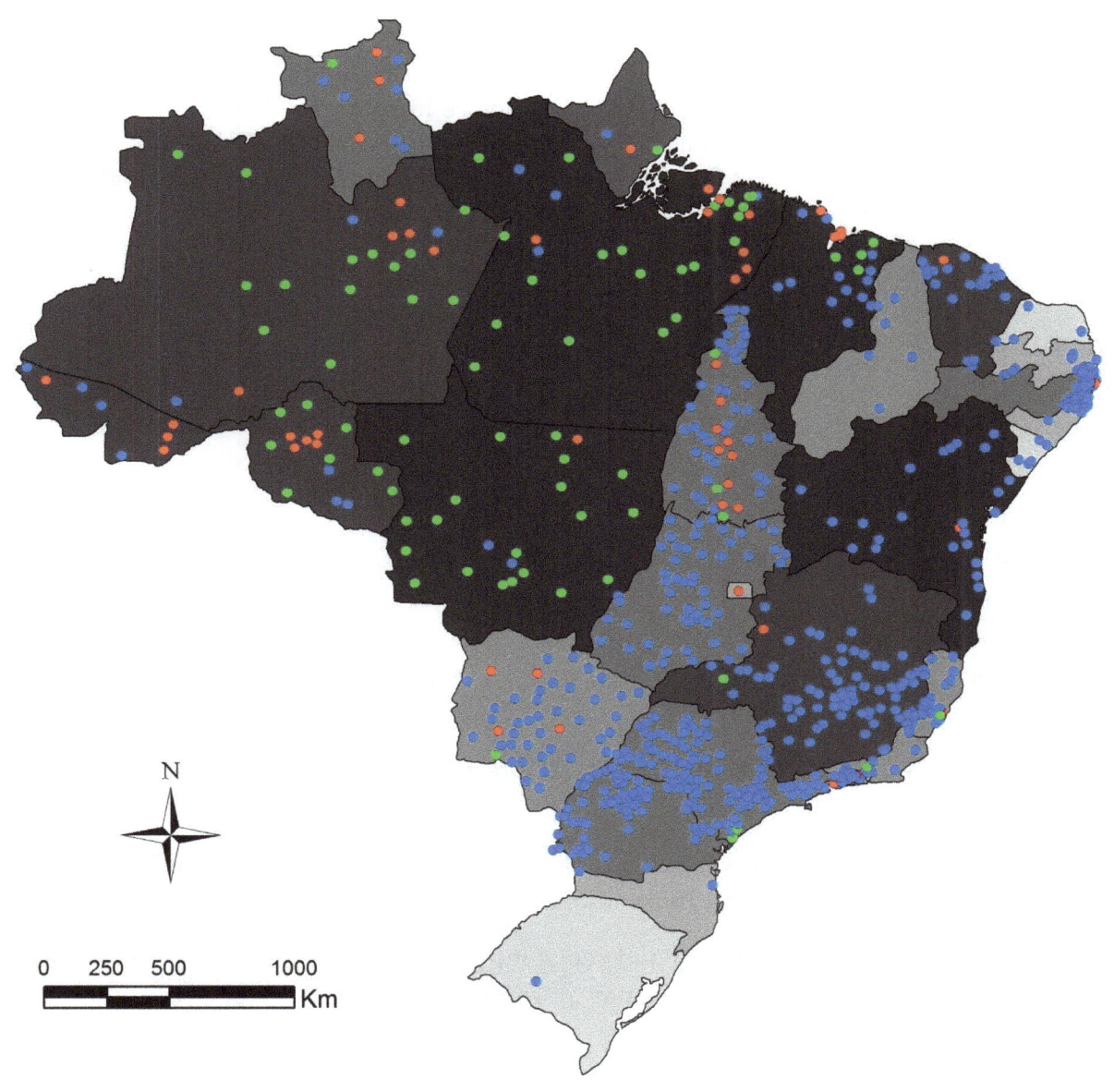

Legend

ACL Human Cases in 2003-2012

- 100 - 220
- 221 - 720
- 721 - 1700
- 1701 - 5450
- 5451 - 6770
- 6770 - 21530
- 21531 - 41774

Municipalities with ACL Vectors

- *Lutzomyia (N.) whitmani*
- *Lutzomyia (N.) flaviscutellata*
- *L. (N.) whitmani* and *L. (N.) flaviscutellata*

Figure 7. Brazilian municipalities with *Lutzomyia (Nyssomyia) whitmani* and *Lutzomyia (Nyssomyia) flaviscutellata* occurrence and American Cutaneous Leishaniasis human cases recorded by state in the past ten years (2003-2012)

Acknowledgements

To Mônica Magalhães, from Instituto de Comunicação e Informação Científica e Tecnológica em Saúde (FIOCRUZ) and Thiago Vasconcelos, from Instituto Evandro Chagas. To Fundação Carlos Chagas Filho de Amparo à Pesquisa do Estado do Rio de Janeiro (FAPERJ) and Instituto Oswaldo Cruz (FIOCRUZ) for financial support.

Author details

Elizabeth F. Rangel, Simone M. da Costa and Bruno M. Carvalho*

*Address all correspondence to: brunomc@ioc.fiocruz.br

Oswaldo Cruz Institute, FIOCRUZ, Rio de Janeiro, Brazil

References

[1] Walsh JF, Molyneux DH, Birley MH. Deforestation: effects on vector-borne disease. Parasitology 1993;106(Suppl) 55-75.

[2] Patz JA, Thaddeus KG, Geller N, Vittor AY. Effects of environmental change on emerging parasitic diseases. International Journal for Parasitology 2000;30 1395-1405.

[3] McMichael AJ. Environmental and social influences on emerging infectious diseases: past, present and future. Philosophical Transactions of the Royal Society London B 2004;359 1049-1058.

[4] Shaw J. How climatic and environmental variations affect the eco-epidemiology of the leishmaniases and their control. In: III Workshop de Genética e Biologia Molecular de Insetos Vetores de Doenças Tropicais; Recife (PE), Brasil 2008; p13.

[5] Ashford RW. The leishmaniasis as emerging and reemerging zoonoses. International Journal for Parasitol 2000;30 1269-1281.

[6] Dujardin JC. Risk factors in the spread of leishmaniases: towards integrated monitoring? Trends in Parasitology 2006;22(1) 4-6.

[7] WHO – World Health Organization. Control of the leishmaniases: report of a meeting of the WHO Expert Committee on the Control of Leishmaniases, Geneva, 22-26 March 2010 (WHO Technical Report Series, nº 949). Geneva: WHO Press; 2010.

[8] Peters W, Killick-Kendrick R. The Leishmaniasis in Biology and Medicine, London: Academic Press; 1987.

[9]   Alvar J, Vélez ID, Bern C, Herrero M, Desjeux P, Cano J, Jannin J, den Boer M. Leish-maniasis worldwide and global estimates of its incidence. PlosOne 2012;7(5) e35671.

[10] Naucke TJ, Pesson B. Presence of *Phlebotomus (Transphlebotomus) mascittii* Grassi, 1908 (Diptera : Psychodidae) in Germany. Parasitolgy Research 2000;86(4) 335-336.

[11] Muzón J, Spinelli GR, Salomón OD, Rossi GC. A first record of Phlebotominae from Argentinean Patagonia (Diptera: Psychodidae: Phlebotominae). Memórias do Instituto Oswaldo Cruz 2002;97(6) 797-798.

[12] Ready PD, Lainson R, Shaw JJ. Habitat and seasonality of *Psychodopygus wellcomei* help incriminate it as a vector of *Leishmania braziliensis* in Amazonia and northeast Brazil. Transactions of the Royal Society of Tropical Medicine and Hygiene 1984;78 543-544.

[13] Alves VR, Freitas RA, Santos FL, Barrett TV. Diversity of sandflies (Psychodidae: Phlebotominae) captured in sandstone caves from Central Amazonia, Brazil. Memórias do Instituto Oswaldo Cruz 2011;106(3) 353-359.

[14] Campbell-Lendrum DH, Brandão-Filho SP, Pinto MC, Vexenat A, Ready PD, Davies CR. Domesticity of *Lutzomyia whitmani* (Diptera: Psychodidae) populations: Field experiments indicate behavioural differences. Bulletin of Entomological Research 2000;90 41-48.

[15] Killick-Kendrick R. The Biology and Control of Phlebotomine Sand Flies. Clinics Dermatology 1999;17(3) 279-289.

[16] Afonso MMS, Chaves SAM, Rangel EF. Evaluation of feeding habits of haematophagous insects, with emphasis on Phlebotominae (Diptera: Psychodidae), vectors of Leishmaniasis - Review. Trends in Entomology 2012;8 125-136.

[17] Ready PD. Biology of Sand Flies as Vectors of Disease Agents. Annual Review of Entomology 2013;58 227-250.

[18] Young DG, Duncan MA. Guide to the identification and geographic distribution of *Lutzomyia* sandflies in Mexico, the West Indies, Central and South America (Diptera:Psychodidae). Memoirs of the American Entomological Institute 1994;54 1-881.

[19] Rangel EF. Tropical Diseases, Society and the Environment. SAREC Documentation/ TDR, 1995; 103-110.

[20] Rangel EF, Lainson R. Ecologia das Leishmanioses: Transmissores de Leishmaniose Tegumentar Americana. In: Rangel EF, Lainson R (eds.) Flebotomíneos do Brasil, Rio de Janeiro: Fiocruz; 2003. p291-310.

[21] Costa, SM, Cechinel M, Bandeira V, Zannuncio JC, Lainson R, Rangel EF. *Lutzomyia (Nyssomyia) whitmani* s.l. (Antunes & Coutinho, 1939) (Diptera: Psychodidae: Phlebotominae) and the Epidemiology of American Cutaneous Leishmaniasis in Brazil. Memórias do Instituto Oswaldo Cruz 2007;102(2) 149-153.

[22] Rangel EF, Lainson R. Proven and putative vectors of American cutaneous leishmaniasis in Brazil: aspects of their biology and vectorial competence. Memórias do Instituto Oswaldo Cruz 2009;104(7) 937-954.

[23] Brasil. Ministério da Saúde. Secretaria de Vigilância em Saúde. Departamento de Vigilância Epidemiológica. Manual de Vigilância da Leishmaniose Tegumentar Americana 2a. ed. Brasília: Editora do Ministério da Saúde; 2007.

[24] Antunes PCA, Coutinho JO. Notas sobre flebótomos sul-americanos. II. Descrição de *Flebotomus whitmani* n. sp. e da armadura bucal de algumas espécies. Boletim de Biologia de São Paulo 1939;4 448-453.

[25] Pessoa SB, Coutinho JO. Infecção natural e experimental dos flebótomos pela *Leishmania braziliensis* no Estado de São Paulo. O Hospital 1941;20 25-35.

[26] Barretto MP. Observações sobre a biologia em condições naturais dos flebótomos do estado de São Paulo (Diptera, Psychodidae). PhD thesis. University of Public Health São Paulo; 1943.

[27] Forattini OP. Entomologia Médica, 4º Volume: Psychodidae. Phlebotominae. Leishmanioses. Bartonelose. São Paulo: Edgard Blücher and Universidae de São Paulo; 1973.

[28] Forattini OP. Novas observações sobre a biologia de flebótomos em condições naturais (Diptera, Psychodidae). Arquivos da Faculdade de Higiene e Saúde Pública 1960;25 209-215.

[29] Costa SM, Cechinel M, Magalhães MAFM, Barcellos C, Rangel EF. Use of geoprocessing techniques in the analysis of the distribution of *Lutzomyia (Nyssomyia) whitmani* (Diptera:Psychodidae:Phlebotominae) in association with vegetation and the epidemiological circuits of American Cutaneous Leishmaniasis (ACL) in Brazil. In: International Symposium on Phlebotomine Sandflies, 25-30 Apr 2011, Kuşadası, Turkey. 2011.

[30] Costa SM, Cordeiro JP, Rangel EF. Distribuição espacial de *Lutzomyia (Nyssomyia) whitmani* (Diptera;Phychodidae;Phlebotominae), vetor de Leishmaniose Tegumentar Americana, em associação com os diferentes biomas brasileiros. In: 1ª Conferência Brasileira em Saúde Silvestre e Humana, 24-26 Oct 2012, Rio de Janeiro, Brazil. 2012.

[31] Taniguchi HH, Tolezano JE, Corrêa FMA, Morales RAP, Veiga RMO, Marassa AM. Epidemiologia da leishmaniose tegumentar americana no Estado de São Paulo, Brasil. I. Composição da fauna flebotomínica no Município de São Roque, Região de Sorocaba. Revista do Instituto Adolfo Lutz 1991;51 23-30.

[32] Taniguchi HH, Tolezano JE. American cutaneous Leishmaniasis in São Paulo State. II Seasonal fluctuation of Phlebotominae sandflies species in São Roque Country. Memórias do Instituto Oswaldo Cruz 1988;83(Supp.1) 201.

[33] Souza NA, Vilela ML, Andrade-Coelho CA, Rangel EF. The Phlebotominae sand fly (Diptera: Psychodidae) fauna of two Atlantic Rain Forest Reserves in the State of Rio de Janeiro,Brazil. Memórias do Instituto Oswaldo Cruz 2001;96(3): 319-324.

[34] Souza NA, Andrade-Coelho CA, Vilela ML, Peixoto AA, Rangel EF. Seasonality of *Lutzomyia intermedia* and *Lutzomyia whitmani* (Diptera: Psychodidae: Phlebotominae), occurring sympatrically in area of Cutaneous Leishmaniasis in the State of Rio de Janeiro, Brazil. Memórias do Instituto Oswaldo Cruz 2002;97(6) 759-765.

[35] Mayrink W, Willians P, Coelho MV, Dias M, Martins AV, Magalhães PA, Costa CA, Falcão AR, Melo MN, Falcão AL. Epidemiology of dermal leishmaniasis in the Rio Doce Valley, State of Minas Gerais, Brazil. Annals of Tropical Medicine and Parasitology 1979;73 123-137.

[36] Falqueto A. Especificidade alimentar de flebotomíneos em duas áreas endêmicas de leishmaniose tegumentar no Estado do Espírito Santo. PhD thesis. Fundação Oswaldo Cruz. Rio de Janeiro; 1995.

[37] Luz E, Membrive N, Castro EA, Dereure J, Pratlong F, Dedet JA, Pandey A, Thomaz-Soccol V. *Lutzomyia whitmani* (Diptera: Psychodidae) as vector of *Leishmania (V.) braziliensis* in Paraná state, southern Brazil. Annals of Tropical Medicine & Parasitology 2000;94(6) 623-631.

[38] Barreto AC, Vexenat JA, Cuba-Cuba CA, Marsden PD. Fauna flebotomínica de uma região endêmica de leishmaniose cutâneo-mucosa, no Estado da Bahia. In: IX Reunião Anual sobre Pesquisa Básica em Doenças de Chagas; 1982. p147.

[39] Vexenat JA, Barretto AC, Rosa AC. Infecção experimental de *Lutzomyia whitmani* em cães infectados com *Leishmania braziliensis braziliensis*. Memórias do Instituto Oswaldo Cruz 1986;81 125-126.

[40] Azevedo ACR, Rangel EF. Study of sandfly species (Diptera: Psychodidae: Phlebotominae) in focus of cutaneous leishmaniasis in the Municipality of Baturité, Ceará, Brasil. Memórias do Instituto Oswaldo Cruz 1991;86(4) 405-410.

[41] Azevedo ACR, Rangel EF, Costa EM, David J, Vasconcelos AW, Lepes VG. Natural infection of *Lutzomyia (Nyssomyia) whitmani* (Antunes & Coutinho, 1939) by *Leishmania* of the braziliensis complex in Baturite, Ceará State, northeast Brazil. Memórias do Instituto Oswaldo Cruz 1990;85: 251.

[42] Queiroz RG, Vasconcelos IA, Vasconcelos AW, Pessoa FA, Souza RN, David JR. Cutaneous leishmaniasis in Ceará State in northeasten Brazil: incrimination of *Lutzomyia whitmani* (Diptera: Psychodidae) as a vector of *Leishmania braziliensis* in Baturité municipality. The American Journal of Tropical Medicine and Hygiene 1994;50 693-698.

[43] Hoch A, Ryan L, Vexenet JA, Rosa AC, Barretto AC. Isolation of *Leishmania braziliensis braziliensis* and other trypanosomatids from Phlebotomines in mucocutaneous

leishmaniases endemic area Bahia, Brazil. Memórias do Instituto Oswaldo Cruz 1986;81(Suppl) BI 44.

[44] Ryan L, Vexenet A, Marsdem PD, Lainson R. The importance of rapid diagnoses of new cases of cutaneous leishmaniasis in pinpointing the sand fly vector. Transactions of the Royal Society of Tropical Medicine and Hygiene 1990;84: 786.

[45] Nunes VLB, Dorval MEC, RC, Oshiro ET, Noguchi Arão LB, Filho GH, Espínola MA, Cristaldo G, Rocha HC, Serafini LN, Santos D. Estudo epidemiológico sobre Leishmaniose Tegumentar (LT) no Município de Corguinho, Mato Grosso do Sul – estudos na população humana. Revista da Sociedade Brasileira de Medicina Tropical1995;28(3) 185-193.

[46] Galati EAB, Nunes VLB, Dorval MEC, Oshiro ET, Cristaldo G, Espínola MA, Rocha HCR, Garcia WB. Estudo dos flebotomíneos (Diptera, Psychodidae), em área de leishmaniose tegumentar, no Estado de Mato Grosso do Sul, Brasil. Revista de Saúde Pública 1996;30 115-128.

[47] Lainson R, Shaw JJ, Ward RD, Ready PD, Naiff RD. Lesmmaniases in Brazil: XIII. Isolation of *Leishmania* from armadillos (*Dasypus novemcinctus*), and observation on the epidemiology of cutaneous leismaniasis in north Pará State. Transactions of the Royal Society of Tropical Medicine and Hygiene 1979;73 239-242.

[48] Ready PD, Lainson R, Shaw JJ, Ward D. The ecology of *Lutzomyia umbratilis* (Ward & Fraiha, 1977) (Diptera: Psychodiade), the major vector to man *Leishmania braziliensis guyanensis* in north-eastern Amazonian Brazil. Bulletin of Entomological Research 1986;76 21-40.

[49] Shaw JJ, Ishikawa EAY, Lainson R, Braga RR, Silveira FT. Cutaneous leishmaniasis of man due to *Leishmania (Viannia) shawi* Lainson, De Souza, Póvoa, Ishikawa & Silveira in Pará State, Brazil. Annales de Parasitologie Humaine et Comparée 1991;66 243-246.

[50] Lainson R, Braga RR, De Souza AA, Pôvoa MM, Ishikawa EA, Silveira FT. *Leishmania (Viannia) shawi* sp. n., a parasite of monkeys, sloths and procyonids in Amazonian Brazil. Annales de Parasitologie Humaine et Comparée 1989;64(3) 200-207.

[51] Mangabeira O. 7a. Contribuição ao estudo dos *Flebotomus* (Diptera: Psychodidae). Descrição dos machos de 24 novas espécies. Memórias do Instituto Oswaldo Cruz 1942;37(2) 111-218.

[52] Sherlock IA, Carneiro M. Algumas fêmeas de *Phlebotomus* do Brasil (Diptera, Psychodidae). Memórias do Instituto Oswaldo Cruz 1962;60(3) 421-435.

[53] Fairchild GB, Theodor O. On *Lutzomyia flaviscutellata* (Mangabeira) and *L. olmeca* (Vargas and Diaz-Najera) (Diptera: Psychodidae). Journal of Medical Entomology 1971;8(2) 153-159.

[54] Floch H, Abonnenc E. Phlébotomes de Guyane Française. V. Institute Pasteur de la Guyane, Publ. No. 61. Cayenne: Institute Pasteur; 1943.

[55] Barreto MP. Sôbre a sinonímia de flebótomos americanos (Diptera, Psychodidae). Primeira nota. Revista Brasileira de Biologia 1946;6: 527-536.

[56] Vargas L, Días-Nájera A. *Phlebotomus farilli* n. sp., *Ph. humboldi* n. sp. y *Ph. olmecus* n. sp. de Mexico (Diptera: Psychodidae). Revista del Instituto de Salubridad y Enfermedades Tropicales1959;19 141-149.

[57] Young DG, Arias JR. A new phlebotomine sand fly in the *Lutzomyia flaviscutellata* complex (Diptera: Psychodidae) from northern Brazil. Journal of Medical Entomology 1982;19(2) 134-138.

[58] Lewis DJ. The *Lutzomyia flaviscutellata* complex (Diptera: Psychodidae). Journal of Medical Entomology 1975;12(3) 363-368.

[59] Galati EAB. Classificação de Phlebotominae. In: Rangel EF, Lainson R (eds.) Flebotomíneos do Brasil. Rio de Janeiro: Editora Fiocruz; 2003. p23-52.

[60] Costa JML, Cunha AK, Gama MEA, Saldanha ACR. Leishmaniose cutânea difusa (LCD) no Brasil: revisão. Anais Brasileiros de Dermatologia 1998;73(6) 565-576.

[61] Lainson R, Shaw JJ. Leishmaniasis in Brazil I. Observations on enzootic rodent leishmaniasis - Incrimination of *Lutzomyia flaviscutellata* (Mangabeira) as the vector in the lower Amazonian Basin. Transactions of the Royal Society of Tropical Medicine and Hygiene 1968;62 385-395.

[62] Shaw JJ, Lainson R. Leishmaniasis in Brazil: II. Observations on enzootic rodent leishmaniasis in the lower Amazon region – the feeding habits of the vector, *Lutzomyia flaviscutellata*, in reference to man, rodents and other animals. Transactions of the Royal Society of Tropical Medicine and Hygiene 1968;62(3) 396-405.

[63] Disney RHL. A trap for phlebotomine sandflies attracted to rats. Bulletin of Entomological Research 1966;56 445-451.

[64] Andrade ARO, Nunes VLB, Galati EAB, Arruda CCP, Santos MFC, Rocca MEG, Aquino RB. Epidemiological study on leishmaniasis in an area of environmental tourism and ecotourism, State of Mato Grosso do Sul, 2006-2007. Revista da Sociedade Brasileira de Medicina Tropical 2009;42(5) 488-493.

[65] Carvalho BM. Aspectos da ecologia de potenciais vetores de leishmanioses (Diptera: Psychodidae: Phlebotominae) na Ilha Grande, Angra dos Reis, Rio de Janeiro. MS dissertation. Instituto Oswaldo Cruz. Rio de Janeiro; 2011.

[66] Vilela ML, Azevedo CG, Carvalho BM, Rangel EF. Phlebotomine fauna (Diptera: Psychodidae) and putative vectors of leishmaniases in impacted area by hydroelectric plant, state of Tocantins, Brazil. PLoS One 2011;6(12) e27721.

[67] Vilela ML, Pita-Pereira D, Azevedo CG, Godoy RE, Britto C, Rangel EF. The phlebotomine fauna (Diptera: Psychodidae) of Guaraí, state of Tocantins, with an emphasis

on the putative vectors of American cutaneous leishmaniasis in rural settlement and periurban areas. Memórias do Instituto Oswaldo Cruz 2013;108(5) 578-585.

[68] Ready PD, Lainson R, Shaw JJ. Leishmaniasis in Brazil. XX: Prevalence of "enzootic rodent leishmaniasis" (*Leishmania mexicana amazonensis*) and apparent absence of pian-bois (*Le. braziliensis guyanensis*), in plantations of introduced tree species and in other non-climax forests in eastern Amazonia. Transactions of the Royal Society of Tropical Medicine and Hygiene 1983;77 775-785.

[69] Lainson R, Shaw JJ, Silveira FT, de Souza AA, Braga RR, Ishikawa EA. The dermal leishmaniases of Brazil, with special reference to the eco-epidemiology of the disease in Amazonia. Memórias do Instituto Oswaldo Cruz 1994;89(3) 435-443.

[70] Shaw JJ, Lainson R. Leishmaniasis in Brazil: VI. Observations on the seasonal variations of *Lutzomyia flaviscutellata* in different types of forest and its relationship to enzootic rodent leishmaniasis (*Leishmania mexicana amazonensis*). Transactions of the Royal Society of Tropical Medicine and Hygiene 1972;66(5) 709-717.

[71] Shaw JJ, Lainson R, Ward RD. Leishmaniasis in Brazil. VII. Further observations on the feeding habitats of *Lutzomyia flaviscutellata* (Mangabeira) with particular reference to its biting habits at different heights. Transactions of the Royal Society of Tropical Medicine and Hygiene 1972;66(5) 718-723.

[72] Feitosa MAC, Castellon EG. Fauna de flebotomíneos (Diptera: Psychodidae) em fragmentos florestais ao redor de conjuntos habitacionais na cidade de Manaus, Amazonas, Brasil. II. Estratificação horizontal. Acta Amazônica 2004;34(1) 121-127.

[73] Lainson R, Shaw JJ, Silveira FT, Fraiha H. Leishmaniasis in Brazil. XIX. Visceral leishmaniasis in the Amazon region, and the presence of *Lutzomyia longipalpis* on the Island of Marajó, Pará State. Transactions of the Royal Society of Tropical Medicine and Hygiene 1983;77(3) 323-330.

[74] Arias JR, Freitas RA. The known geographical distribution of sand flies in the State of Acre, Brasil (Diptera: Psychodidae). Acta Amazonica 1982;12 401-408.

[75] Azevedo ACR, Costa SM, Pinto MCG, Souza JL, Cruz HC, Vidal J, Rangel EF. Studies on the sandfly fauna (Diptera: Psychodidae: Phlebotominae) from transmission areas of American Cutaneous Leishmaniasis in state of Acre, Brazil. Memórias do Instituto Oswaldo Cruz 2008;103(8) 760-767.

[76] Castellón EG, Arias JR, Freitas RA, Naiff RD. Os flebotomíneos da região amazonica, estrada Manaus-Humaitá, Estado do Amazonas, Brasil (Diptera: Psychodidae; Phlebotominae). Acta Amazônica 1994;24(1-2) 91-102.

[77] Castellón EG, Fé NF, Buhrnheim PF, Fé FA. Flebotomíneos (Diptera, Psychodidae) na Amazônia. II. Listagem das espécies coletadas na bacia petrolífera no Rio Urucu, Amazonas, Brasil, utilizando diferentes armadilhas e iscas. Revista Brasileira de Zoologia 2000;17(2) 455-462.

[78] Silva DF, Freitas RA, Franco AMR. Diversidade e abundância de flebotomíneos do gênero *Lutzomyia* (Diptera: Psychodidae) em áreas de mata do nordeste de Manacapuru, AM. Neotropical Entomology 2007;36(1) 138-144.

[79] Alves VR, Freitas RA, Santos FL, Oliveira AFJ, Barrett TV, Shimabukuro PHF. Sand Flies (Diptera, Psychodidae, Phlebotominae) from Central Amazonia and four new records for the Amazonas state, Brazil. Revista Brasileira de Entomologia 2012;56(2) 220-227.

[80] Freitas RA, Naiff RD, Barrett TV. Species diversity and flegellate infections in the sand fly fauna near Porto Grande, state of Amapá, Brazil (Diptera: Psychodidae. Kinetoplastida: Trypanosomatidae). Memórias do Instituto Oswaldo Cruz 2002;97(1) 53-59.

[81] Ryan L. Flebótomos do Estado do Pará, Brasil (Diptera: Psychodidae: Phlebotominae). Tech Doc No. 1, Instituto Evandro Chagas, Belém, Pará, Brazil; 1986.

[82] Gil LHS, Basano AS, Souza AA, Silva MGS, Barata I, Ishikawa EA, Camargo LMA, Shaw JJ. Recent observations on the sand fly (Diptera: Psychodidae) fauna of the state of Rondônia, Western Amazonia, Brazil: the importance of *Psychodopygus davisi* as a vector of zoonotic cutaneous leishmaniasis. Memórias do Instituto Oswaldo Cruz 2003;98(6) 751-755.

[83] Gil LHS, Araújo MS, Villalobos JM, Camargo LMA, Ozaki LS, Fontes CJF, Ribolla PEM, Katsuragawa TH, Cruz RM, Silva AA, Silva LHP. Species structure of sand fly (Diptera: Psychodidae) fauna in the brazilian western Amazon. Memórias do Instituto Oswaldo Cruz 2009;104(7) 955-959.

[84] Castellón EG, Araújo Filho NA, Fé NF, Alves JMC. Flebotomíneos (Diptera: Psychodidae) no Estado de Roraima, Brazil. II. Espécies coletadas na região Norte. Acta Amazônica 1991;21 45-50.

[85] Castellón EG, Araújo Filho NA, Fé NF, Alves JMC. Flebotomíneos (Diptera: Psychodidae) no Estado de Roraima. III. Listagem das espécies no Estado. Acta Amazônica 1991;21 51-54.

[86] Vilela ML, Azevedo ACR, Costa SM, Costa WA, Motta-Silva D, Grajauskas AM, Carvalho BM, Brahim LRN, Kozlowsky D, Rangel EF. Sand fly survey in the influence area of Peixe Angical hydroeletric plant, state of Tocantins, Brazil. In: 6th International Symposium on Phlebotomine Sandflies, 27-31 Oct 2008, Lima, Peru; 2008.

[87] Dorval MEC, Cristaldo G, Rocha HC, Alves TP, Alves MA, Oshiro ET, Oliveira AG, Brazil RP, Galati EAB, Cunha RV. Phlebotomine fauna (Diptera: Psychodidae) of an American cutaneous leishmaniasis endemic area in the state of Mato Grosso do Sul, Brazil. Memórias do Instituto Oswaldo Cruz 2009;104 695-702.

[88] Dorval MEC, Alves TP, Cristaldo G, Rocha HC, Alves MA, Oshiro ET, Oliveira AG, Brazil RP, Galati EAB, Cunha RV. Sand Fly Captures with Disney traps in area of occurrence of *Leishmania (Leishmania) amazonensis* in the State of Mato Grosso do Sul,

mid-western Brazil. Revista da Sociedade Brasileira de Medicina Tropical 2010;43(5) 491-495.

[89] Galati EAB, Nunes VLB, Dorval MEC, Cristaldo G, Rocha HC, Gonçalves-Andrade RM, Naufel G. Attraction of black Shannon trap for phlebotomines. Memórias do Instituto Oswaldo Cruz 2001;96 641-647.

[90] Araújo Filho NA, Sherlock IA, Coura JR: Leishmaniose Tegumentar Americana na Ilha Grande, Rio de Janeiro. V. Observações sobre a biologia dos transmissores em condições naturais. Revista da Sociedade Brasileira de Medicina Tropical 1981;14(4-6) 171-183.

[91] Azeredo-Coutinho RB, Conceição-Silva F, Schubach A, Cupolillo E, Quintela LP, Madeira MF, Pacheco RS, Valete-Rosalino CM, Mendonça SC. First report of diffuse cutaneous leishmaniasis and *Leishmania amazonensis* infection in Rio de Janeiro State, Brazil. Transactions of the Royal Society Tropical Medicine and Hygiene 2007;101 735-737.

[92] Campbell-Lendrum D, Dujardin JP, Martinez E, Feliciangeli MD, Perez JE, Silans LNMP, Desjeux P. Domestic and peridomestic transmission of American cutaneous leishmaniasis: Changing epidemiological patterns present new control opportunities. Memórias do Instituto Oswaldo Cruz 2001;96(2) 159-162.

6

Geographical and Environmental Variables of Leishmaniasis Transmission

Roqueline A.G.M.F. Aversi-Ferreira,

Jucimária Dantas Galvão, Sylla Figueredo da Silva,

Giovanna Felipe Cavalcante,

Ediana Vasconcelos da Silva, Naina Bhatia-Dey and

Tales Alexandre Aversi-Ferreira

1. Introduction

Leishmaniasis, an infectious disease is not contagious. It belongs to the group of tropical neglected diseases [1, 2] that are ignored as priority in terms of eradication. It is estimated to be the ninth largest cause of disease among infected individuals [3, 4] ; it can cause intense epidemics that are primarily associated with the nutritional and the migratory factors [5, 6].

Most likely leishmaniasis originated in East Africa, however, it has been reported in ancient Egypt and in Christian Nubian approximately 4,000 B.C. In fact, it appears that Egyptians got the disease in the trade, as Egyptian Nile Valley is not a niche to sand flies [7]. Currently it has been reported in more than 80 countries, primarily in the developing countries in 4 continents, reaching indices around 500,000 new cases/year, with relatively higher incidence in India, Bangladesh, Nepal, Sudan and Brazil; approximately 200 million people have been estimated to get the exposure to the risk of its transmission [8].

Protozoan *Leishmania*, a unicellular flagellate, is the root cause of the disease; the parasite is transmitted to humans via female sand flies and manifests into two main forms: visceral [LV], and tegumentary [LT], the later divides into cutaneous [LC] and mucocutaneous [LMC] sub forms [7] (figure 1). Leishmaniasis has different clinical forms depending on the parasite, immune responses of the infected individuals and additional still unknown factors. Indeed, studies on leishmaniasis could be focused on both unknown and known factors to eradicate this disease.

The LV, also known as Kala-azar (Indian name), black fever or DumDum fever, is the most severe form of leishmaniasis (figure 1) caused by *Leishmania donovani* and *Leishmania infantum* (*Leishmania infantum chagasis*, a subspecies typical of Brazil), both protozoans belonging to the same family, *Trypanossomatidae*. These species have different geographical distribution: *Leishmania infantum* is typical of South America, Europe and Northern Africa, while *Leishmania donovani* is commonly found in Eastern Africa.

LV is a chronic and systemic disease characterized by anemia, mucosal ulcers, fever, hepatomegaly and splenomegaly, lymphadenopathy, pancytopenia, weight loss, weakness and, eventually death due to lack of treatment [9].

The most common form of leishmaniasis in the world is LC, it can progress to other forms and is caused by about 20 different species of *Leishmania*; it is known with various different names, such as Aleppo boil, Chiclero ulcer, Bauru's ulcer, Bay sore, Biskra button, Lahore sore, Oriental sore, Pian bois, Uta and leishmaniasis tropica.

LMC produces destructive and disfiguring lesions in the body, especially in the face (figure 1), they are primarily caused by *Leishmania braziliensis* and rarely by *Leishmania aethiopica*.

Regardless of the type of leishmaniasis this disease is transmitted through the bite of the female sand flies and the geographical distribution of this disease is directly associated with the habitat of its vector. Phlebotomine sand flies primarily inhabit hot and wet tropical regions with regular pluvial index [10], however, sometimes they also inhabit the dry and hot places; therefore, the environmental and geographical niches of this vector that are associated with its natural vertebrate hosts are determinants of the disease transmission.

The association of the vector with natural reservoir became a propitious factor towards keeping an endemic status for leishmaniasis. In fact, there are many natural reservoirs such as canine, avian (chicken), bovine, equine, caprine, ovine, swine and feline [11-14] ; all of them inhabit the same regions as Phlebotomine.

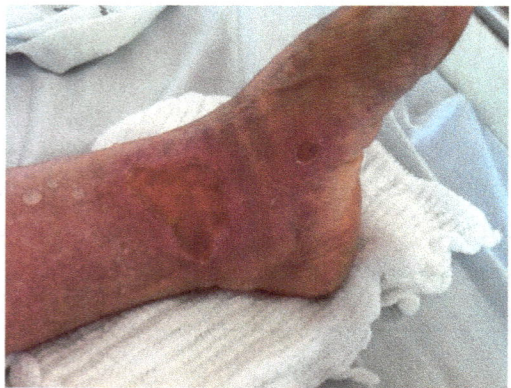 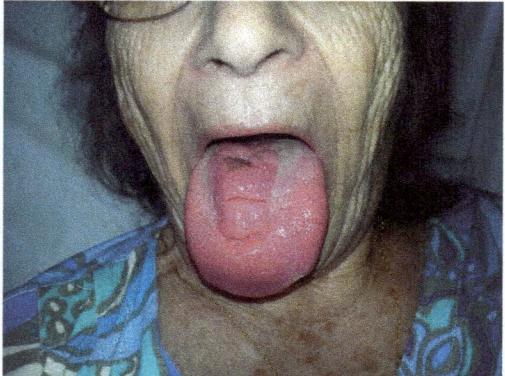

Figure 1. Clinical features of *cutaneous leishmaniasis* (left), and *mucocutaneous leishmaniasis* (right).

In addition, an important factor associated with leishmaniasis occurrence is the canine leishmaniasis (figure 2), a zoonosis that indirectly indicates the prevalence of this disease in humans at a specific site.

Indeed, leishmaniasis is associated with the tropical and the equatorial zones, poor sanitary conditions and surveillance in the areas where the parasites and the vectors are close to the reservoir and the humans, therefore, the most important point to understand the cause of epidemic and the transmission of the disease is the knowledge on the geographical and the environmental variables. Nevertheless, both these variables will be considered here into two categories: the worldwide and the regional.

In the geographic terms, the worldwide variables represent the geographic area where the vector has its niches and where the climate is favorable to its development. However, there are places and the environmental factors that are relatively propitious to the transmission of leishmaniasis than other factors such as higher population of the sand flies; these are considered.as the regional variables that would be accountable for the frequency of the disease.

In the environmental terms, the worldwide variables indicate the global climate and the associated landscape; however, the anthropomorphic factors and the climate peculiarities in a specific region represent the regional variables.

This chapter will present the worldwide and the regional aspects of geographical and environmental variables associated with leishmaniasis transmission.

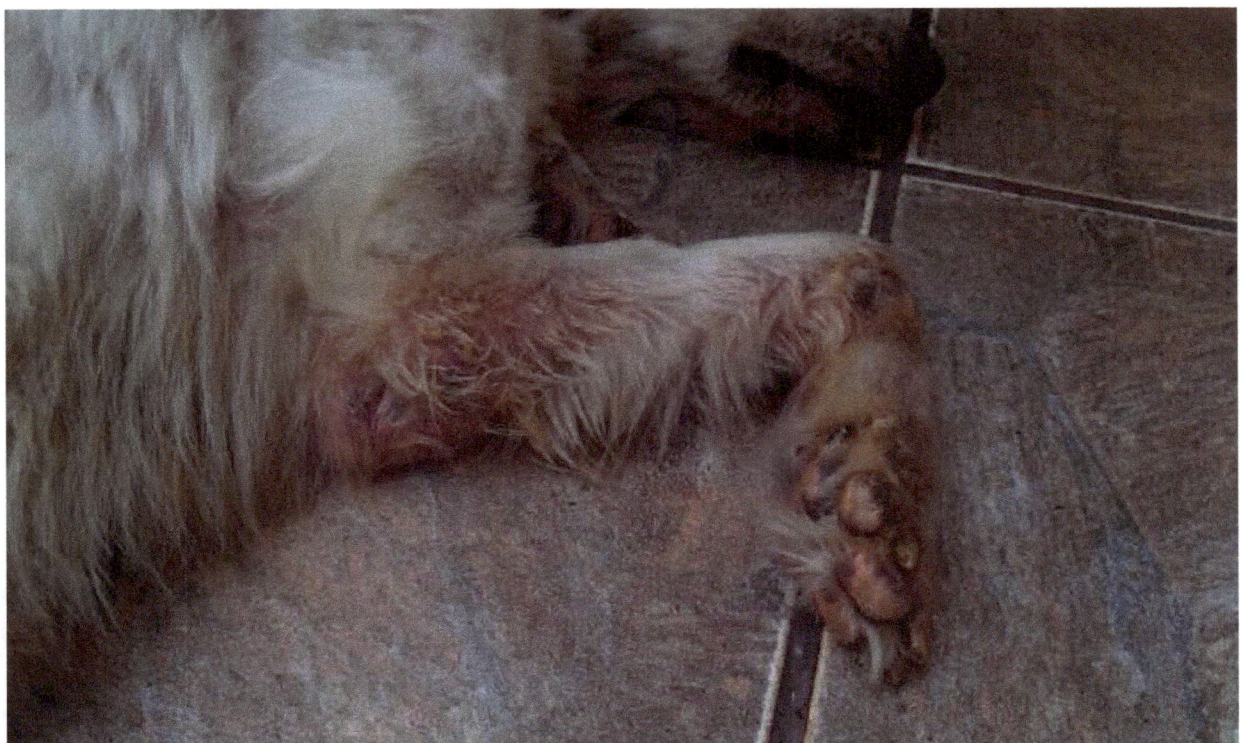

Figure 2. A photographic representation of a dog displaying clinical symptoms of canine leishmaniasis.

2. Materials and methods

The goal of this chapter is to collect the information from an extensive literature using the followings electronic databases: MEDLINE, Plos, PubMed, LILACS, CAPES periodic, Open Journal System, Scielo and Google Academic. The descriptors used were: *leishmaniasis, leishmaniasis visceral, leishmaniasis cutaneous, leishmaniasis mucocutaneous, Phlebotomine, the sand flies, the geographical aspects of leishmaniasis* and the *environmental aspects of leishmaniasis*.

2.1. Inclusion criteria

Indexed papers published in the last 20 years; classic indexed papers on more ancient and severe areas. Some textbooks have also been used to elaborate this chapter.

2.2. Exclusion criteria

Papers that did not mention the main ideas used in this chapter and the texts with the same contents as the most recent papers used here.

3. Geographical variables

3.1. Worldwide variables

In the terms of biosphere, geographical variables of leishmaniasis transmission are associated with tropical zone as well as hot and the wet climates with regular pluvial index [10]. The countries that are underdeveloped as well as the developing countries show the highest incidence of leishmaniasis transmission (figures 3 and 4).

Indeed, both human LV and LC follow the geographical distribution of the insect vector (see [15]); it is found globally between tropics but has also been detected in some regions with relatively rigorous winter such as in France [16], Portugal, Russia and China [3].

Based on the information available since past ten years, in Africa, the data on reported cases of LV are sparse and the reported cases in sub-Saharan African region are scarce (table 1); Nigeria had just one reported case within this period [3]. However, in Eastern African countries, LV is endemic and the reported cases have increased above predicted expectation in the last 20 years [9]. The countries with the most infections are Sudan [17, 18], Ethiopia [2, 9], South Sudan [3], Somalia, Uganda, Kenya [9] and Eritrea [3] (table 1, figures 3 and 4).

As for LC, Sub-Saharan region (figures 3 and 4) showed elevated number of the reported cases than cases for LV, i.e., 154 cases of LC in comparison to 1 case of LV; whereas the countries with higher number of LC cases are Cameroon and Nigeria respectively. In Eastern Africa, interestingly, Eritrea is the country with the lowest cases of LV and the highest cases of LC, while other countries in this region have no reported cases in the past ten years (table 1). In general, in African subcontinent, the number of reported cases of LV is much higher than those of LC, i.e., 8,571 of LV in comparison to 204 of LC.

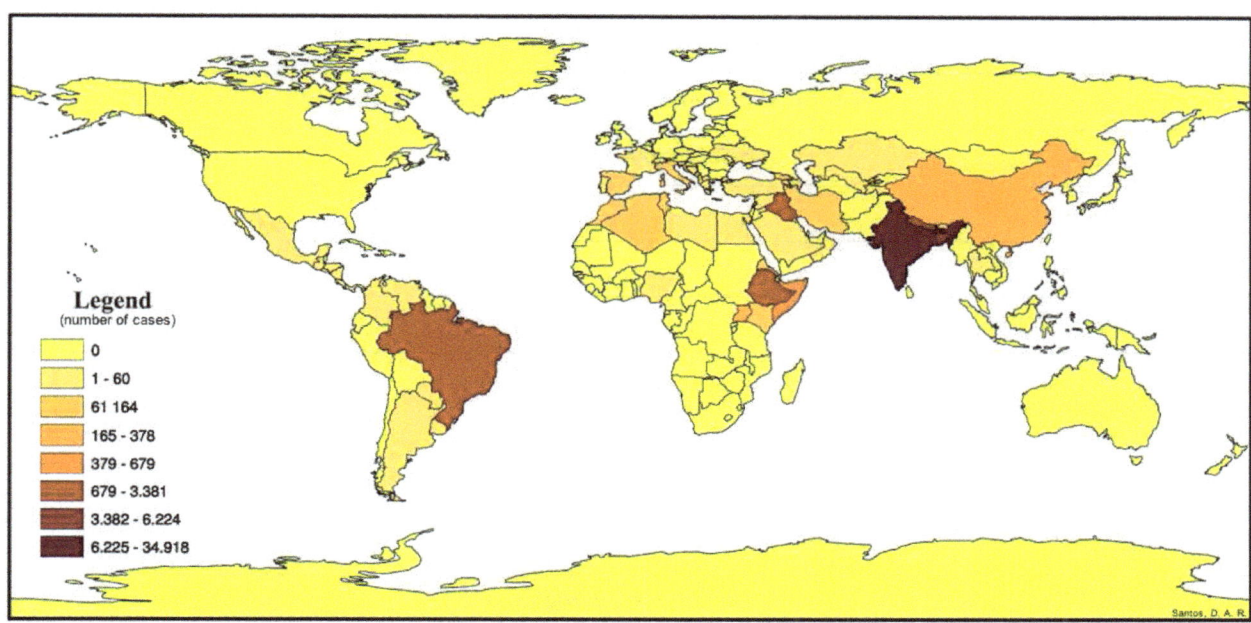

Figure 3. World LV distribution in the last 10 years.

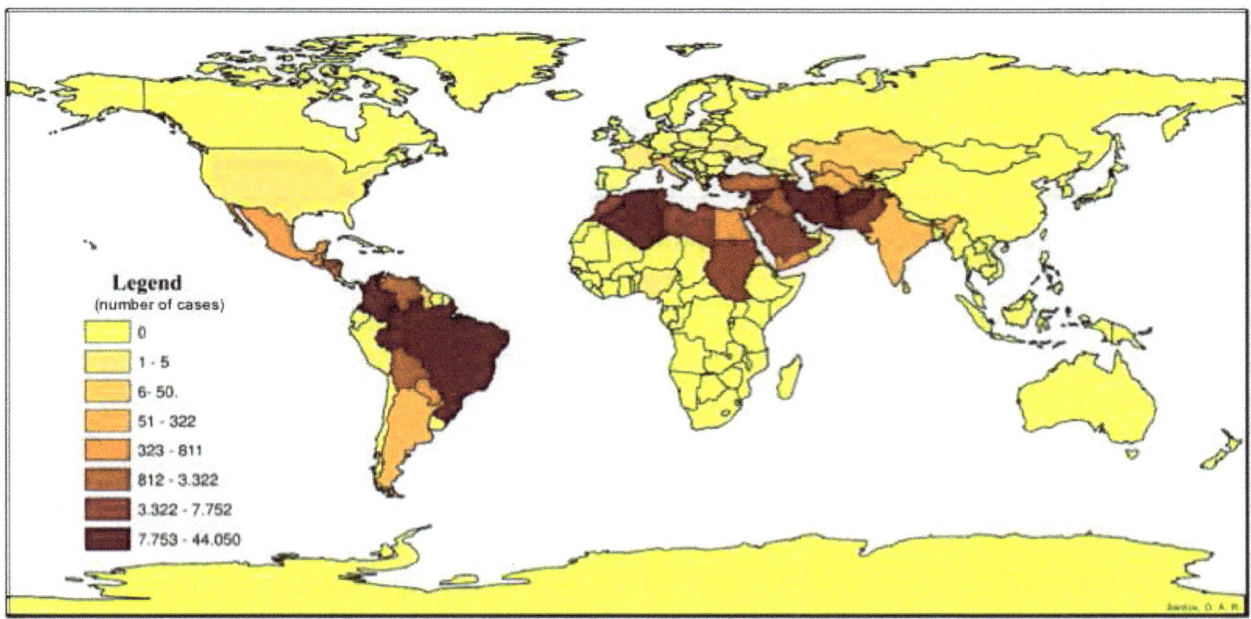

Figure 4. World LC distribution in the last 10 years.

	Reported cases in Africa	
	Visceral leishmaniasis	**Cutaneous leishmaniasis**
Sub-Saharan African region		
Cameroon	0	55
Cote d'Ivore	0	1
Ghana	0	27
Mali	0	58
Nigeria	1	5
Senegal	0	8
Total	**1**	**154**
Eastern African region		
Eritrea	100	50
Ethiopia	1860	0
Kenya	145	0
Somalia	679	0
Sudan	3742	0
South Sudan	1756	0
Uganda	288	0
Total	**8570**	**50**

Table 1. Geographical distribution of LV and LC in Africa based on reference [3].

In Asian subcontinent from the Middle East to Central Asia, significant LV prevalence was only found in Iraq with more than 1,000 reported cases; in China, Georgia and Iran the reported cases ranged at little over 100. In this Asian region, the reported cases of LC are much higher than those of LV, i.e., 61,015 of LC in comparison to 2,497 of LV. As regards to LC, more than 1,000 cases were reported in Iran, Afghanistan, Pakistan, Saudi Arabia and Iraq; and in Yemen and Uzbekistan the number of reported cases was over 100 (table 2) (figures 4 and 5).

In Indian subcontinent [3, 20] and in Southwestern Asia [3, 21], there are more than 1,000 reported LV cases in countries like India, Bangladesh and Nepal; in this same territory LC cases higher than 100 in number have only been reported in Sri Lanka and India. The reported total LV cases are higher than LC cases in Indian Subcontinent and in Southeastern Asia, i.e., 42,623 of LV in comparison to 478 of LC (table 2, figures 4 and 5).

In Asia, overall number of the reported LC cases is higher than those of LV cases, i.e., 61,493 of LC while 45,120 of LV.

	Reported cases in Asia	
	Visceral leishmaniasis	Cutaneous leishmaniasis
Middle East to Central Asia		
Afghanistan	0	22620
Armenia	7	0
Azerbaijan	28	17
China	378	0
Georgia	164	5
Iran	149	24630
Iraq	1711	1655
Kazakhstan	1	15
Oman	1	5
Pakistan	0	7752
Saudi Arabia	34	3445
Tajikistan	15	25
Turkmenistan	0	99
Ukraine	2	2
Uzbekistan	7	142
Yemen	0	603
Total	2497	61015
Indian Subcontinent and Southeastern Asia		
Bangladesh	6224	0
Bhutan	2	0
India	34918	156
Nepal	1477	0
Sri Lanka	0	322
Thailand	2	0
Total	42623	478

Table 2. Geographical distribution of LV and LC in Asia based on reference [3].

In the Mediterranean region, countries with more than 100 reported LV cases are Morocco, Italy, Spain, Albania and Algeria; for LC, the countries with more than 1,000 reported cases are Algeria, Syria, Tunisia, Libya, Morocco and Turkey (table 3, figures 3 and 4). Israel, Egypt, Jordan and Palestine are on lower tier of LC prevalence, in these countries, over 100 LC cases have been reported (table 3, figures 3 and 4). Thus in this region, overall number of the reported

LC cases is much higher than LV cases, i.e., 85,886 of LC in comparison to 874 of LV in the last ten years.

	Reported cases in the Mediterranean region	
	Visceral leishmaniasis	Cutaneous leishmaniasis
Albania	114	6
Algeria	111	44050
Bosnia and Herzegovina	2	0
Bulgaria	7	0
Croatia	5	2
Cyprus	2	1
Egypt	1	471
France	18	2
Greece	42	3
Israel	2	579
Italy	134	49
Jordan	0	227
Libya	3	3540
Macedonia	7	0
Malta	2	0
Montenegro	3	0
Morocco	152	3430
Palestine	5	218
Portugal	15	0
Spain	117	0
Syria	14	22882
Tunisia	89	7631
Turkey	29	2465
Total	**874**	**85556**

Table 3. Geographical distribution of LV and LC in the Mediterranean region based on reference [3].

In Latina America, the number of LV cases have increased in northern Argentina [22], in areas bordering Brazil and Paraguay, in Colombia [23], in Venezuela [24] as well as in North America [25] ; recently one case has been recorded in Uruguay as well [19] (table 4).

Brazil is the only country in the Americas with over 1,000 reported cases of LV, in other countries the reported cases of LV are lower than 100 (table 4). In contrast, LC is relatively widespread with 10 countries that have over 1,000 reported cases, these are Brazil, Colombia, Peru, Nicaragua, Bolivia, Venezuela, Panama, Ecuador, Costa Rica and Honduras in descending order of prevalence. Additionally, 5 countries show over 100 reported cases, they are Mexico, Guatemala, Paraguay, Argentina and French Guyana respectively (table 4).

An interesting aspect in the Americas is the inclusion of the United States in the world scenario with 42 reported cases of LC [25].

The overall number of the reported cases of LC is much higher than those of LV, i.e., 66,983of LC in comparison to only 3,668 of LV in the American subcontinent.

Specifically in Brazil, and mostly in other developing countries, leishmaniasis was restricted to rural areas; however, currently the disease has advanced to other regions and has reached urban peripheries [26-28]. This demonstrates that the urbanization process is one of the major factors for the scattering of leishmaniasis.

	Reported cases in America	
	Visceral leishmaniasis	Cutaneous leishmaniasis
Argentina	8	261
Bolivia	0	2647
Brazil	3481	26008
Colombia	60	17420
Costa Rica	0	1249
Ecuador	0	1724
French Guyana	0	233
Guatemala	15	684
Guyana	0	16
Honduras	6	1159
Mexico	7	811
Nicaragua	3	3222
Panama	0	2188
Paraguay	48	431
Peru	0	6405
Suriname	0	3
Venezuela	40	2480
Uruguay	1	0
United States	0	42
Total	**3668**	**66983**

Table 4. Geographical distribution of LV and LC in the Americas, based on references [3], [19] and [25].

The geographical distribution of leishmaniasis in the world appears to be changing, firstly, the variation of global climate [25, 29] could be increasing the area of Phlebotomine niches; and secondly, the globalization of economy increases the migration of the people among countries thereby increasing the contact of people with Phlebotomine niche where leishmaniasis is either incipient or non-existent. The former hypothesis could be explained by the growing economy in BRIC countries, such as Brazil, Russia, India and China; among these India and Brazil are endemic to leishmaniasis.

Nowadays, the geographical distribution of leishmaniasis is similar for LC and LV in the continents; however, differences exist among the countries. Indeed, approximately 57% of countries studied here showed both LC and LV. Nevertheless, in the last ten years the number of the reported LV cases in the world is approximately 58,413 with 77.2% in Asia. In contrast, the number of the reported LC cases in the world is approximately 214,082 with almost 40% of those in the Mediterranean region.

In fact, the reported LC cases are much higher than those reported for LV. A possible explanation for this scenario is the number of LC parasites, there are over 20 parasites causing LC whereas only just few parasites cause LV. Although there are only few sand fly species that are vectors for both LV and LC, both conditions have the same kind of reservoir hosts [30].

The above problems that have emerged from studying the worldwide geographical distribution must be resolved with the collaborative prevention measures by the countries where leishmaniasis is endemic; such cumulative force would lead to the global solutions to eradicate this disease.

3.2. Regional variables

Regional variables represent areas of the countries where the probability of existence of leishmaniasis has increased. In fact, there are internal regions in different countries such as the rural zone and the urban periphery where the incidence of leishmaniasis has increased (figure 6). A plausible explanation for such increase is the higher density of Phlebotomine and natural reservoir hosts of the parasites inhabiting these areas; these areas in the developing countries are infused with poverty where people live and work close to the forests or the woodlands.

In the developing countries, leishmaniasis was a rural disease, however, it was found to be associated with the growing urbanization. This disease began to develop in the urban periphery in Brazil and it was noted around 1970s [31]. A probably explanation of such spreading is the internal migration of the people from the rural zone to the urban areas [30].

People that arrive from the rural zones to the urban areas usually have limited and scant financial resources and therefore, they inhabit the periphery of the towns that are regions with the woodland and he forest remnants; they are basically inter topical zones. Such city periphery is a risk zone for the dissemination of leishmaniasis since here the contact among humans, Phlebotomine and their hosts is maximized. Indeed, some reservoir hosts are used as the pets and others are raised in peridomicile to feed these people.

This regional geographical distribution of leishmaniasis incidence must be analyzed by public health agencies to identify and verify the risk zone for leishmaniasis. Additional studies are also required to identify all the causative factors; specifically the data on Phlebotomine niches, presence of natural reservoir hosts of *Leishmania* and the sanitary quality of the habitat for the people are of utmost importance.

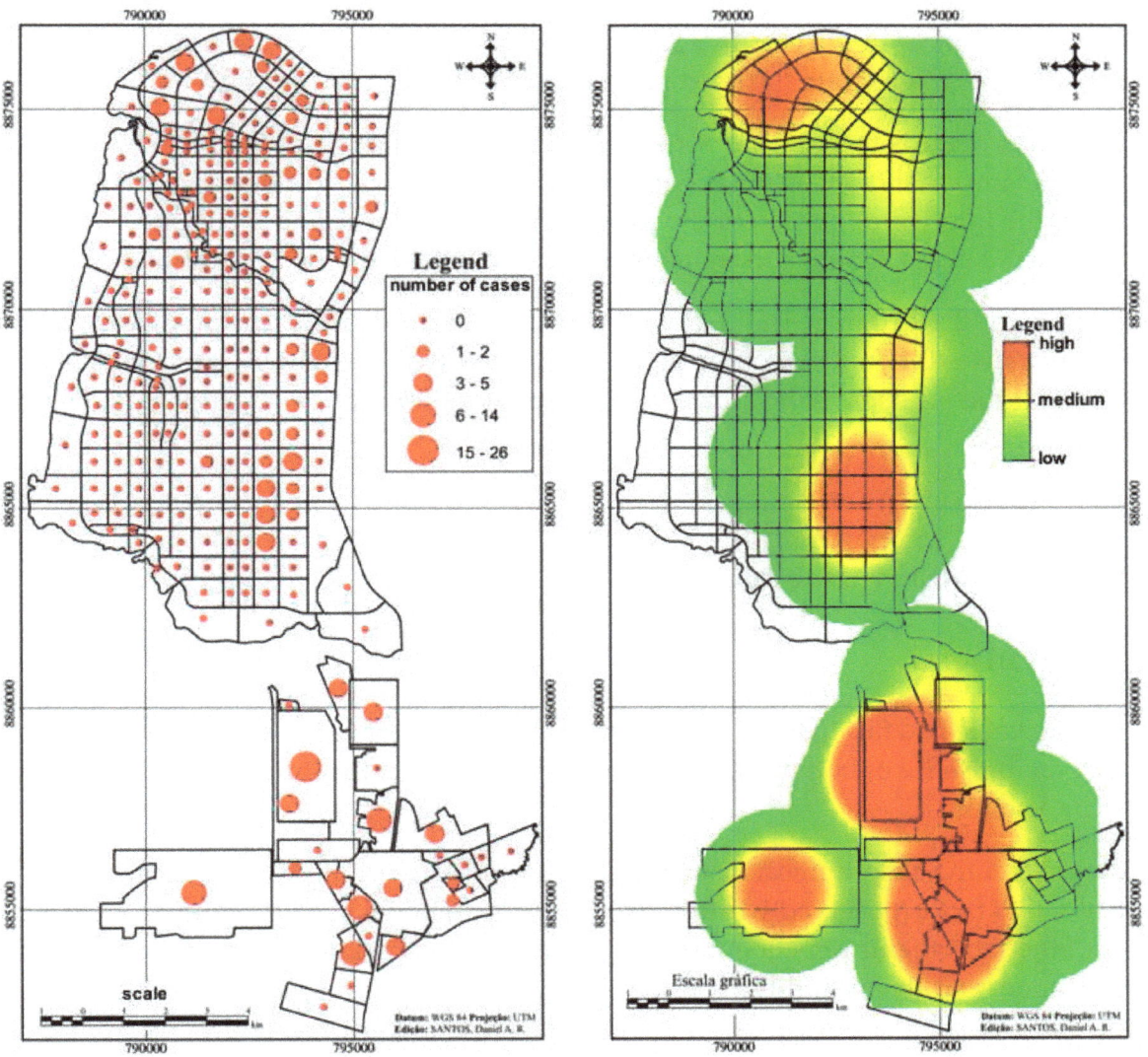

Figure 5. The map of city of Palmas, northern Brazil, is shown. On the left the dots represent reported cases fo leishmaniasis in this municipality from 2007 to 2012. The Kernel map of the same locality is demonstrated on the right, where darker/stronger color indicates the higher number of cases. The bigger dots (left) and the dark color distribution (right) are present in periphery of the town, that is closest to the forest.

Briefly, the geographical areas of leishmaniasis dissemination are the rural zones and the urban peripheries.

In geographical and regional terms the best way to start the fight against this disease, is the construction of a risk map for each municipality where leishmaniasis is endemic; it will indicate the points where the eradication effort should be focused. Such approach would include the elimination of Phlebotomine along with the complete removal and killing of the natural reservoir hosts of *Leishmania* from the population. We shall not address these specific problems in this chapter, however, georeferencing studies using adequate maps such as Kernel maps (figure 5), utilizing the new technologies for geographical representation along with spatial analysis of databases [32] appear to be the principle strategies to combat leishmaniasis.

Leishmaniasis is a complex multi-systemic disease [33], and therefore, it requires multidisciplinary team effort of public health agencies working together with the health professionals and the scientists to generate the most positive results towards its eradication.

Specifically as regards to the topic of this chapter, the monitoring of the reported cases from the data is an important tool on the geographical variables to control leishmaniasis since it may spread by the internal migration of the people to endemic areas and increasing its incidence due to elevated person-to-person transmission in the crowded living conditions [32].

The analysis of the geographical region is the first step to monitor leishmaniasis, however, majority of causes for endemic outbreak are associated with the natural environment as well as man-made factors such as the human migration, the deforestation, the urbanization and the malnutrition [34].

4. Environmental variables

4.1. World variables

It is a well-established fact that the maintenance of LV is related to the environmental variables favoring the presence of both the vectors and the vertebrate hosts at the same site [24], and it can occur also for LC.

It is known that the geographical distribution of leishmaniasis follows the distribution of sand fly niches, this fact is observed worldwide and in the regional analyses. However, the distribution of the sand flies is dependent on the environmental variables such as the temperature, the vegetation, and the humidity.

Indeed, the geographical variables are directly associated with the environmental variables in the biosphere and are inter-dependent. The geographical distribution of leishmaniasis generally occurs in the tropical and the equatorial regions, where warm and rainy weather prevails [10, 35, 36] favoring Phlebotomine reproduction [37, 38].

In fact, the analysis of the planet temperature map compared to the maps of reported cases of leishmaniasis (figures 4 and 5) demonstrates that these regions are parallel (figure 7).

In general, leishmaniasis is primarily present in the tropics, however, its incidence is increasing in other areas as well, and most likely this increase is associated with the global climate changes [25].

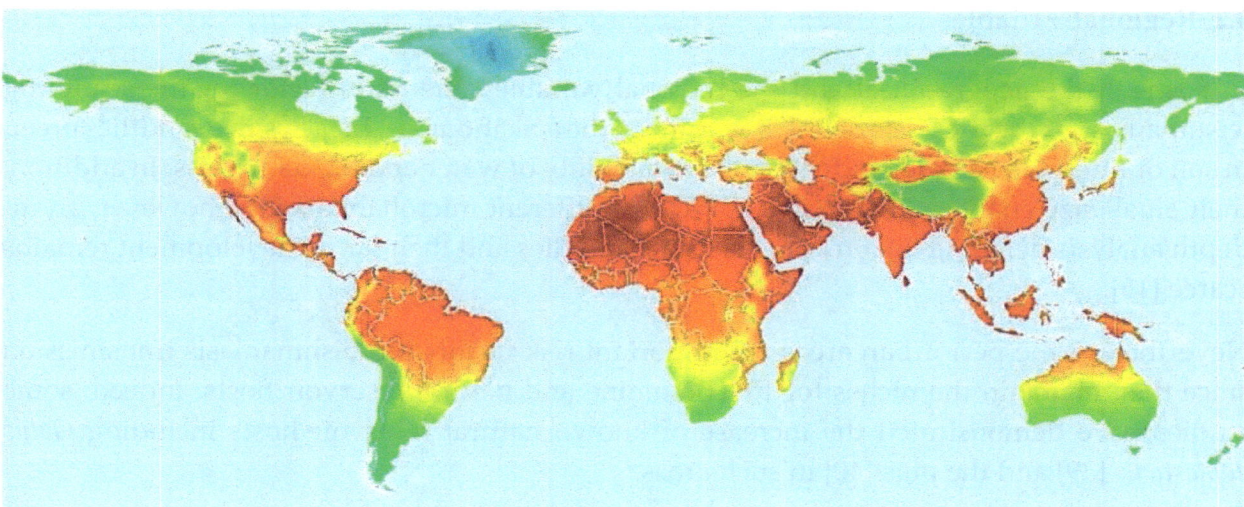

Figure 6. World temperature map where darker colors indicate higher temperatures

The world climate changes are implicated with physical consequences [21] as well as with the alterations of the vector niches and the reservoir species for the infectious diseases [21, 25].

According to Gonzalez *et al* [25], leishmaniasis is expanding to northern United States from Mexico and Texas, where it is considered autochthonous, primarily due to the increase in the niches of the sandflies associated with the reservoir hosts to *Leishmania*; however, other associated reasons could be dog importation [30] and the increase in human migration and/or travel in the recent years.

The movement of people occurs from countries where leishmaniasis is endemic to countries where climate is temperate. The people move from the temperate areas to the tropical and the equatorial climates, particularly for the holidays, sometimes they carry their dogs and other pets [30].

Climate is not the only factor associated with the vector niches, the vegetation also has some impact. In fact, in some regions, the climate indicates the existence of certain kind of vegetation, i.e., it is usual to think of the tropical forest in the tropical climate and the equatorial forest in the equatorial climate, however, it is possible to find desert, savanna, Cerrado (Brazilian savanna) and Atlantic forest in the same regions where the tropical and the equatorial climates prevail.

Phlebotomine prefers the forest areas, but, interestingly, it can also be found in open and urban areas [35].

In summary, the world environmental variables linked to Phlebotomine niche exist mainly in Latina America and some parts of Africa and Asia. The hot and the wet climates are associated with the forest and the woodlands areas; however, some species prefer open and the dry areas. In all these regions, it is possible to find some kind of host to *Leishmania*, nevertheless, the density of sand flies in some areas depends on the regional environmental variables.

4.2. Regional variables

In terms of the geographical and the regional variables, the main factor for the scattering leishmaniasis is the presence of Phlebotomine in the specific areas. In fact, since sandflies breed in soil or litter, they are dependent on the availability of water and the dampness. In addition, their small size enables them to live in various different microhabitats [36], however, an in-depth analysis detailing the breeding sites of sand flies and their larval development remains scarce [15].

Nevertheless, the peri-urban areas are important risk factors for leishmaniasis transmission since they maintain the niches for Phlebotomine and natural reservoir hosts. Indeed, some studies have demonstrated the increase of known natural reservoir hosts including *Galus domesticus* [39] and the pigs [40] in such areas.

In relation to the local environment, the urban periphery is frequently inhabited by poor populations, they are forced to live far from downtown and these habitats grow as the people arrive there from the rural areas. This is a common case in the poor and developing countries. Such lesser-developed areas are comprised of the forests or the woodlands and become a favorable place to increase contact of sandflies with the people as well as domestic and wild reservoir hosts of leishmaniasis.

At the same time, this population has limited access to basic sanitation and sewage treatment, and therefore, it generates exclusionary urbanization [41].

In fact, the deforestation linked to unplanned urbanization seems to be the cause of peak incidence of leishmaniasis in some regions [32]. Urbanization parameters associated with the growing cities and the deforestation areas generate ecological changes [41] that could modify the forest flora; this in turn generates trunks of dead trees thereby increasing the amount of decomposed organic material as well as the microorganisms on the ground that positively affect Phlebotomine cycle [38, 42-45].

These findings justify that in the peri-urban areas there is increase in number of the infected people carrying leishmaniasis and other infectious diseases that are dependent on the vector transmission, the people in those areas get higher exposure to vectors and reservoir hosts.

The reservoir hosts to *Leishmania* are the rodents, the marsupials, the monkeys, wild canines [30], the domestic dogs, chickens, the cattle, the equine, the caprine, the bovine, the swine and the feline species [11-14, 30], they all inhabit the areas populated with the sand flies.

Indeed, the presence of the swine species in the peridomicile is an important risk of the contamination [40], and the contamination has also been found associated with the presence of chickens as wild predators that are potential wild reservoirs hosts of *Leishmania* and *feed* on them, thereby intensifying the parasite cycle to the human and the canine populations [39].

The life cycle of Leishmania is mainly associated with the ecological factors in the rural or the peridomicile areas that harbor the sand fly niches and the reservoir hosts with human habitation (figure 7).

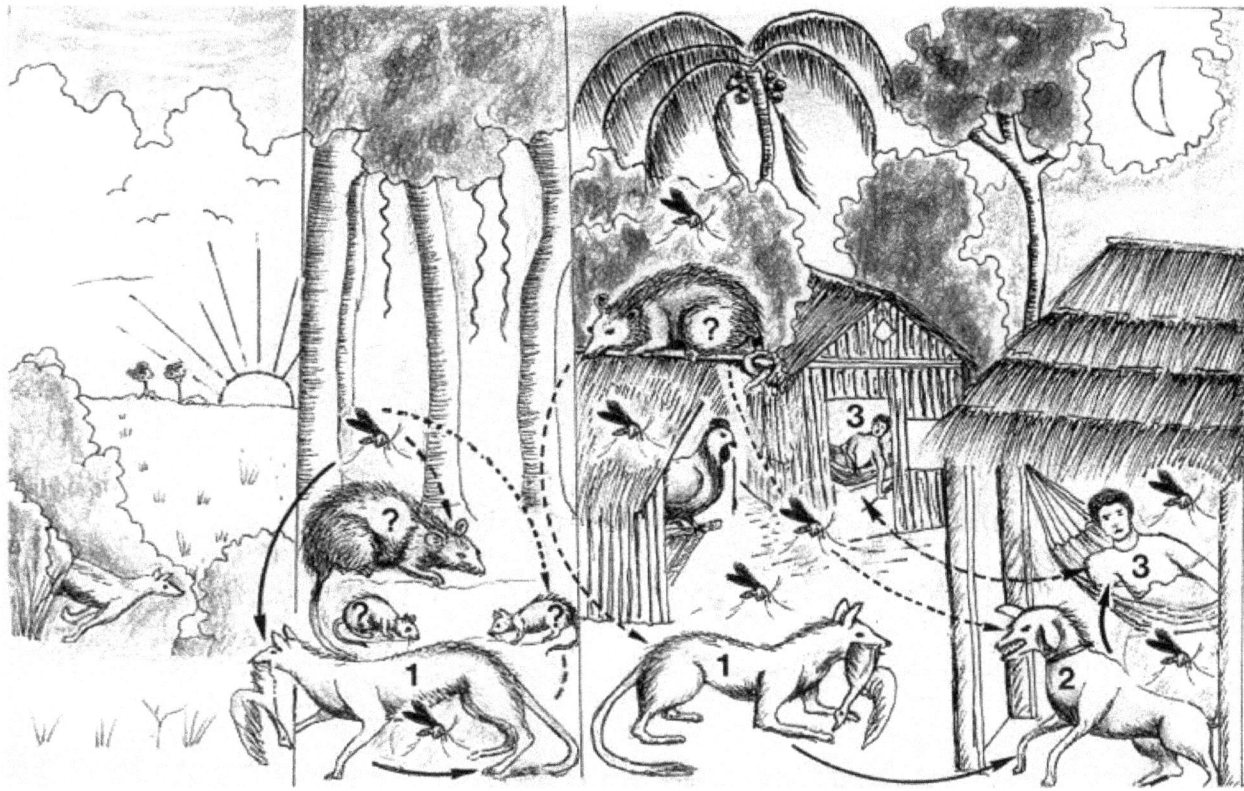

Figure 7. Scheme showing the life cycle of sandflies, reservoir hosts and humans, based on [46].

The human knowledge about leishmaniasis is not complete; many factors are still unknown or only partially known. Nevertheless, the current knowledge on this disease is adequate to develop accurate eradication strategies for the government and the public to work together developing specific protections with control of Phlebotomine by using insecticides, by removing organic material in the peridomicile areas [47, 48] and exterminating the contaminated reservoir hosts.

5. Conclusions

The aim of this chapter was simply to put together the collected information about the geographical and the environmental variables of leishmaniasis transmission. Leishmaniasis transmission is dependent on the association of contaminated sandflies with the reservoir hosts of *Leishmania* and the humans. In geographical terms association is favored in inter tropical regions, where the environmental factors such as the warm and the wet climate and certain types of the forest vegetation are predominant. In regional terms, the vicinity of the forest remnants or the woodland in the respective local periphery increases the density of sandflies thereby creating favorable conditions for the propagation of *Leishmania* life-cycle and its exposure to the people inhabiting that area.

Accurate and adequate public health policies and the proper dissemination of relevant information to the populations living in the endemic areas along with the severe control and the surveillance would be helpful in eliminating the contamination of humans and reservoir hosts by sandflies.

Author details

Roqueline A.G.M.F. Aversi-Ferreira[1,2,4], Jucimária Dantas Galvão[2,3], Sylla Figueredo da Silva[2,3], Giovanna Felipe Cavalcante[2], Ediana Vasconcelos da Silva[2,3], Naina Bhatia-Dey[1] and Tales Alexandre Aversi-Ferreira[1,2,3]

1 Department of Anatomy, Howard University, Washington, DC, USA

2 LABINECOP, Federal University of Tocantins, Palmas, state of Tocantins, Brazil

3 Graduate Program in Health Sciences, Federal University of Tocantins, Palmas, state of Tocantins, Brazil

4 Graduate Program in Animal Biology, University of Brasilia, Brasilia, DF, Brazil

References

[1] Feitosa MM, Ikeda FA, Luvizotto MCR, Perri SHV. Aspectos clínicos de cães com leishmaniose visceral no município de Araçatuba São Paulo (Brasil). Clínica Veterinária 2000; 2836-4.

[2] Custodio E, Gadisa E, Sordo L, Cruz I, Moreno J, Nieto J, Chicharro C, Aseffa A, Abraham Z, Hailu T, Canãvate C. Factors Associated with Leishmania Asymptomatic Infection: Results from a Cross-Sectional Survey in Highland Northern Ethiopia. PLOS Neglected Tropical Diseases 2012; 9(6) e1813.

[3] Alvar J, Velez ID, Bern C, Herrero M, Desjeux P, Cano J, Jannin J, Den Boer M. Leishmaniasis Worldwide and Global Estimates of Its Incidence. PLOS One 2012; 5(7) e35671.

[4] Hotez PJ, Molyneaux DH, Fenwick A, Ottesen E, Ehrlich, Sachs SE, Sachs, JD. Incorporating a rapid impact package for neglected tropical disease with programs for HIV/AIDS, tuberculosis and Malaria. Plos Med. 2006; 5(3) e102.

[5] Silva, ES, Roscoe EH, Arruda, LQ. Leishmaniose visceral canina: estudo clínico-epidemiológico e diagnóstico. Revista Brasileira de Medicina Veterinária 2001; 23(3) 111-16.

[6] Marins, JRP. Leishmaniose Visceral: uma doença em expansão: 15ª Reunião de Pesquisa Aplicada em Leishmaniose. Centro Educacional e Administrativo da Universidade Federal do Triângulo Mineiro, Uberaba, Brasil. 2011.

[7] Zink RA, Spigelman M, Schraut, B Greenblatt CL, Nerlich AG, Donoghue, HD. Leishmaniasis in Ancient Egypt and Upper Nubia. Emerg Infect Dis. 2006; 12(10) 1616-17.

[8] WHO (World Health Organization). Leishmaniasis: Burden of Disease. Geneva: World Health Organization 2013.

[9] Kolaczinski JH, Reithinger R, Dagemlider TW, Ocheng A, Kasimiro J, Kabatereine N, Brooker S. Risk factors of visceral leishmaniasis in East Africa: a case-control study in Pokot territory of Kenya and Uganda. International Journal of Epidemiology 2008; 2(37) 344-52.

[10] Rebelo JMM, Oliveira ST, Silva FS, Barros VLL, Costa JML. Sandflies (diptera:psychodidae) of the Amazonia of Maranhao v. seasonal occurrence in ancient colonization area and endemic for cutaneous leismaniasis. Rev Brasil Biol. 2001; 1(61) 107-15.

[11] Aguiar GM, Medeiros WM, De Marco TS, Santos SC, Gambardella S. Ecologia dos flebotomíneos da Serra do Mar, Itaguaí, Estado do Rio de Janeiro, Brasil. I - A fauna. flebotomínica e prevalência pelo local e tipo de captura (Diptera, Psychodidae, Phlebotominae). Caderno de Saúde Pública 1996; 2(12) 195-06.

[12] Domingos MF, Carreri-Bruno GC, Ciaravolo RMC, Galati EAB, Wanderley DMV, Corrêa FMA. Leishmaniose tegumentar americana: flebotomíneos de área de transmissão, no município de Pedro de Toledo, região sul do Estado de São Paulo, Brasil. Revista Sociedade Brasileira de Medicina Tropical 1998; 31(5) 425-32.

[13] Freitas JS, Santana RG, Melo SR. Levantamento dos casos de leishmaniose registrados no município de Jussara, Paraná, Brasil. Arquivo Ciências Saúde Unipar 2006; 1(10) 23-7.

[14] Moraes-Silva E, Antunes FR, Rodrigues MS, Silva FJ, Dias-Lima AG, Lemos-de-Sousa V, Alcantara AC, Reis EAG, NakataniM, Badaró R, Reis MG, Pontes-de-Carvalho L, Frankeb CR. Domestic swine in a visceral leishmaniasis endemic area produce antibodies against multiple *Leishmania infantum* antigens but apparently resist to *L. infantum* infection. Acta Tropica. 2006; 98176-82.

[15] Feliciangeli MD. Natural breeding places of phlebotomine sandflies. Med Vet Entomol. 2004; 18(4) 71-80.

[16] Hartemink N, Vanwambeke SO, Heesterbeek H, Rogers D, Morley, Pesson B, Davies C, Mahamdallie S, Ready P. PLoS ONE 2011; 8(6) e20817.

[17] Thomson MC,Elnaiem DA, Ashford RW, Connor SJ. Towards a kalaazar risk map for Sudan: mapping the potential distribution of *Phlebotomus orientalis* using digital data

of environmental variables. Tropical Medicine and International Health.1999; 4105-13.

[18] Elnaiem DE, Schorscher J, Bendall A, Obsmer V, Osman ME, Mekkawi AM, Connor SJ, Ashford RW, Thomson MC. Risc mapping of visceral leishmaniasis: the role of local variation in rainfall and altitude on the presence and incidence of kala-azar in eastern Sudan. Am J Trop Med Hyg. 2003; 68(1) 10-7.

[19] Salomón OD, Basmajdian Y, Fernández MS, Santini MS. *Lutzomyia longipalpis*in Uruguay: the first report and the potential of visceral leishmaniasis transmission. Mem Inst Oswaldo Cruz. 2011; 106(3) 381-382.

[20] Bhunia GS, Chatterjee N, Kumar V, Siddiqui NA, MandalR, Das P, Kesari S. Delimitation of kala-azar risk areas in the district of Vaishali in Bihar (India) using a geo-environmental approach. Mem Inst Oswaldo Cruz. 2012; 107(5) 609-20.

[21] Cross ER, Hyams KC. The potential effect of global warming on the geographic and seasonal distribution of *Phlebotomus papatasi* in Southwest Asia. Environment Health Perspectives 1996; 7(104) 724-27.

[22] Santini MS, Salamón OD, Acardi SA, Sandoval EA, Tartaglino L. *Lutzomyia longipalpis* behavior and control at an urban visceral leishmaniasis focus in Argentina. Rev Inst Med Trop. 2010; 52(4) 187-91.

[23] King RJ, Campbell-Lendrum DH, Daview CR. Predicting Geographic Variation in Cutaneous leishmaniasis, Colombia. Emerging Infectious Diseases 2004; 4(10) 598-07.

[24] Feliciangeli MD, Delgado O, Suarez B, Bravo A. *Leishmania* and sand flies: proximity to woodland as a risk factor for infection in a rural focus of visceral leishmaniasis in west central Venezuela. Tropical Medicine and International Health 2006; 12(2) 1785-91.

[25] Gonzales C, Wang O, Strutz SE, Gonzalez-Salazar C, Sanchez-Cordeiro V, Sarkar S. Climate change and risk of leishmaniasis in North America: predicitions from ecological niche models of vector and reservoir species. Plos Neglected Tropical Diseases 2010; 1(4) e585.

[26] Monteiro EM, Silva JCF, Costa RT, Costa DC, Barata RA, Paula EV, Machado-Coelho GLL, Rocha MF, Fortes-Dias CL, Dias ES. Leishmaniose Visceral: Estudo de Flebotomíneos e Infecção canina em Montes Claros. Revista Sociedade Brasileira de Medicina Tropical 2005; 2(38) 147-52.

[27] Sangioni LA, Gebara CMS, Aragão GM, Bezerra CAA, Almeida CC. Busca ativa de casos de leishmaniose cutânea em humanos e cães em area periférica do município de Campo Mourão - PR, Brasil. Ciência Rural 2007; 5(37) 1492-94.

[28] Zanzarini PD, Santos DR, Santos AR, Oliveira O, Poiani LP, Lonardoni MVC, Teodoro U, Silveira TGV. Leishmaniose tegumentar Americana canina em municípios do norte do Estado do Paraná, Brasil. Caderno de Saúde Pública 2005; 6(21) 1957-61.

[29] Barcellos C,Monteiro AMV, Corvalán C,Gurgel HC, Carvalho MS, Artaxo P, Hacon S,RagoniV. Mudançasclimáticas e ambientais e as doenças infecciosas: cenários e incertezas para o Brasil. Epidemiologia e Serviços de Saúde 2009; 3(18) 285-04.

[30] Ready PD. Leishmaniasis emergence and climate change. Rev Sci Tech Off Int Epiz. 2008; 2(27) 399-12.

[31] Cerbino Neto J, Werneck GL, Costa CHN. Factors associated with the incidence of urban visceral leishmaniasis: an ecological study in Teresina, Piauí state, Brazil. Caderno Saúde Pública. 2009; 7(25) 1543-51.

[32] Mott KE, Nuttal I, Desjeux P, Cattand P. New geographical approaches to control of some parasitic zoonoses. Bull World Health Organ. 1995; 2(73) 247-57.

[33] Nieto P, Malone JB, Bavia ME. Ecological niche modeling for visceral leishmaniasis in the state of Bahia, Brazil, using genetic algorithm for rule-set prediction and growing degree day-water budget analysis. Geospat Health. 2006; 1(1) 115-26.

[34] Desjeux P. The increase in risk factors for leishmaniasis worldwide. Transactions of the Royal Society of Tropical Medicine and Hygiene 2001; 3(95) 239-43.

[35] Oliveira EF, Silva EA, Fernandes CES, Paranhos Filho AC, Gamarra RM, Ribeiro AA, Brazil RP, Oliveira AG. Biotic factors and occurrence of *Lutzomya longipalpis* in endemic area of visceral leishmaniasis, Mato Grosso do Sul, Brazil. Mem Inst Oswaldo Cruz. 2012; 3(107) 396-401.

[36] Lewis DJ. Plebotomid Sandflies. Bull World Health Organ.1971; 44(4)535–51.

[37] Guerra JAO, Onety AC, Santos SL, Santos FGC, Talhari S, Paes MG. Situação da Leishmaniose em Manaus na última década. Revista Sociedade Brasileira de Medicina Tropical 2001; 34 Suppl244.

[38] Dias-Lima AG, Castéllon EG, Sherlock I. Flebotomíneos (*Diptera: Psychodidae*) de uma floresta primária de terra firme da estação experimental de silvicultura tropical, estado do amazonas, Brasil. Acta Amazônica 2003; 2(33) 303-16.

[39] Alexander B, Carvalho RL, Mccallum H, Pereira MH.Role of the domestic chicken (*Gallus gallus*) in the epidemiology of urban visceral leishmaniasis in Brazil. Emerging Infectious Diseases 2002; 12(8) 1480-85.

[40] Barboza DCPM, Gomes Neto CMB,Leal DC, Bittencourt DVV, Carneiro AJB, Souza BMPS, Oliveira LS, Julião FS, Souza VMM, Franke CR. Estudo de coorte em áreas de risco para leishmaniose visceral canina, em municípios da Região Metropolitana de Salvador, Bahia, Brasil. Revista Brasileira de Saúde e Produção Animal 2006; 2(7) 152-63.

[41] Kran FS, Ferreira FPM. Qualidade de Vida naCidade de Palmas TO: uma Análise Através de Indicadores Habitacionais e Ambientais Urbanos. Ambiente e Sociedade 2006; 2(9) 123-41.

[42] Rutledge LC, Ellenwood DA. Production of Phlebotomine sandflies on the open forest floor in Panama: The species complement. EnvEntomol. 1975; 471-7.

[43] Hanson WJ. The immature stages of the subfamily Phlebotominae in Panama (Diptera: Psychodidae). PhD thesis.University of Kansas; 1968.

[44] Geoffroy B, Dedet JP, Lebbe J, Esterre P, Trape JF. Note sur les relations des vecteurs de leishmaniose avec les essences forestieres en Guyane Française. Ann Parasitol Hum Com. 1986; 61(4) 491-05.

[45] Cabanillas MRS, CastellónEG. Distribution of sandflies (*Diptera: Psychodidae*) on Tree-trunks in a Non-flooded area of the Ducke Forest Reserve, Manaus, AM, Brazil. Memórias do Instituto Oswaldo Cruz 1999; 94(3) 289-96.

[46] Apostila UFPE 2013.http://www.ufpe.br/biolmol/Leishmanioses-Apostila_on_line/infogerais.htm.

[47] Teodoro U, Vicent LSF, Lima EM, Misuta NM, Silveira TGV, Ferreira MEMCF. American cutaneous leishmaniasis: phlebotominae of the area of transmission in the North of Paraná, Brazil. Revista de Saúde Pública 1991;2(25) 129-33.

[48] Teodoro U, Thomaz-Soccol V, Kühl JB, Santos DR, Santos ES, Santos AR, Abbas M, Dias AC. Reorganization and cleaness of peridomiciliar area to control sand flies (Diptera, Pschodidae, Phlebotominae) in South Brazil. Arquivos Brasileiros de Biolo-giaTecnológica 2004; 2(47) 205-12.

7

Metal-Based Therapeutics for Leishmaniasis

Ana B. Caballero, Juan M. Salas and
Manuel Sánchez-Moreno

1. Introduction

1.1. Metal-based drugs and their growing application to the treatment of parasitic diseases

When we speak of metals in medicine, many of us still associate them almost unconsciously with toxic rather than curative effects. However, despite the known toxic effect of some metal ions in humans, many metal ions (in adequate dosages) are required for many critical functions in our organism. Scarcity of some of them even can lead to a disease. Well-known examples include anemia resulting from iron deficiency, growth retardation arising from insufficient zinc, and heart disease in children owing to copper deficiency.

Metals have been used for medicinal purposes since ancient times. The earliest evidence of their therapeutic application has been dated back to 1500BC in Ebers Papyrus, Egypt. Among 700 magical formulas and remedies, this ancient manuscript describes the use of copper to reduce inflammation and the use of iron to treat anemia. Later on, the alchemical practice in the Middle Age made a significant use of metals like gold or arsenic to prepare medicinal compounds and elixirs. In the 16th century, antimony was introduced by Paracelsus as a general panacea and was considered as one of the Seven Wonders of the World.

In the early 20th century, the physician Paul Elhrich (Nobel Prize 1908) discovered an impresive therapeutic effect of the compound arsenophenylglycine to treat sleeping sickness (Trypanosoma disease) and developed the first effective medicinal treatment for syphilis, also arsenium-containing drug Arshphenamine, which was commercialized under the name Salvarsan. The concept of chemotherapy was born. At this time, other metallodrugs appeared. Sodium vanadate and derivatives of bismaltolato oxovanadium(IV) complexes started to be applied to lower levels of blood sugar in diabetic patients, and gold(I) complexes such as Auranofin, sodium aurothiomalate and aurothioglucose were prescribed to treat rheumatoid arthritis

(Figure 1). In 1987, sodium aurothiomalate was also used to treat 10 patients with kala-azar and showed an excellent clinical response.[1]

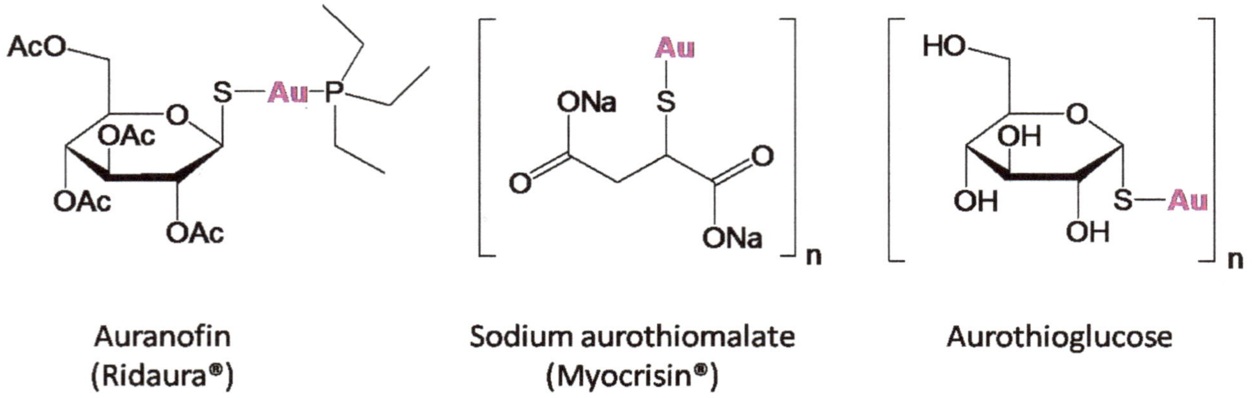

Auranofin
(Ridaura®)

Sodium aurothiomalate
(Myocrisin®)

Aurothioglucose

Figure 1. Gold-based drugs most commonly used for the treatment of rheumatoid arthritis. Sodium aurothiomalate has also shown chemotherapeutic effect against kala-azar.

Despite these early demonstrations of the potential of metals to treat diseases, organic drugs have traditionally dominated modern medicinal chemistry and pharmacology. It was the serendipitous discovery in 1969 of the anticancer properties of cisplatin, a Pt(II) complex, which propelled dramatically the research on metal ions in modern medicine until nowadays, not only in therapy but also in diagnosis. Examples of the latter are radiolabeling of compounds with ^{99m}Tc for X-ray imaging and use of Gd(III) complexes as MRI agents. Moreover, this event marked the change from an empirical discovery into a rational design of new metallodrugs and the consequent development of medicinal inorganic chemistry as a mature research discipline.

The increasing interest in the research of metal compounds with potential applications in medicine along the last decades has come along to a deeper understanding of the reactivity of metal ions and their interaction with a wide range of biomolecules such as DNA and proteins. [2] Scientific community has realized that either coordination or organometallic chemistry offer wide possibilities to develop novel metal-based drugs bearing quite different mechanisms of action aiming at different targets.

The dramatic incidence and economic impact of cancer diseases in modern world and especially in developed countries has led research on medicinal inorganic chemistry (and still is) to focus mainly on development of antitumoral compounds of different metals. This includes their design to specifically attack cancer cells and interact directly with DNA, with protein active sites or with smaller biomolecules of key importance in cancer development, as well as improving their biodistribution. As a result, a number of metal complexes with antitumoral potential have been developed in the last years, mostly of platinum and ruthenium, and some of them have provided excellent results. In fact, drugs like oxaliplatin are currently used to treat colorrectal cancer. Moreover, the antimetastatic drug NAMI-A is under the last phase of clinical evaluation.

On the other hand, a comparatively smaller progress has been made in the discovery of new metal compounds to treat tropical parasitic diseases, which has been mostly based on an empirical use. Various inorganic salts have been administered against the major tropical diseases, sometimes with very good results.

The best-known example is a series of antimony compounds such as sodium stibogluconate (Pentostam) and meglumine antimoniate (Glucantime). These compounds were developed more than 60 years ago and still constitute the treatment of choice for some forms of leishmaniasis. However, antimonial-based treatments usually present toxicity problems, limited efficacy and emerging resistance. This leads scientists to explore other metal ions in search of improved therapies. In addition no structure-function correlation studies have yet been performed on antiparasitic metal-based compounds. These arguments open the way to new mechanistic investigations in this research area for optimization of the identified metal leads and development of new ones.

But what can metals offer towards improved antiparasitic therapies? Metal ions offer a wide range of coordination numbers and geometries, redox states, and thermodynamic and kinetic characteristics. This, along with the possibility to rationally combine the intrinsic properties of a metal ion with a bioactive ligand/s bearing therapeutic interest, provides innumerable possibilities for drug design and an extremely wide spectrum of therapeutic activity not readily available to organic compounds.

One of the most used design approaches is grounded in the metal-drug synergism that results from the attachment of a metal moiety to the structure of an organic drug. [3] This synergy gives rise to two main effects:

a. An enhancement of biologic activity of the organic drug caused by the presence of the metal ion, possibly due to a longer time of residence of the drug in the organism allowing it to reach the biological targets more efficiently, or due to formation of reactive oxygen species (ROS), among other effects.

b. A decrease in the toxicity of the metal ion towards host cells due to the fact that complexation with organic drugs carries the metal ion to the specific site of action and makes it less readily available for undesired reactions such as inhibition of enzymes, or other damaging reactions leading to a malfunction in the organism.

The work of Williamson and Farrell in 1976 was the first in applying and demonstrate this concept for a tropical disease, trypanosomiasis. [4]

Among other illustrative examples of this approach, it should be mentioned the ferroquine (FQ), in which insertion of a Fe(II) ion in the form of ferrocene into the scaffold of the antimalarial drug chloroquine enhanced the pharmacology of the drug. [5] FQ is being developed by Sanofi-Aventis and entered phase II clinical trials in September 2007. Other example is a ruthenium(II) complex with the antitrypanocidal compound benznidazole, $trans$-[Ru(Bz)(NH$_3$)$_4$SO$_2$](CF$_3$SO$_3$)$_2$, which shows higher hydrosolubility and activity than the free antiparasitic drug. [6] (Figure 2)

Other advantages of using metal compounds are their pronounced selectivity for selected parasites biomolecules compared to the host biomolecules,[7] and the possibilities they offer to targeted therapies as targeting molecules may be reversibly appended and prodrugs can be developed to deliver highly reactive metal specia in the parasite target while minimising non-specific interactions.

In the last years, nanotechnology has revolutioned the medicine field by opening novel and promising approaches for drug design, in particular regarding use of nanoparticles (1-100 nm) as drug delivery vehicles. Despite being liposomes and polymeric particles the most investigated systems to deliver antiparasitic drugs, metal nanoparticles have also emerged as interesting alternative carriers. [8] Furthermore, use of nanoforms of antiparasitic metals like antimony and selenium as alternatives to molecular forms [9,10] has also been recently reported.

In summary, there is a clear need for research in this largely neglected area of medicinal chemistry that is tropical parasitic diseases, and use of metal complexes as possible chemotherapeutic agents arises as a very attractive alternative to tackle this immense problem. However, despite the obvious potential of metal complexes as diagnostic and chemotherapeutic agents, few pharmaceutical or chemical companies have serious in-house research programs that address these important bioinorganic aspects of medicine, which contrast tremendously with the case of purely organic drugs.

The following sections will focus on diverse examples of metal compounds with current or potential applications for leishmaniasis treatment.

2. Metal compounds as a new generation of leishmanicidal agents. Design strategies

2.1. Metal-based drugs for leishmaniasis

Currently, there is no vaccine against leishmaniasis yet, either purely organic or containing metals. Disease treatment relies solely on chemotherapy. After an intensive revision of the literature, we have found a wide range of metal-containing compounds that are currently used to treat different varieties of leishmaniasis or present a strong antileihsmanial activity and hence potential to be part of a new generation of chemotherapeutic agents with high efficacy and minimal toxicity for the patient. All of them are described in detail in this section.

2.1.1. Pentavalent antimonials: a (still) unbeatable classic in leishmanicidal therapy

Antimony-based compounds started to be used a century ago. Trivalent antimonials -Sb(III)- were first used, e.g. tartar emetic, which was first reported for treatment of cutaneous leishmaniasis in 1913. But the high toxicity of Sb(III) compounds and their unstability in tropical climate, led to discovery of pentavalent antimonials –Sb(V)- and in 1920 the Sb(V) compound urea stibamine emerged as an effective agent against visceral leishmaniasis (kala azar) while being less toxic than the trivalent antimonials.

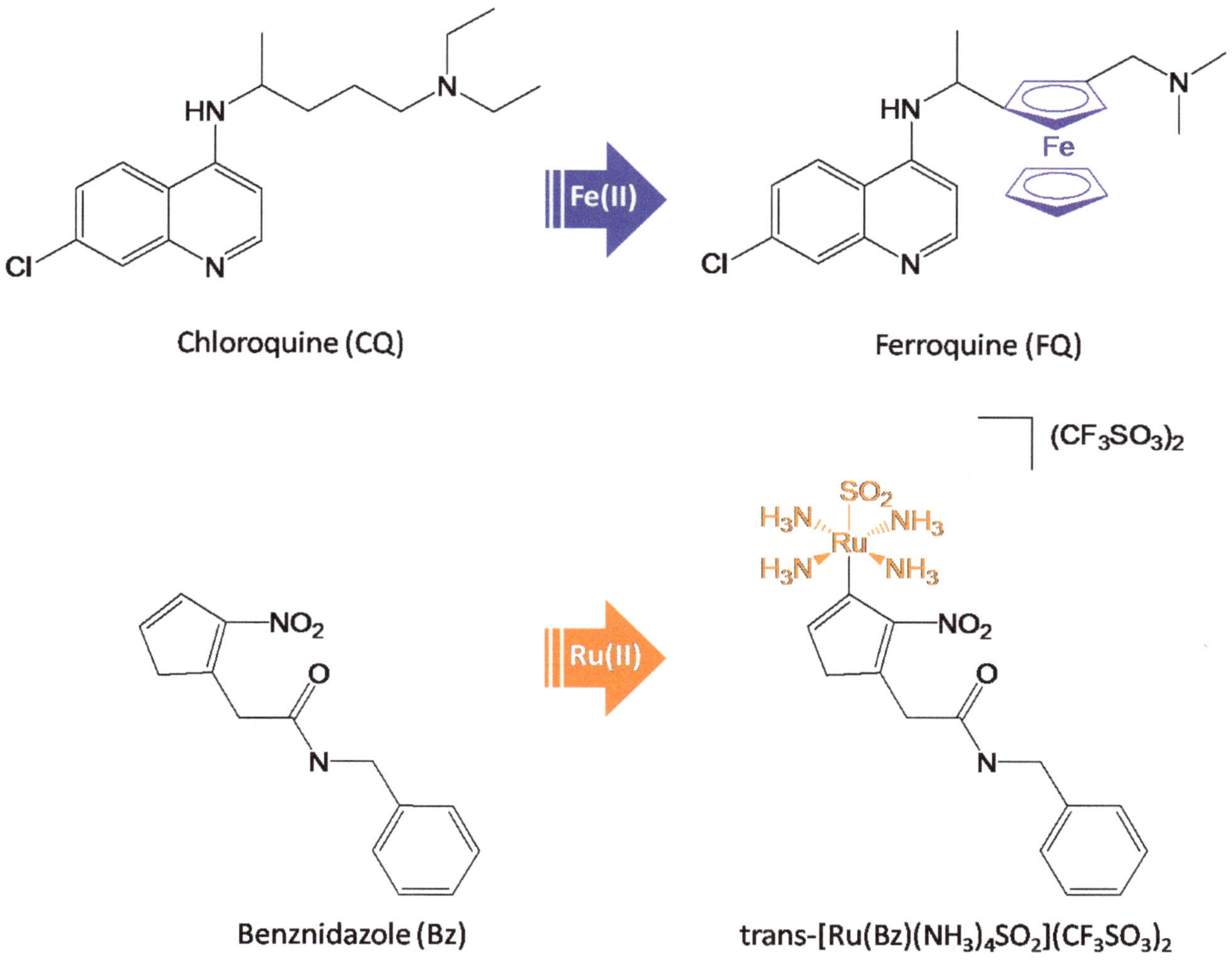

Figure 2. Structures of antimalarial drug chloroquine and antitrypanocidal drug benznidazole, and their respective metallo-derivatives, which show enhanced antiparasitic properties.

Nowadays pentavalent antimonials still constitute the first-line treatment for leishmaniasis. The most commonly used organic salts of Sb(V) are sodium stibogluconate (Pentostam) and meglumine antimoniate (Glucantime). See figure 3.

However, a significant increase in clinical resistance has been reported for this class of drugs in recent years. In some parts of the world like North East India, the percentage of cases of resistance development is so high (up to 65%) that these drugs are becoming obsolete.

Although acquired resistance is the most limiting factor for the application of pentavalent antimonials, these drugs present other important drawbacks such as low efficacy for some forms of leishmaniasis and toxic effects (e.g. cardiotoxicity, pancreatitis, anemia and leucopenia). Their toxicity is aggravated by usually required long periods of therapy (up to 4-6 weeks).

Even though antimonials have been in clinical use against leishmaniasis for more than 60 years, their molecular and cellular mechanisms of action are not well understood yet. [11] What is clear is that to be active, antimony has to enter the host cell, cross the phagolysomal membrane and act against the intracellular parasite. By analogy to pentavalent arsenate, it has been

sodium stibogluconate   meglumine antimoniate

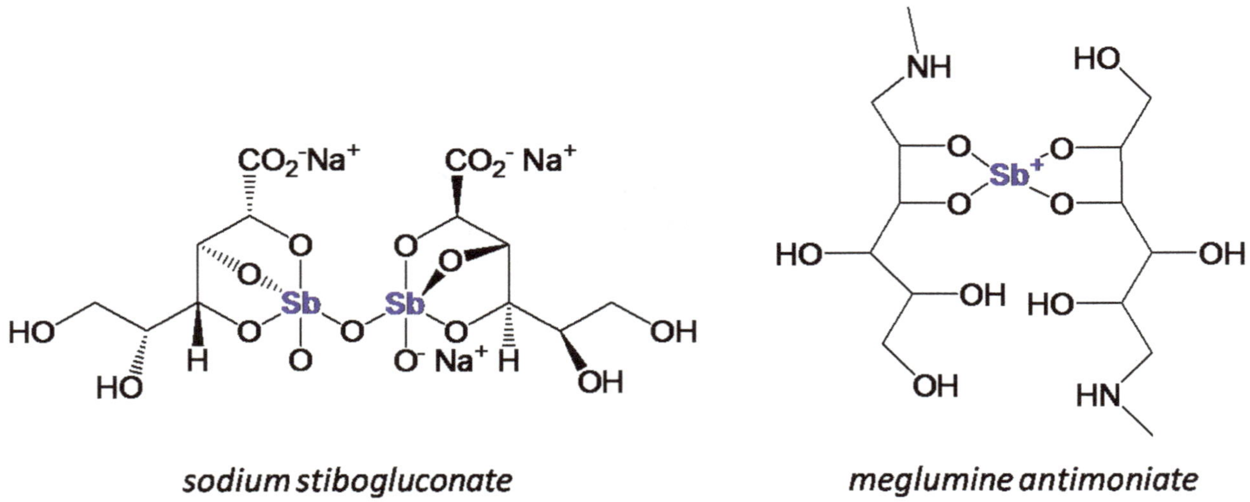

Figure 3. Chemical structure of sodium stibogluconate (Pentostam) and meglumine antimoniate (Glucantime).

suggested that they enter the cell via a phosphate transporter. Two main models have been proposed to explain the mechanism of action of pentavalent antimonials (Figure 4):

Prodrug model. Recent studies suggest that antimony compromises the thiol redox potential of the cell by inducing efflux of intracellular thiols and by inhibiting trypanothione reductase. Because Sb(III) is highly active against both stages of the parasite, extra- and intracellular on one hand, and Sb(V) is active mostly against amastigotes on the other, it is generally accepted that Sb(V) needs to be reduced to Sb(III) in order to be active. However, the site and the mechanism of reduction are unclear. Recent results suggest that activation occurs inside macrophages as well as inside parasites (amastigotes). [12] Both reduced glutathione (GSH) and reduced trypanothione (T(SH)$_2$) have been found to be responsible for non-enzymatic reduction of Sb(V) to Sb(III). Other studies have suggested the participation of a parasite-specific enzyme, namely thiol-dependent reductase (TDR1), in the reduction process of Sb(V) to Sb(III). Recent crystal structure studies display the mechanism of *Leishmania* trypanothione reductase (TR) inhibition by Sb(III). These studies show that trivalent antimony binds the protein active site with high affinity, and strongly inhibits enzyme activity. Metal binds directly to Cys52, Cys57, Thr335 and His461, thereby blocking hydride transfer and trypanothione reduction. Also evidence suggests that the active specia Sb(III) may interact with zinc-finger proteins by binding Cys residues. The interaction with TR would affect the metabolism of T(SH)$_2$ and induce rapid efflux of intracellular T(SH)$_2$ and GSH in *Leishmania* cells. [13] Moreover, the lowering of concentration of intracellular trypanothione in its reduced form T(SH)$_2$, increases the chances for oxidative damage and decreases the disposal of reducing equivalents for DNA synthesis. Sereno *et al.* found that Sb(III) induces DNA fragmentation after treating amastigotes of *L. infantum* at low concentrations of drug, which suggests appearance of late events of apoptosis.[14]

Active Sb(V) model. According to this model, Sb(V) would present intrinsic anti-leishmanial activity. It has been shown that sodium stibogluconate, but not Sb(III), specifically inhibits type I DNA topoisomerase by binding the enzyme, thus inhibiting unwinding and cleavage.[15]

Formation of Sb(V) complexes with ribonucleosides has been reported, which would be kinetically favored in acidic biological compartments. Moreover, stability constants are consistent with the formation of such a complex in the vertebrate host following treatment with pentavalent antimonial drugs. It is hypothesized that formation of this complex might act as an inhibitor of the *Leishmania* purine transporters or that, once inside the parasite, this complex interferes with the purine salvage pathway. [16] The formation of these complexes with ribonucleosides might explain as well the depletion of ATP and GTP, as reported previously with sodium stibogluconate. [17]

When antimonials fail, amphotericin B and pentamidine are the recommended second-line treamtent for visceral, cutaneous and mucocutaneous leishmaniasis.However, they are not fully effective either and, additionally,produce toxic side effects. On the other hand, new formulations such as liposomal amphotericin B have been found to be very effective, but its high cost limits its availability to patients.

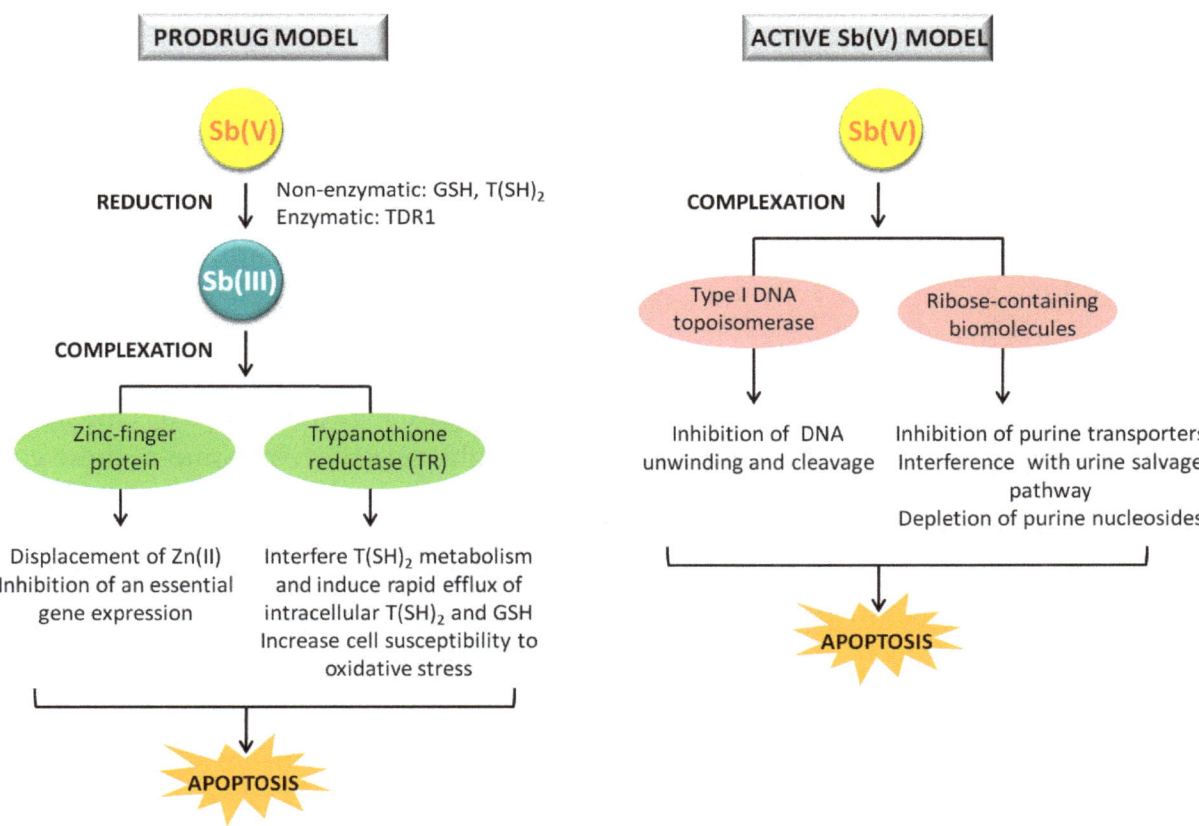

Figure 4. Main models proposed for the mechanism of action of pentavalent antimonials against leishmaniasis.

2.1.2. Metal complexes of organic drugs: Following the metal-drug synergism approach

Metal-drug synergism has led to several attempts to develop new potent antiparasitic agents. This approach involves combination of a compound of known antiparasitic activity and a metal in a single molecule. One example is complexation of antileishmanial drug pentamidine with

Rh(I) and Ir(I) to form binuclear complexes of general formula $[M_2(L_2)(pentamidine)]^{2+}$, where L_2= 1,5-cyclooctadiene (COD), 1,3,1,5-cyclooctatetraene (COT) or $(CO)_2$. Some of these compounds were found to be more active than the uncomplexed drug pentamidine isethionate. The complex $[Ir(COD)(pentamidine)][BPh_4]$ exhibits the same *in vitro* activity as free pentamidine, but its *in vivo* activity reaches 23% and 32% of parasite suppression for *L. donovani* and *L. major*, respectively, under conditions where pentamidine isethionate is inactive. The related compound $[Ir_2(COT)_2(pentamidine)][alizarin red]_2$ showed to be at least twice as active as pentamidine isethionate against amastigotes of *L. donovani* and synergistic effect was observed when this complex was administered in combination with pentamidine, amphotericin B or paromomycin. [18]

Other metal-drug synergy-based strategies make use of diverse chemotherapeutic targets such as sterol 14-demethylases by attaching azole-type sterol biosynthesis inhibitors (SBIs) such as clotrimazole (CTZ) and ketoconazole (KTZ), to a metal-containing fragment. For example, compound $[Ru(\eta^6$-p-cymene)Cl_2(CTZ)]$ shows an enhancement of the activity of CTZ by a factor of 110 against *L. major* promastigotes, resulting in low nanomolar lethal doses. In addition, this Ru(II) compound does not exhibit any appreciable toxicity toward human osteoblasts when assayed up to 7.5 µM, which translates into excellent selectivity indexes higher than 500. This compound also significantly inhibited the proliferation of intracellular amastigotes of *L. major* in infected intraperitoneal mouse macrophages (IC_{70}=29 nM). *In vivo* testing and detailed mechanistic studies of these ruthenium–CTZ complexes are currently in progress.[19] Likewise, a series of Ru(II) complexes with KTZ have recently been synthesized: *cis,fac*-$[RuCl_2(DMSO)_3(KTZ)]$, *cis*-$[RuCl_2(bipy)(DMSO)(KTZ)]$, $[Ru(\eta^6$-p-cymene)Cl_2(KTZ)]$, $[Ru(\eta^6$-p-cymene)(en)(KTZ)][BF_4]_2$, $[Ru^{II}(\eta^6$-pcymene)(bipy)(KTZ)][BF_4]_2$, and $[Ru(\eta^6$-p-cymene)(acac)(KTZ)][BF_4]$. They showed a marked increase of the activity against promastigotes and intracellular amastigotes of *L. major* when compared with free KTZ or with similar ruthenium compounds not containing KTZ. Interestingly, selectivity of some of these compounds toward *Leishmania* parasites in relation to normal human cells was also higher than selectivities of the individual constituents of the drug. Hydrolysis of the chloride ligands to form cationic aqua species appears to be a prerequisite for biological activity, and dissociation of KTZ probably occurs but only on further interactions of the active species with biomolecules within the parasite cell. Authors relate the antiparasitic activity to a combination of the SBI action of dissociated KTZ and the ability of the nitrogen-containing ligands on the remaining ruthenium fragment to promote interactions with DNA through hydrogen bonding or by π–stacking interactions. [20]

Other metal ions like Pt(II), Rh(I) or Os(III) have been used to obtain organometallic compounds with ligands derived from benzothiazole, a compound of which some derivatives have shown promising antimicrobial, antifungus and antiparasite activity. The obtained compounds were active against promastigotes and amastigotes of *L. donovani* by targeting different biochemical pathways: $[cis$-[Pt(da)(2,5-dihydroxybenzenesulfonate)_2]$ (da = 1,2-diaminocyclohexane), $[Ru(CO)_2(2$-aminobenzothiazole)]$, $[Ru(CO)_2(2$-methylbenzothiazole)]$, [21] and a series of dithiocarbamate complexes with formula $[Os(L)]$ where L= nitroimidazole, dinitroimidazole, benznidazole. Osmium complexes clearly inhibited DNA, RNA and protein synthesis, as well as enzymatic activities of succinate dehydrogenase, malate dehydrogenase and pyruvate kinase. [22]

Apart from vanadium compounds ability to exert different insulin-mimetic and antidiabetic effects, it has been recently proved that vanadium also offers interesting chemical and biochemical properties for the development of antiparasitic drugs. Noleto *et al.* combined the oxovanadium(IV) core with the antileishmanial compound galactomannan (GMPOLY), isolated from southern Brazil lichen *Ramalina celastri*. [23] Complexation highly increased leishmanicidal effect of galactomannan on amastigotes of *L. amazonensis* infecting peritoneal macrophages. This effect of GMPOLY on amastigotes could be attributed to the activation of the nitric oxide pathway. Nitric oxide is secreted by macrophages in response to IFN-γ (interferon γ) stimulation and it is regulated by tyrosine phosphatase events. Since the effect detected for GMPOLY oxovanadium(IV) complex occurred at concentrations where GMPOLY was non active, authors suggested the involvement of oxovanadium(IV) ion in the anti-parasite action.

2.1.3. Targeting cysteine proteases

Cysteine proteases have been found to play multiple roles in parasitic life cycles including nutrition, host invasion, protein processing, and evasion of the host immune response. In fact, there is an abundance of data to suggest that parasite cysteine proteases represent valid drug targets. For example, it was shown that an inhibitor of cathepsin B-like cysteine protease of *L. major*, cpB, inhibited parasite growth *in vitro* and ameliorated the pathology associated with a mouse model of leishmaniasis. [24] Since cysteine proteases found in *Leishmania* and *T. cruzi* have similarities to mammalian cathepsins B and L, the latter ones have been used as models to study the bioactivity of diverse metallic compounds. Cyclometallated gold, palladium, and rhenium derivatives have displayed cathepsin B inhibitory ability against cathepsin B and also similar order activity against the corresponding parasite enzyme cpB. These compounds have also shown growth inhibition of extracellular promastigotes of *L. major*, *L. mexicana* and *L. donovani* (see figure 5 and table 1). [25]

2.1.4. Vanadium compounds and their interaction with protein tyrosine phosphatases

Peroxovanadium compounds have shown potent inhibitors of protein tyrosine phosphatases and inducers of antileishmania effects like ROS and NO. Treatment of infected mice with bisperoxovanadium-1,10-phenanthroline or bis-peroxovanadiumpicolinate completely controlled progression of leishmaniasis in a NO-dependent manner. After injection, compounds rapidly triggered expression of inducible NO synthase in liver of mice infected with *L. major*. *In vivo* functional and immunological events associated with this peroxovanadium protective process have been identified. More recently, three dinuclear triperoxovanadate complexes, two mononuclear diperoxovanadate complexes with aminoacids or dipeptides as ancillary ligands and bis-peroxovanadate have been tested for their ability to kill *Leishmania* parasites *in vitro*, being $K[VO(O_2)_2(H_2O)]$ the most potent one. Combined administration of the latter with sub-optimal doses of sodium antimony gluconate on BALB/c mice experimentally

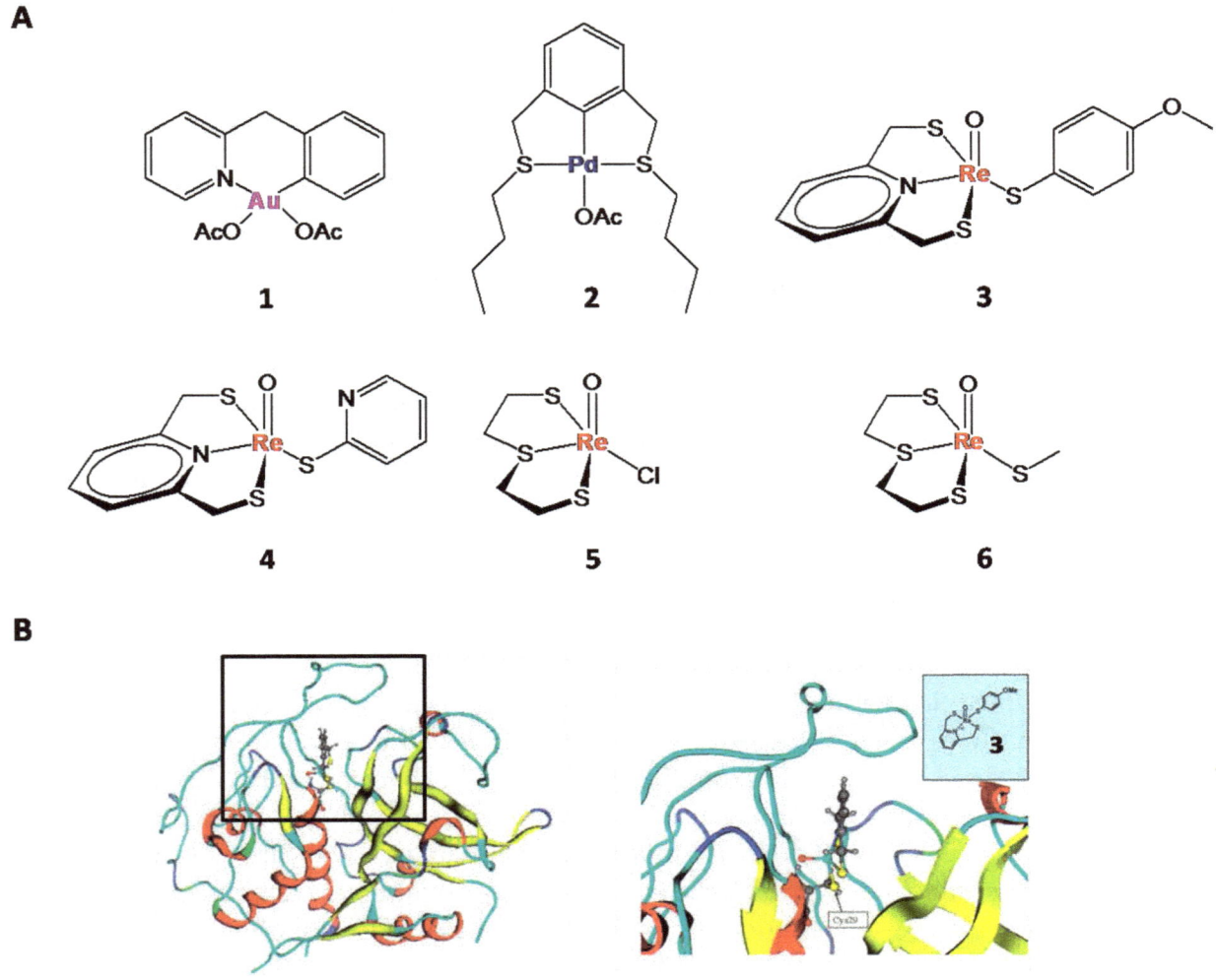

Figure 5. A) Structures of metal complexes with antileishmanial activity via inhibition of parasite cysteine proteases: (**1**) diaceto [2-[(2-pyridinyl-κN)methyl] phenyl-κC] gold(I), (**2**) aceto [2,6-bis [(butylthio-κS)methyl]-phenyl-κC] palladium(II), (**3**) (p-methoxyphenylthiolato-S) [2,6-bis[(mercapto-κS)methyl] pyridine-κN¹] oxorhenium(V), (**4**) (2(1H)-pyridinethiona-to-κS²)[2,6-bis [(mercapto-κS)-methyl] pyridine-κN¹] oxorhenium(V), (**5**) chloro [2,2'-(thio-κS)bis [ethanethiolato-κS)]] ox-orhenium(V), (**6**) (methanethiolato) [2,2'-(thio-κS)bis [ethanethiolato-κS)]] oxorhenium(V). B) Hypothetical model of oxorhenium(V) complex 3 binding to the active site cysteine of cathepsin B. Adapted from Ref. [25].

Compound	1	2	3	4	5	6
Cat B	1.29	0.40	6.51	0.12	0.0088	1.26
L. Major cpB	1.7	2.1	1.0	0.07	0.2	"/> 10

Table 1. Inhibitory effect of metal compounds 1-6 against mammalian cathepsin B and cathepsin B-like cystein protease of L. major. Results expressed as IC_{50} (μM). [25]

infected with antimony resistant *L. donovani* was highly effective in reducing the organ parasite burden. The effect was mainly associated with generation of ROS and nitrogen species that could kill intracellular parasites.

2.1.5. DNA-metallointercalators are not only to fight cancer

As the metabolic pathways of kinetoplastid parasites are similar to those of tumor cells, it has been proposed that compounds which efficiently interact with DNA in an intercalative mode could also show anti-trypanosomatid activity. [26] Based on this hypothesis, some work has been carried out on design of metallointercalators as anti-leishmania drugs, including metals of pharmacological interest. It has been found that certain DNA intercalating drugs which have potent trypanocidal action, such as ethidium, acriflavine, and ellipticines, inhibit the DNA topoisomerases. These enzymes thus may represent another potential target for DNA-intercalating trypanocidal metallodrugs.

DNA-intercalating metal complexes with potential leishmanicidal activity are generally made up of metals of known clinical application such as platinum, copper, silver and gold with planar polyaromatic ligands such as dppz (dipyrido[3,2-a:2',3'-c]phenazine) and dpq (dipyrido[3,2-a:2',3'-h]quinoxoline). Figure 6. Copper complexes with dppz and dpq ligands, $[Cu(L)_n(NO_3)_{2-n}](NO_3)_n$ where L = dppz or dpq (Fig. 6) have shown activity against *Leishmania braziliensis* (causative of the muco-cutaneous mode of the disease), and it has been demonstrated that their action is related to their ability to interact with DNA. $[Cu(dppz)_2](NO_3)_2$ was the most effective complex in this series, and the activity order was $[Cu(dppz)_2](NO_3)_2 > [Cu(dppz)(NO_3)](NO_3) > [Cu(dpq)_2](NO_3)_2 > [Cu(dpq)(NO_3)](NO_3)$. [27]

Among the most effective complexes is $[Au(dppz)_2]Cl_3$. This complex induced a dose dependent antiproliferative effect with a minimal inhibitory concentration (MIC) of 3.4 nM and lethal doses LD_{26} of 17 nM at 48 h. This strong *in vitro* activity against *L. mexicana* could be related to their ability to interact with DNA through an intercalative mode. Also, preliminary ultra-structural studies using transmission electron microscopy carried out with treated parasites at a sublethal concentration (IC_7 = 0.34 nM for 24 h) showed polynucleated cells with DNA fragmentation and drastic disorganization of the mitochondria. [28]

Several years ago, a DNA metallointercalator (2,2':6'2''-terpyridine) platinum showed a remarkable antileishmanial activity, causing complete growth inhibition of *Leishmania donovani* amastigotes at 1 μM concentration.[29] This complex exploits simultaneous DNA intercalation of terpyridine and platinum(II) binding to the enzyme active site. The highest activity against *L. donovani* was found for the case of *p*-bromophenyl substituents in 4'-terpyridine position, and NH_3 as the ancillary hydrolysable ligand.[18]

Various DNA-intercalating organic ligands, have also been bound to vanadium ions. Although the potentiality of vanadium compounds in medicinal chemistry and medicinal applications has been extensively explored, work on vanadium compounds for treatment of some parasitic diseases of high incidence in human health has only arisen in a systematic way in recent years. [30] Benítez *et al.* obtained a series of oxovanadium complexes combining the aromatic planar polycyclic system 1,10-phenanthroline (phen) and tridentate salicylaldehyde semicarbazone derivatives as ligands, $[VO(L^1-2H)(phen)]$ and $[VO(L^2-2H)(phen)]$, where L^1 = 2-hydroxybenzaldehyde semicarbazone and L^2= 2-hydroxy-3-methoxybenzaldehyde semicarbazone. These compounds were active against *Leishmania* parasites showing low toxicity on mammalian cells. In addition, they showed cytotoxicicity on human promyelocytic leukemia HL-60 cells with

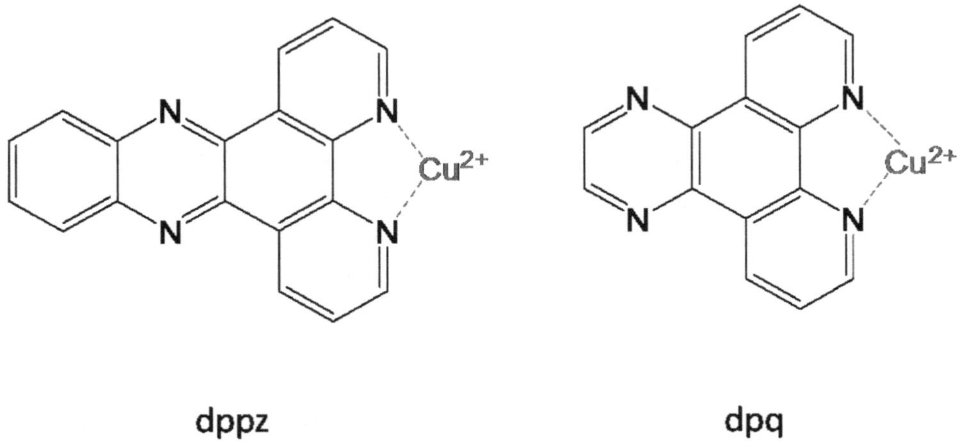

Figure 6. Structures of dppz (dipyrido[3,2-a:2′,3′-c]phenazine) and dpq (dipyrido[3,2-a:2′,3′-h]quinoxoline).

IC_{50} values of the same order of magnitude as cisplatin. Their interaction with DNA was demonstrated and studied by different techniques, suggesting that this biomolecule could be one of the potential targets for activity either in parasites or in tumor cells. [31]

2.1.6. Zinc sulphate against cutaneous leishmaniasis: The privilege of simplicity

Since zinc sulphate administered orally has been used in the last decades in medicine and dermatology, [32] then its use as an oral therapy for cutaneous leishmaniasis has appeared recently as an important addition to the armamentarium of antileishmanial drugs.

In vitro sensitivities of *L. major* and *L. tropica* strains to zinc were reported to be higher than those to pentavalent antimony, and these data were confirmed on mice. Zinc sulphate was also delivered intralesionally with success in cutaneous leishmaniasis. It is been suggested that oral zinc might not only affect directly to the parasite but also to macrophages function. Also it could have immunomodulatory effect (including T-lymphocytes), and help wound-healing. [33]

More recently, zinc sulphate was orally administered to Iraqi patients suffering from parasitologically confirmed cutaneous leishmaniasis. The species was not identified but it is known that only *L. major* and *L. tropica* are present in Iraq. This salt showed very promising cure rates (96.9%) against cutaneous leishmanaisis in a 45-days treatment with oral daily doses of 10 mg/kg. After a comparative study between oral zinc sulfate and meglumine antimoniate in the treatment of cutaneous leishmaniasis, it was suggested that systemic antimonial injections in cutaneous leishmaniasis treatment were better than zinc sulphate but oral administration of zinc sulphate makes it cheaper, more convenient its consumption, and nearly close cure percentage to systemic meglumine antimoniate injections without serious side effects. However at the moment zinc sulphate therapeutic effects should be confirmed by a greater sample volume. [34] Nevertheless, reported studies suggest that antileishmanial effect of zinc may result, partially or entirely, from inhibition of enzymes that are necessary for the parasites' carbohydrate metabolism and virulence. [35]

2.1.7. Selenium and the key role of antioxidants in disease

Selenium is an important and potent antioxidant in cells. Selenium compounds like selenites and selenates have strong inhibitory effects particularly on mammalian tumor cell growth. What is more, the nutritional deficiency of this essential trace metal may inhibit initiation and post-initiation phases of chemically induced mammary carcinogenesis and expression of some viruses, and it is important for optimal functioning of the immune system. [36]

Compounds of this metal have been reported to control human malaria if used in combination with vitamin E. [37] *In vitro* studies have shown that sodium selenite can inhibit *Leishmania donovani* growth although the mechanism of action is not clear yet. [38] Some authors have suggested that selenium has an important role in the pathophysiologic processes of cutaneous leishmaniasis, and that decreasing levels of this metal may be a host defense strategy of the organism against cutaneous leishmaniasis infection. Lack of selenium leads to a decrease of GSH-Px enzyme activity (it degrades H_2O_2), leading to increased amounts of hydroperoxides to kill protozoa as a host defense strategy.

2.1.8. Triazolopyrimidines and their metal complexes: Mimicking the nature

Triazolopyrimidines are purine analogues that have attracted much pharmaceutical interest during last decades. The most widely known derivative is the simple molecule Trapidil or Rocornal, a clinically used antiischemic and cardiatonic agent which acts as a platelet-derived growth factor (PDGF) antagonist and as a phosphodiesterase inhibitor. [39] This family of compounds have also found interesting applications as antipyretic, analgesic and anti-inflammatory, herbicidal, fungicidal agents with about 200 relevant patents. For example, 2-arenesulfonamido triazolopyrimidines were tested as leishmanicides showing some of them similar *in vitro* activity than pentamidine against *L. donovani* (Figure 7).

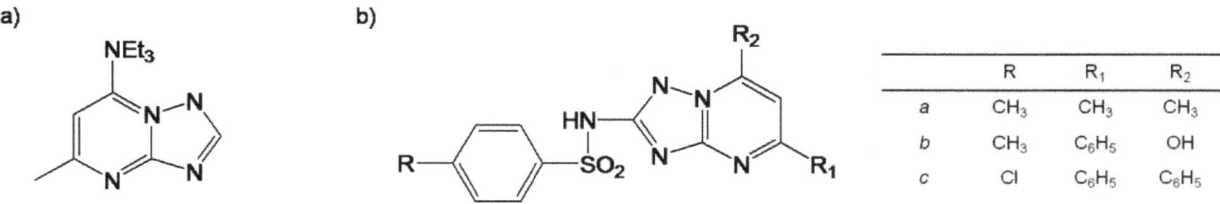

	R	R$_1$	R$_2$
a	CH$_3$	CH$_3$	CH$_3$
b	CH$_3$	C$_6$H$_5$	OH
c	Cl	C$_6$H$_5$	C$_6$H$_5$

Figure 7. Structures of triazolopyrimidine drugs: a) the anticoagulant drug Trapidil; b) a series of leishmanicidal derivatives.[39]

The biological activity of this family of organic compounds has led to investigating their coordination chemistry with the aim to develop new drugs with enhanced leishmanicidal activity and selectivity towards the parasites. Recently our group developed a series of transition metal complexes containing 1,2,4-triazolo[1,5-a]pyrimidines with high antiproliferative activity and extremely high selectivity indexes (see section 3). Studies revealed that apart from being all of them active *in vitro* against both extracellular and intracelular forms of *L. infantum* and *L. braziliensis*, these compounds are not toxic towards the host cells and are effective at lower concentrations than the drug used as a reference, Glucantime.[40] In the following section, we will present a case study in which our latest findings of our research with triazolopyrimidine metal complexes are described.

2.1.9. Nanoparticles: a promise for the future

A vast array of intriguing nanoscale particulate systems capable of targeting different cells and extracellular elements in the body to deliver drugs, genetic materials and diagnostic agents have been developed in the last years. Currently, antiparasitic delivery via nanosized particles is at the forefront of the research in this area. Liposomes and polymeric nanoparticles are the best studied nanosystems for evaluating antileishmania activity of compounds like amphotericin B or pentamidine. [41]

But nanosized metal particles are also emerging as promising antiparasitic agents. In recent studies it was determined that metal nanoparticles possess effective antimicrobial activities due to their unique properties and large surface areas. Moreover, metal nanoparticles are capable of producing reactive oxygen species (ROS), which would be able to kill parasites and other infectious agents.

Use metal of metal nanoparticles against *Leishmania* has followed two main approaches:

a.   As antiparasitic drug carriers. Nano-bioconjugate gold has recently been conceived as a stratagem against macrophage-infested leishmanial infections. One example is the functionalization of gold nanoparticles with the flavonoid quercetin, reported as one of the most powerful leishmanicidal among all plan flavonids tested so far. [8] This flavonoid inhibits synthesis of parasite DNA by inhibition of topoisomerase II mediated linearization of kDNA. Quercetin in addition can chelate iron and then limit availability of this metal for ribonucleotide reductase during DNA synthesis. On the other hand, gold nanoparticles as such can cause impairments in parasite oxygen metabolism.

Quercetin functionalized gold nanoparticles showed to be effective against *L. donovani* promastigotes and amastigotes. They were also effective against drug resistant strains with a very high selectivity index. A synergistic effect was considered by the authors as a possible reason for the higher activity of the nanoconjugate related to the free quercetin.

b.   As antiparasitic administration nanoforms. Because of the larger surface area of nanoparticles, they are more reactive and thus chemotherapeutic properties of a metal with antiparasitic activiy would be enhanced for its nanoform.

Selenium, for example, is a bioactive metal as it has antioxidant, cancer preventing, and antiviral activities. [37] Beheshti *et al.* prepared biogenic selenium nanoparticles, in this case, biosynthesized by *Bacillus sp.* MSh-1 and tested their *in vitro* and *in vivo* activity against *Leishmania major*. The particles showed antiproliferative activity against promastigote and amastigote forms of *L. major* and limited localized cutaneous leishmaniasis in animal model. These results present this kind of particles as novel therapeutic agents for treatment of the localized lesions typical of cutaneous leishmaniasis. However further studies are needed to investigate the mechanism of action of these Se NPs.[9]

Antimony sulfide NPs (Sb_2S_5), obtained also by green synthetic methods, proved to be effective on proliferation of promastigote forms of *L. infantum* and can induce apoptosis in promastigotes. [10]

The capability of metal nanoparticles to generate ROS and their potential use as leishmanicidal agents have also been explored. This is the case of silver nanoparticles, which have shown to be able to produce high amounts of ROS independently of the host cells. *In vitro* effects of AgNPs against promastigotes and amastigotes of *Leishmania tropica* were investigated. In order to increase the amount of ROS that are generated, AgNPs were irradiated with UV light which enhanced their antileishmanial effects without affecting host cells. [42]

2.2. Strategies for the design of new metal-based leishmanicidal drugs

To address the need for new, cost-effective metal-based leads for chemotherapy of leishmaniasis, different strategies of structure-based drug design have been applied so far. Four main strategies may be identified along revision in section 2.1:

2.2.1. Antitumoral activity implies antiparasitic activity

This strategy is based on the knowledge that highly-proliferative cells such as kinetoplastid parasites and tumor cells show metabolic similarities that lead in many cases to a correlation between antitrypanosomal and antitumor activities.[4] In this sense, use of metal complexes which have previously shown antitumoral activity, or synthesis of new metal complexes with ligands bearing activity could be a promising approach towards development of new agents against protozoa like *Leishmania*. A good correlation between antitumor and trypanostatic properties of several metal-based drugs has already been observed.

2.2.2. Metal-drug synergism approach

Perhaps one of the most popular strategies to develop new antiparasitic drugs consists on using an established antiparasitic drug as scaffold for the inclusion of a metal centre, either via direct coordination to the drug or by binding a metal complex. This way an enhancement of the drug pharmacological properties is pursued and resistance mechanism might be circumvented. See section 2.1.2.

2.2.3. Delivery nanovehicles

In finding innovative parasite-specific formulations, established but deficient drugs might be optimised by using drug delivery systems, in order to enhance their efficiency and reduce negative side effects at relatively low cost. Antiparasitic efficacy of drugs already in clinical use might be significantly improved by the adaptation of a new drug formulation. Use of nanocarriers to deliver established metal-based drugs such as antimonials would be both cost-effective and the quickest way to produce effective results. New drug formulations like liposomes for other drugs like amphotericin B (Ambisome) have been successfully developed for treating visceral leishmaniasis.

On the other hand, use of metal-based nanosystems as drug carriers, e.g. noble metal nano-particles, might provide additional advantages such as the possibility for diagnosis by imaging techniques and the combined effect of producing ROS as it is the case for silver. ROS can induce oxidative stress, DNA damage, alkylation of target proteins and eventually apoptosis of the parasite.

In order to inhibit *Leishmania* parasites with a ROS-based treatment, these oxygen derivatives must be produced in a physical way rather than in an enzymatic way that can be blocked by parasites. Metal nanoparticles are able to produce high amounts of ROS, as they are more reactive than the corresponding bulk metal (see example of AgNPs in section 2.1.9).

Nanocarriers also offer the possibility to specifically target the parasites by attaching appro-piate targeting molecules onto their surface. This way side effects to the host would be minimised. In addition, drug delivery vehicles such as nanoparticles allow prompt interactions with biomolecules present within as well as on the surface of the cell and may be tuned into different sizes to get the optimal uptake rate and blood circulation times of the drug.

2.2.4. Specifically targeted drugs: Metal inhibitors of parasite enzymes and DNA-binders

Recent advancements in molecular biology have identified a few parasite targets that are likely to be very sensitive to metal-based compounds. These targets usually are enzymes, some of them bearing free thiols at their active sites that manifest a high propensity to react with soft Lewis acids, i.e. metal ions such as Ag(I), Au(III) or Zn(II). Therefore these parasite targets will be susceptible to strong and selective inhibition by this kind of metals. This is the case of dithiol reductases like trypanothione reductase (T(SH)$_2$), which have been shown to play a key role in the *Leishmania* metabolism (see Section 2.1.1) and therefore constitute primary targets for metal compounds. Cysteine proteases, such as cathpesin L-like or cathepsin B-like, are another example of proteins with thiol-containing active sites and thus responsive to inhibition by metal compounds. Inhibitors that would effectively target both types of cysteine proteases in *Leishmania*, while maintaining some selectivity versus homologous host enzymes, would be ideal drug leads.

Regarding DNA interaction, previous studies have shown that DNA-binding metal com-pounds such as cisplatin display antiparasitic activity. These findings along with the obser-vation that many antiparasitic drugs bind to DNA, have led to propose that in general every DNA interacting compound is potentially active against parasites.

Therefore DNA-intercalating molecules have been used as ligands to form metal complexes showing antiparasitic activity. Intercalating ligands are usually polyaromatic systems with two or more donor atoms in close disposition to "chelate" metal ions. These ligands would not only be responsible for interaction of the metal compound with DNA but also they could act as carriers of the metal, increasing interaction of complexes with DNA by minimizing exposure of metal to inactivating cellular nucleophiles such as thiols.

3. Case study: Evaluation of the chemotherapeutic potential of metal complexes containing nucleobase-analogues against *Leishmania infantum* and *Leishmania braziliensis*

In this section we will describe some of our latest findings, which have been published recently. [40] Through this case study, we seek to provide the reader with an useful insight on our research, which is aimed at the rational design of new biomimetic metal-based systems as potential antiparasitic agents. Our research activity can be summarized in the following tasks:

a. Study of the interaction of a series of purine analogs, namely 1,2,4-triazolopyrimidines, with a wide range of metal ions, mainly from the first and second transition series.

b. Based on the coordination properties of triazolopyrimidine derivatives, design and synthesize new metal complexes showing structural and physical properties such as photoluminescent or magnetic properties that might be of interest for further applications.

c. Evaluate their *in vitro* activity against *Trypanosoma cruzi* and different species of *Leishmania* spp. Studies with *T. cruzi* are complemented with *in vivo* assays (murine model) for the most active compounds.

d. Analyze possible structure-activity correlations and investigate mechanism of action.

3.1. Transition metal complexes with 1,2,4-triazolo[1,5-a]pyrimidines

1,2,4-triazolopyrimidines are bicyclic heterocycles that are formed from the condensation of a ring of 1,2,4-triazole and another one of pyrimidine. Depending on the relative orientation of both rings, four different isomeric families can arise: 1,2,4-triazolo[1,5-a]pyrimidines, 1,2,4-triazolo[1,5-c]pyrimidines, 1,2,4-triazolo[4,3-a]pyrimidines, and 1,2,4-triazolo[4,3-c]pyrimidines. Among them, 1,2,4-triazolo[1,5-a]pyrimidine derivatives are the most stable thermodynamically and, because of this, the object of our present studies.

In previous works, 1,2,4-triazolo[1,5-a]pyrimidines have proved to be excellent ligands for a wide range of transition metal ions. [43] This fact is due to their, at least, three coordination positions, N1, N3 and N4, which can lead to several coordination modes. The coordination capability of these derivatives can be increased by the presence of heteroatoms as ring-substituents. However, a systematic revision on the existing results indicates a clear trend of these ligands to coordinate monodentately by N3, followed by N3,N4-bidentate and N1,N3-bidentate bridging modes (Figure 8).

The rich coordination chemistry of these derivatives has led in the last years to a great variety of multidimensional coordination compounds showing interesting properties, especially from the magnetic and biological viewpoints.

In addition, the biomimetic character of 1,2,4-triazolo[1,5-a]pyrimidines with purine nucleobases confers a potential biological activity to these derivatives and to their metal complexes, which can be used for therapeutic aims. Our studies have revealed the high potential of this kind of compounds for acting as leishmanicidal agents.

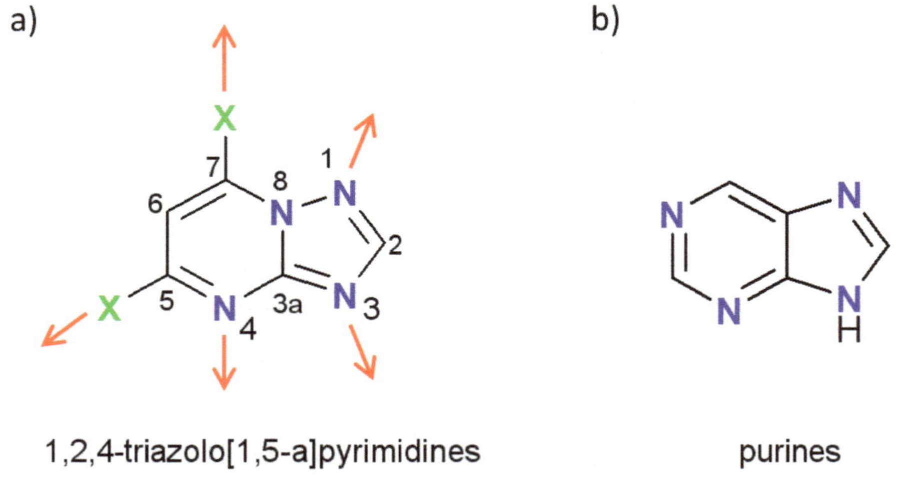

Figure 8. Basic structure of 5,7-substituted 1,2,4-triazolo[1,5-a]pyrimidines (a) and purines (b). Numbering scheme and possible binding sites to metal ions are also depicted for triazolopyrimidines. X=donor atom (N, O, S, etc.)

Herein we report the results obtained with three of the most promising metal compounds we have obtained so far: $[Cu(HmtpO)_2(H_2O)_3](ClO_4)_2 \cdot H_2O$ (1), $\{[Cu(HmtpO)_2(H_2O)_2](ClO_4)_2 \cdot 2HmtpO\}_n$ (2) and $\{Co(HmtpO)(H_2O)_3](ClO_4)_2 \cdot 2H_2O\}_n$ (3), Figure 9. All of them contain the neutral form of 5-methyl-1,2,4-triazolo[1,5-a]pyrimidin-7(4H)-one (HmtpO) and perchlorate as counteranion. The three compounds show different topology and dimensionality. Compound 1 is a monomeric complex in which HmtpO shows both N3 monodentate and N1,O71 bidentate modes; compound 2 is a two-dimensional framework in which HmtpO ligand shows an N3,O71 bidentate bridging mode; and the structure of compound 3 consists of one-dimensional chains in which HmtpO displays an N1,N3,O71 tridentate bridging mode. The structural diversity of these compounds is mainly due to the mode of the triazolopyrimidine ligand.

As depicted in Figure 9, the compounds 1-3 were synthesized by mixing their corresponding metal perchlorate salts with HmtpO derivative in aqueous media and bringing to reflux for 30 min before acidification with HCl. In all cases, compounds were isolated as crystals from their respective solution after several days standing at room temperature. Obtention of single crystals allowed to determine their crystal structure by X-ray analysis and their characterization was completed by elemental and thermal analysis (thermogravimetry and differential scanning calorimetry), and spectroscopic techniques such as FTIR and UV-Vis. Magnetic studies indicate that compound 1 exhibits simple paramagnetism in 2-300 K while the overall behaviour of 2 and 3 corresponds to weak ferromagnetically and antiferromagnetically coupled systems, respectively. [44]

3.2. *In vitro* antiproliferative activity against promastigote forms (extracellular forms) and toxicity against a mammalian host cell model

Firstly we evaluated the toxic activity of the free triazolopyrimidine compound HmtpO and its Cu(II) and Co(II) complexes 1-3 against promastigotes of two species of *Leishmania* (*L.*

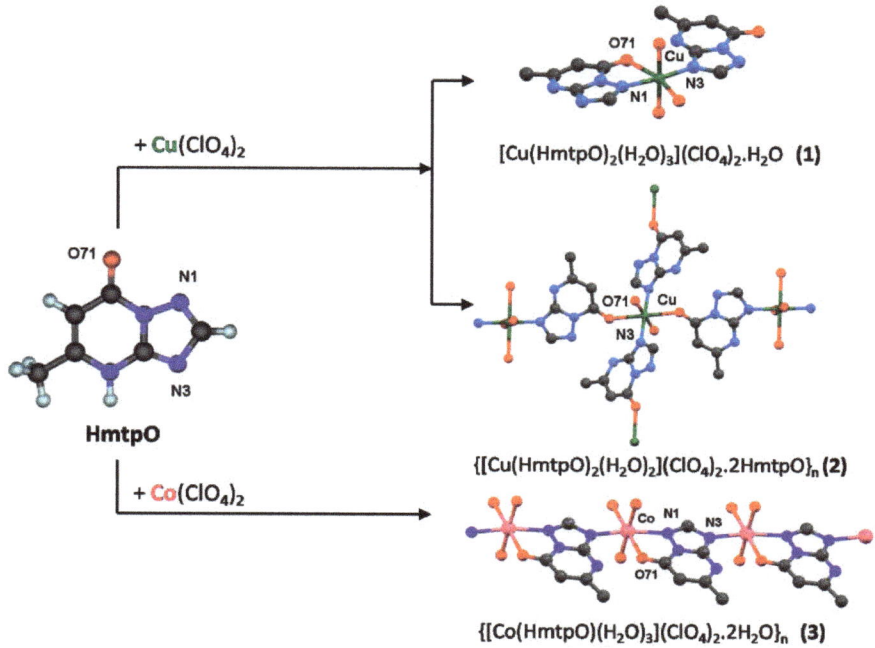

Figure 9. Synthetic scheme and structures of triazolopyrimidine derivative HmtpO and its metal complexes 1-3. Please note that the graphs of 1-3 correspond only to the cationic part of the metal compounds.

infantum and *L. braziliensis*). IC_{50} values registered after 72 h of exposure are shown in Table 2, including Glucantime as reference drug. Antileishmanial activity of metal complexes 1-3, expressed as IC_{50}, was similar to that found for Glucantime for both *L. infantum* and *L. braziliensis*. In contrast, the free derivative HmtpO is significantly less active than its metal compounds.

To evaluate toxicity on the host, J774.2 macrophages (mammalian cells) were used as cell model. Cytotoxic studies showed that metal complexes 1-3 are much less toxic than Glucantime and the free HmtpO derivative (Table 2).

On the other hand, selectivity and thus efficacy of assayed compounds towards parasite cells was evaluated and quantified by using the selectivity index (SI). This parameter is defined as the cocient between IC_{50} for cells and IC_{50} for parasites. A value greater than 1 is considered more selective for activity against parasites, and a value less than 1 is considered more selective for activity against cells.[45] SI of these derivatives was 30-fold or more higher than SI of Glucantime and HmtpO. These results are indicative of the higher potential of metal compounds 1-3 as antiparasitic agents compared with the current treatments, in this case Glucantime. Moreover it is evident that the presence of the metal ion in the scaffold enhances significantly triazolopyrimidine derivative activity and selectivity. This example constitutes another proof of the validity of the metal-drug synergism approach.

3.3. Effects on the infection rate and the intracellular replication of the amastigote forms

Most studies on *in vitro* biological activity of new compounds against *Leishmania* spp. are performed on promastigote forms because it is much easier to work with these forms *in vitro*.

Compound	IC50 (µM)		Toxicity J774.2 macrophages IC_{50} (µM) [a]	SI [b]	
	L. infantum	L. braziliensis		L. infantum	L. braziliensis
Glucantime	18.0	25.6	15.2	1	1
HmtpO	63.4	60.6	99.8	1.6	1.6
1	20.0	22.1	723.8	36	33
2	24.4	31.5	945.5	39	30
3	29.0	23.5	843.3	29	36

[a] Towards J774.2 macrophages after 72 h of culture. IC_{50} is the concentration required to give 50% inhibition, calculated by linear regression analysis from the K_c values at concentrations employed (1, 10, 25, 50 and 100 µM).

[b] Selectivity index (SI) = IC_{50} macrophages/IC_{50} parasite

Table 2. *In vitro* activity of reference drugs, free HmtpO derivative and metal compounds 1, 2 and 3 against promastigote forms of *Leishmania* spp.

However, in our studies we also include the effects of these compounds on the forms that develop in the host (amastigotes). This study is of great importance to determine effects in the definitive host and thus it gives a better idea of the potential application as antiparasitic drugs.

To predict the effect of metal complexes 1-3 on the capacity for infection and growth inhibition of intracellular forms of *L. infantum* and *L. braziliensis*, adherent J774.2 macrophages (1×10⁵ macrophages) were incubated for two days and then infected with 1×10⁶ promastigote forms of *L. infantum* and *L. braziliensis* for 12 h. Non-phagocytosed parasites were afterwards removed and culture was kept in fresh medium for 10 days. Parasites invaded cells and then converted into amastigotes within one day after infection. On the 10th day, the rate of host-cell infection reached the maximum. When drugs 1-3 were added at their respective IC_{25} concentration to macrophages infected with *Leishmania* spp. promastigote forms in exponential growth phase, infection rate decreased significantly after 12 h with respect to control measurements, following the trend 1>3>2 for *L. infantum* and 3>1>2 for *L. braziliensis*, with percentages of infestation-inhibition capacity of 84%, 79% and 67%, respectively, in the case of *L. infantum* and 86%, 79% and 75%, respectively, in the case of *L. braziliensis*. These values are remarkably higher than those for inhibition by Glucantime (56% and 36% for *L. infantum* and *L. braziliensis*, respectively). The three complexes inhibited *Leishmania* spp. amastigote replication in macrophage cells *in vitro*, following a similar pattern to that for infection rate inhibition and again being more effective than reference drug. Although not always it is possible to establish a direct relationship between drug action on extracelular promastigote and intracellular amastigote forms, in case of compound 3, it was effective against both forms.

3.4. Studies on the mechanism of action

In order to investigate the possible mechanism of action of metal compounds 1-3 on the parasite, their effect on metabolite excretion is analyzed, and microscopy studies on the treated parasites are carried out to visualize any ultrastructural alteration that may be provocked by the compounds.

3.4.1. Metabolite excretion effect

To the best of our knowledge, none of the trypanosomatids studied is capable of completely degrading glucose to CO_2 under aerobic conditions, so they excret a great part of the carbon skeleton into medium as fermented metabolites, which can differ according to the employed species.[46] *Leishmania* spp. have a high rate of glucose consumption, thereby acidifying culture medium due to incomplete oxidation to acids. ^{1}H-NMR spectra enable us to determine fermented metabolites that are excreted by the parasites during their *in vitro* culture. One of the major metabolites excreted by *Leishmania* spp. is succinate, the main role of which is probably to maintain the glycosomal redox balance by providing two glycosomal oxidoreductase enzymes. These enzymes allow reoxidation of NADH that is produced by glyceraldehyde-3-phosphate dehydrogenase in the glycolytic pathway. Succinic fermentation offers one significant advantage, since it requires only half of the produced phosphoenolpyruvate (PEP) to maintain the NAD^+/NADH balance. The remaining PEP is converted into acetate, depending on the species being considered. Figure 10 (on the left) shows ^{1}H-NMR spectrum of cell-free medium four days after inoculation with *L. infantum*. Additional peaks, corresponding to the major metabolites that were produced and excreted during growth, could be detected when this spectrum was compared with the one made in fresh medium. Taking into account that *L. infantum* excretes mainly succinate and acetate, ^{1}H-NMR spectra show that only compound 2 significantly altered excreted metabolites by *L. infantum*. When promastigote forms of *L. infantum* were treated with compound 2 at IC_{25} doses, the excretion of catabolites (succinate and acetate) was clearly disturbed and a new peak, identified as pyruvate, appeared (Figure 10). These results mean that compound 2 inhibits glycosomal enzymes, causing pyruvate to be excreted as a final metabolite. On the other hand, compounds 1 and 3 inhibit excreted metabolites only slightly. In the case of *L. braziliensis*, compounds 1-3 showed a similar behavior as for *L. infantum*, being again compound 2 the most inhibitory.

3.4.2. Ultrastructural alterations

Transmission electron microscopy images showed that compounds 1-3 induced morphological alterations in *L. infantum* and *L. braziliensis* promastigotes when parasites were treated with the respective IC_{25}. Compound 2 was the most effective against both parasite species.

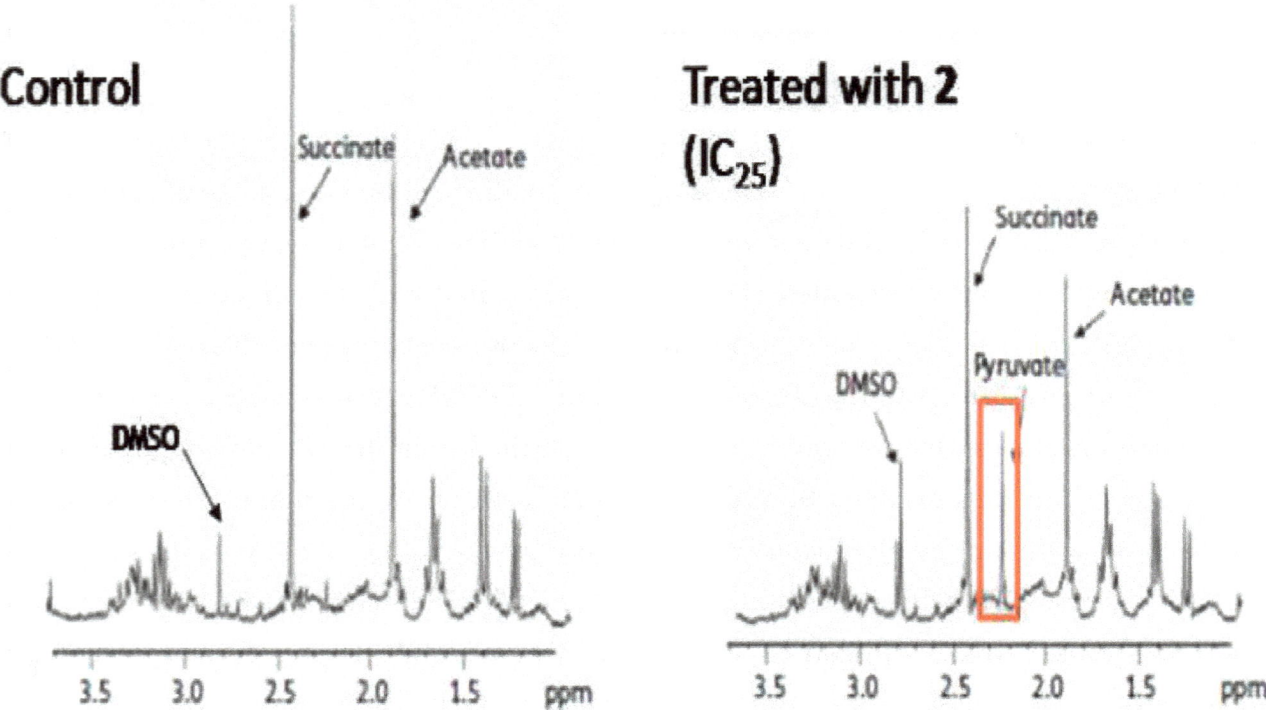

Figure 10. NMR spectra of promastigote forms of *L. infantum*, which show the characteristic peaks of the major excreted metabolites of non-treated parasites (left) and parasites that have been treated with IC_{25} of compound 2 (right) for four days.

After treating *L. braziliensis* promastigotes with compound 2, many of the parasites appeared dead and others adopted distorted shapes, while in others a uniformly electrodense cytoplasm was formed, in which no cytoplasmic organelles were visible. Parasites vacuolization was pronounced and many of these vacuoles contained strongly electrodense inclusions. In case of *L. infantum*, compound 2 led mostly to cell destruction (Figure 11c), which was evident from

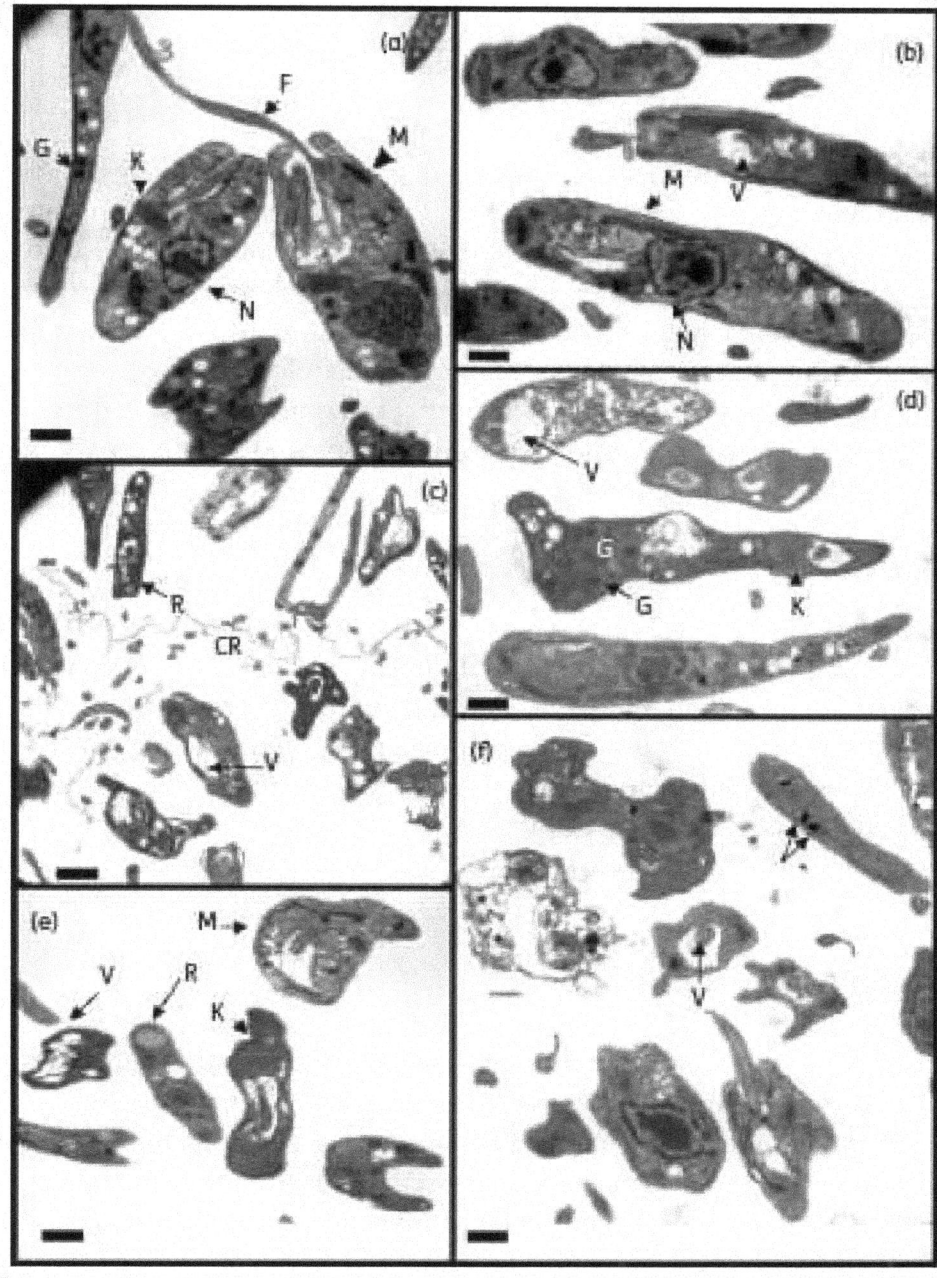

Figure 11. TEM images showing ultrastructural alterations in *L. infantum* and *L. braziliensis* after being treated with compounds 1, 2 and 3 (at IC_{25} concentrations) for 72h. (a) Control parasite of *L. infantum* showing organelles with their characteristic aspect, such as nucleus (N), kinetoplast (K), flagellum (F), glycosomes (G) and mitochondrion (M). Bar=1.00 μm. (b) Control parasite of *L. braziliensis* with structures such as nucleus (N), vacuoles (V) and mitochondrion (M). Bar=1.00 μm. (c) *L. infantum* treated with compound 2, showing cellular rest (CR), intense vacuolization (V) and reservosomes (R). Bar=1.59 μm. (d) *L. infantum* treated with compound 3, showing electrodense cytoplasm, vacuoles (V), glycosomes (G) and kinetoplast (K). Bar=1.00 μm. (e) *L. braziliensis* treated with compound 1, showing intense vacuolization (V), giant reservosomes (R) and kinetoplast (K) and swelling mitochondrion (M). Bar=1.00 μm. (f) Promastigotes of *L. braziliensis* treated with compound 2, with vacuoles (V) and electrodense organelles (arrows). Bar=1.00 μm.

the presence of a great quantity of cell remains in supernatant. Likewise parasites had strongly electrodense cytoplasm with intense vacuolization, with both empty vacuoles and membranes, and reservosomes, which appeared in greater numbers than in non-treated promastigotes (Figure 11a).

On the other hand, compound 1 was again very effective against L. braziliensis as some parasites appeared dead and others completely altered (Figure 11e), replete with reservosomes and enormous vacuoles. Some promastigotes appeared to be distorted and strongly electrodense, and showed condensed kinetoplast and very swollen mitochondria. In contrast, compound 3 was effective against L. infantum (Figure 11d), whose alterations were similar to those already described, with unrecognizable parasites, filled with vacuoles, which distorted their morphology, as well as a great quantity of reservosomes that occupied practically the entire cytoplasm. In these parasites kinetoplast and mitochondria also appeared swollen, resulting in a strongly electrodense cytoplasm. Dead parasites were also visible.

3.5. Final remarks

In addition to these studies, it should be noted that compounds 1-3 have displayed a high *in vitro* activity against both extra and intracellular forms of *T. cruzi* and are effective at concentrations similar to those of benznidazole. At the same time, they are much less toxic for host cells than the latter. Moreover antileishmanial activity of metal compounds is much higher than that of isolated HmtpO ligand, which is an evidence of the critical role of metal ions in antiparasitic activity. Furthermore, promising *in vivo* activity was observed for all of them, with results consistent with those observed *in vitro*.

4. Conclusion and future trends

In comparison with economically more attractive diseases like cancer, cardio-vascular problems and allergies, commercial interest in developing new antiparasitics is still rather low. Low income of most of the people affected by leishmaniasis, as it is the case for other tropical diseases, discourages big pharmaceutical companies from investing in developing new therapies. Therefore there is an urgent need to investigate into new drugs with low cost of production but also with high efficacy and selectivity.

Research on metal-based compounds to treat leishmaniasis has resurged in the last years and significant progress has been made. The possibility to finely tune their reactivity through a change of the metal ion and appropiate choice of the ligand/s makes of metal compounds promising alternatives to fight this disease in a cost-effective way.

Optimization of currently available metal-based drugs such as antimonials through use of nanovehicles and attachment of targeting moieties may be an interesting option to overcome antimonials resistance problems and maybe the quickest way to produce effective results. Therapeutic effects might be enhanced by using e.g. metal nanoparticles as delivery carriers, which depending on the metal, might be able to produce high amounts of reactive oxygen species and induce oxidative stress to the parasites.

On the other hand, significant advances in parasite genoma sequences and identification of targets in the last years along with an increasing understanding of metals interactions with a wide range of biomolecules, will contribute to development of highly efficient target-specific metal-based drugs in the future while avoiding recurring to time-consuming drug screening methodologies.

Meanwhile some authors have pointed at the metal-drug synergism approach as a very useful alternative for drug design at the moment.

Author details

Ana B. Caballero[1], Juan M. Salas[2] and Manuel Sánchez-Moreno[3]

1 School of Chemistry, University of Birmingham, Birmingham, United Kingdom

2 Department of Inorganic Chemistry, School of Sciences, University of Granada, Granada, Spain

3 Department of Parasitology, School of Sciences, University of Granada, Granada, Spain

References

[1] Singh MP, Mishra M, Khan AB, Ramdas SL, Panjiyar S. Gold treatment for kala-azar. Br. Med. J. 1989; 299 1318.

[2] Bruijnincx PC, Sadler PJ. New Trends for Metal Complexes with Anticancer Activity. Curr Opin Chem Biol. 2008; 12(2) 197–206.

[3] Sánchez-Delgado RA, Anzellotti A. Metal complexes as chemotherapeutic agents against tropical diseases: trypanosomiasis, malaria and leishmaniasis. Mini-Reviews in Medicinal Chemistry 2004; 423-30.

[4] Farrell NP. Transition Metal Complexes as Drugs and Chemotherapeutic Agents. In: R. Ugo, B. R. James (eds.) Catalysis by Metal Complexes. Vol 11. Dordrecht: Kluwer Academic Publishers; 1989. p. 222-242.

[5] Dubar F, Khalife J, Brocard J, Dive D, Biot C. Ferroquine, an Ingenious Antimalarial Drug –Thoughts on the Mechanism of Action. Molecules 2008; 13 2900-2907.

[6] Nogueira-Silva JJ, Pavanelli WR, Salazar Gutierrez FR, Chagas Alves Lima F, Borges Ferreira da Silva A, Santana Silva J, Wagner Franco D. Complexation of the anti-*Trypanosoma cruzi* Drug Benznidazole Improves Solubility and Efficacy. J. Med. Chem. 2008; 51 4104–4114.

[7]   Navarro M, Gabbiani C, Messori L, Gambino D. Metal-based drugs for malaria, try-
      panosomiasis and leishmaniasis: recent achievements and perspectives. Drug Dis-
      covery Today 2010; 15 1070-1078.

[8]   Das S, Roy P, Mondal S, Bera T, Mukherjee A. One pot synthesis of gold nanoparti-
      cles and application in chemotherapy of wild and resistant type visceral leishmania-
      sis. Colloids and Surfaces B: Biointerfaces 2013; 107 27-34.

[9]   Beheshti N, Soflaei S, Shakibaie M, Yazdi MH, Ghaffairfar F, Dalimi A, Shahverdi
      AR. Efficacy of biogenic selenium nanoparticles against *Leishmania major*: *In vitro* and
      in vivo studies. Journal of Trace Elements in Medicine and Biology 2013; 27 203-207.

[10] Soflaei S, Dalimi A, Ghaffarifar F, Shakibaie M, Shahverdi AR, Shafiepour M. In Vitro
      Antiparasitic and Apoptotic Effects of Antimony Sulfide. Nanoparticles on Leishma-
      nia infantum. Journal of Parasitology Research 2012; doi 10.1155/2012/756568.

[11] Ouellette M, Drummelsmith J, Papadopoulou B. Leishmaniasis: drugs in the clinic,
      resistance and new developments. Drug Resistance Updates 2004; 7 257-266.

[12] Ashutosh, Sundar S, Goyal N. Molecular mechanisms of antimony resistance in
      Leishmania. Journal of Medical Microbiology 2007; 56 143-153.

[13] Baiocco P, Colotti G, Franceschini S, Ilari A. Molecular Basis of Antimony Treatment
      in Leishmaniasis. J. Med. Chem. 2009; 52 2603–2612.

[14] Sereno D, Holzmuller P, Mangot I, Cuny G, Ouaissi A, Lemesre J. Antimonial-medi-
      ated DNA fragmentation in *Leishmania infantum* amastigotes Antimicrob. Agents
      Chemother. 2001;45 2064-2069.

[15] Chakraborty AK, Majumder K. Mode of action of pentavalent antimonials: Specific
      inhibition of type I DNA topoisomerase of Leishmania donovani. Biochemical and
      Biophysical Research Communications 1988; 152(2) 605-611.

[16] Haldar AK, Sen P, Roy S. Use of Antimony in the Treatment of Leishmaniasis: Cur-
      rent Status and Future Directions. Molecular Biology International 2011, Article ID
      571242. DOI: 10.4061/2011/571242

[17] Berman, J.D.; Waddell, D.; Hanson, B.D. Biochemical mechanisms of the antileishma-
      nial activity of sodium stibogluconate. Antimicrob. Agents Chemother. 1985, 27,
      916-920.

[18] Sánchez-Delgado RA, Anzellotti A, Suárez L. Metal complexes as chemotherapeutic
      agents against tropical diseases: malaria, trypanosomiasis and leishmaniasis. In: Sigel
      A and Sigel H (eds). Metal Ions in Biological Systems Volume 41: Metal Ions and
      Their Complexes in Medication. FontisMedia and Marcel Dekker; 2004, p. 379-420.

[19] Martinez A, Carreon T, Iniguez E, Anzellotti A, Sanchez A, Tyan M, Sattler A, Her-
      rera L, Maldonado RA, Sanchez-Delgado RA. Searching for New Chemotherapies for
      Tropical Diseases: Ruthenium–Clotrimazole Complexes Display High in Vitro Activ-

ity against *Leishmania major* and *Trypanosoma cruzi* and Low Toxicity toward Normal Mammalian Cells. J Med Chem 2012; 55 3867–3877.

[20] Iniguez E, Sanchez A, Vasquez MA, Martınez A, Olivas J, Sattler A, Sanchez-Delgado RA, Maldonado RA. Metal–drug synergy: new ruthenium(II) complexes of ketoconazole are highly active against *Leishmania major* and *Trypanosoma cruzi* and nontoxic to human or murine normal cells. J Biol Inorg Chem 2013. DOI 10.1007/s00775-013-1024-2

[21] Mesa-Valle CM, Moraleda-Lindez V, Craciunescu D, Osuna A. Antileishmanial Action of Organometallic Complexes of Pt(II) and Rh(I). Mem. Inst. Oswaldo Cruz, Rio de Janeiro 1996, 91, 625-633.

[22] Castilla JJ, Mesa-Valle MC, Sánchez-Moreno M, Arnedo T, Rosales MJ, Mascaro C, Craciunescu D, Osuna A. In vitro activity and biochemical effectiveness of new organometallic complexes of osmium(III) against *Leishmania donovani* and *Trypanosoma cruzi*. Arzneim.-Forsch.-Drug Res. 1996, 46, 990-996.

[23] Noleto GR, Mercê ALR, Iacomini M, Gorin PAJ, Soccol VT, Oliveira MBM. Effects of a lichen galactomannan and its vanadyl (IV) complex on peritoneal macrophages and leishmanicidal activity. Mol. Cell. Biochem. 2002; 233 73-83.

[24] Selzer PM, Pingel S, Hsieh I, Ugele B, Chan VJ, Engel JC, Bogyo M, Russell DG, Sakanari JA, McKerrow JH. Cysteine protease inhibitors as chemotherapy: Lessons from a parasite target. Proc. Natl. Acad. Sci. U. S. A. 1999; 96 11015–11022.

[25] Fricker SP. Cysteine proteases as targets for metal-based drugs. Metallomics 2010; 2 366–377.

[26] a) Kinnamon K, Steck EA, Rane ES. Activity of antitumor drugs against African trypanosomes. Antimicrob. Agents Chemother. 1979; 15 (2) 157-160. (b) Farrell NP, Williamson J, McLaren DJM. Trypanocidal and antitumour activity of platinum-metal and platinum-metal-drug dual-function complexes. Biochem. Pharmacol. 1984; 961-971.

[27] Navarro M, Cisneros-Fajardo EJ, Sierralta A, Fernández- Mestre M, Silva P, Arrieche D, Marchán E. Design of copper DNA intercalators with leishmanicidal activity. J. Biol. Inorg. Chem. 2003;8 401-408.

[28] Navarro M, Hernandez C, Colmenares I, Hernandez P, Fernandez M, Sierraalta A, Marchan E. Synthesis and characterization of [Au(dppz)$_2$]Cl$_3$. DNA interaction studies and biological activity against *Leishmania (L) Mexicana*. Journal of Inorganic Biochemistry. 2007; 101 111–116.

[29] Lowe G, Droz AS, Vilaivan T, Weaver GW, Tweedale L, Pratt JM, Rock P, Yardley V, Croft SL. Cytotoxicity of (2, 2′:6′, 2″-terpyridine) platinum (II) complexes to *Leishmania donovani, Trypanosoma cruzi* and *Trypanosoma brucei*. J. Med. Chem. 1999; 42, 999–1006.

[30] Gambino D. Potentiality of vanadium compounds as anti-parasitic agents.Coordination Chemistry Reviews 2011; 255 (19–20) 2193–2203.

[31] Benítez J, Becco L, Correia I, Milena Leal S, Guiset H, Costa Pessoa J, Lorenzo J, Aviles F, Escobar P, Moreno V, Garat B, Gambino D. Vanadium polypyridyl compounds as potential antiparasitic and antitumoral agents: new achievements. J. Inorg. Biochem. 2011; 105 303-312.

[32] Neldner KH, Hambidge KM, Walravens PA. Acrodermatitis enteropathica. Int J Dermatol. 1978;17(5) 380-387.

[33] Minodier P, Parola P. Cutaneous leishmaniasis treatment. Travel Medicine and Infectious Disease 2007; 5, 150–158.

[34] Yazdanpanah MJ, Banihashemi M, Pezeshkpoor F, Khajedaluee M, Famili S, Rodi IT, Yousefzadeh H. Comparison of Oral Zinc Sulfate with Systemic Meglumine Antimoniate in the Treatment of Cutaneous Leishmaniasis. Dermatology Research and Practice 2011, doi 10.1155/2011/269515.

[35] Al-Mulla Hummadi YM, Al-Bashir NM, Najim RA. The mechanism behind the antileishmanial effect of zinc sulphate. II. Effects on the enzymes of the parasites. Annals of Tropical Medicine and Parasitology 2005; 99(2) 131-139.

[36] Combs Jr GF. Selenium and cancer. In: Garewal HS, editor. Antioxidants and disease prevention. New York, NY: CRC Press; 1997. p. 97–113.

[37] Levander OA. Selenium and sulfur antioxidant protective systems, relationships with vitamin E and malaria. Proc Sot Exp Biol Med 1992; 200 255-259.

[38] Mukhopadhyay R, Madhubala R. Effect of antioxidants on the growth and polyamine levels of *Leishmania donovani*. BiochemicalPharmacology 1994; 47(4) 611-615.

[39] Fischer G. Recent Progress in 1, 2, 4-Triazolo[1, 5-a]pyrimidine Chemistry. Adv. Heterocycl. Chem. 2008; 95 143-219.

[40] Ramirez-Macias I, Marin C, Salas JM, Caballero A, Rosales MJ, Villegas N, Rodriguez-Dieguez A, Barea E, Sanchez-Moreno M. Biological activity of three novel complexes with the ligand 5-methyl-1, 2, 4-triazolo[1, 5-a]pyrimidin-7(4H)-one against *Leishmania* spp. J Antimicrob Chemother 2011; 66 813–819.

[41] Venier-Julienne MC, Vouldoukis I, Monjour L, Benoit JP. In vitro study of the antileishmanial activity of biodegradable nanoparticles.*Journal of Drug Targeting* 1995; 3(1) 23–29. (b) Durand R, Paul M, Rivollet D, Fessi H, Houin R, Astier A, Deniau M. Activity of pentamidine-loaded poly (D, L-lactide) nanoparticles against *Leishmania infantum* in a murine model, " *Parasite 1997;* 4(4) 331–336.

[42] Allahverdiyev AM, Abamor ES, Bagirova M, Ustundag CB, Kaya C, Kaya F, Rafailovich M. Antileishmanial effect of silver nanoparticles and their enhanced antiparasit-

ic activity under ultraviolet light. International Journal of Nanomedicine 2011; 6 2705–2714.

[43] a) Salas JM, Romero MA, Sánchez MP, Quirós M. Metal complexes of [1, 2, 4]triazolo-[1, 5-a]pyrimidine derivatives. Coord. Chem. Rev. 1999; 193-195 1119-1142. (b) Caballero AB, Maclaren JK, Rodríguez-Diéguez A, Vidal I, Dobado JA, Salas JM, Janiak C. Dinuclear silver(I) complexes for the design of metal-ligand networks based on triazolopyrimidines. Dalton Trans. 2011; 40(44) 11845-55; (c) Caballero AB, Rodríguez-Diéguez A, Barea E, Quirós M, Salas JM. Influence of pseudohalide ligands on the structural versatility and properties of novel ternary metal complexes with 1, 2, 4-triazolo[1, 5-a]pyrimidine. CrystEngComm 2010; 12 3038; (d) Abul Haj M, Quirós M, Salas JM, Dobado JA, Molina J, Basallote MG, Máñez MA. Structurally different dinuclear copper(II) complexes with the same triazolopyrimidine bridging ligand. Eur. J. Inorg. Chem. 2002; 811-818.

[44] Caballero AB, Rodriguez-Dieguez A, Lezama L, Barea E, Salas JM. Structural and magnetic properties of three novel complexes with the versatile ligand 5-methyl-1, 2, 4-triazolo[1, 5-a]pyrimidin-7(4H)-one. Dalton Transactions 2011; 40(19), 5180-5187.

[45] Tiuman TS, Ueda-Nakamura T, Garcia Cortez DA, Dias Filho BP, Morgado-Díaz JA, de Souza W, Nakamura CV. Antileishmanial activity of parthenolide, a sesquiterpene lactone isolated from *Tanacetum parthenium*. Antimicrob. Agents Chemother. 2005; 49 176-182.

[46] Bringaud F, Riviere L, Coustou V. Energy metabolism of trypanosomatids: adaptation to available carbon sources. Mol BiochemParasitol 2006; 149 1–9.

8

Molecular Diagnosis of Leishmaniasis, Species Identification and Phylogenetic Analysis

Constantina N. Tsokana, Labrini V. Athanasiou,
George Valiakos, Vassiliki Spyrou,
Katerina Manolakou and Charalambos Billinis

1. Introduction

Leishmaniases are vector-borne infections caused by protozoa of genus *Leishmania*, affecting various mammals, mainly carnivores and humans. Clinical patent disease is relatively easy to be diagnosed and laboratory-confirmed by direct detection of the parasite in clinical samples. However, in subclinical cases detection of the causative agent is possible by highly sensitive diagnostic techniques such as molecular assays. Different molecular methods have been developed and evaluated including multilocus enzyme electrophoresis, conventional polymerase chain reaction (PCR) based assays, quantitative Real Time PCR as well as simplified PCR methods.

More than 30 *Leishmania* species have been recognized, of which 20 are considered infective for humans and animals. The ability to distinguish between *Leishmania* species is crucial for differentiation of various forms of disease (visceral, cutaneous, mucocutaneus) at least in humans in order to establish correct diagnosis and prognosis of the disease as well as to support decision-making regarding application of the appropriate treatment protocols.

Available tools for species identification and phylogenetic analysis include DNA sequencing analysis, restriction fragment length polymorphism (RFLP) analysis, and PCR-fingerprinting techniques as well as novel methods such as multilocus sequence typing (MLST) and multilocus microsatellite typing (MLMT). MLST is regarded as the most powerful phylogenetic approach and will be a better alternative to Multilocus Enzyme Electrophoresis (MLEE) in the future. Various studies showed that the same target genomic regions can be used to compare distances among species but also to evaluate genetic diversity within species.

This review aims to critically present current molecular approaches for leishmaniasis diagnosis, species identification and phylogenetic analysis.

2. Molecular diagnosis

PCR is being used for the diagnosis of parasitic diseases, including leishmaniasis. PCR is considered to be the most sensitive and specific technique among the methods applied so far for the direct detection and identification of the causative agent. The procedure is rapid and can be applied to a variety of clinical samples. Regarding the efficacy of the assay, it depends on the target selected for amplification (conserved or variable target region), the number of the target copies, the extraction technique used, the biological sample tested and the PCR protocol adapted or developed [1,2].

The PCR-based assays are advantageous over immunological techniques such as enzyme linked immunosorbent assay (ELISA) and immunofluorescence antibody test (IFAT) as host species specific reagents are not required. The increased PCR sensitivity over serology for the detection of infection is of great interest in certain cases such as in patients with cutaneous, muco-cutaneous leishmaniasis (CL or MCL) and the immunocompromised ones (e.g. coinfected with HIV, under chemotherapy etc). The former have low or no concentrations of antibodies against *Leishmania* due to the localized character of the disease while the latter present limited antibody production both resulting in negative serological tests [3]. In particular, in chronic CL patients, who constitute the greater diagnostic challenge due to their low parasite density, PCR assays for the detection of *Leishmania* DNA presented 100% sensitivity. Moreover, the fact that antibodies remain detectable for years after successful treatment makes the application of PCR a necessity[4].

PCR has been also proved to be valuable in the diagnosis of post-kala-azar dermal leishmaniasis (PKDL) [5]. Additionally, the detection of parasite DNA has been shown to be a useful prognostic marker for the disease relapse or the development of PKDL even after successful treatment outcome. [6]. Furthermore, persistent infection has been found in apparently healed scars from MCL patients [7], the presence of *Leishmania braziliensis* was reported in patients previously treated by immunotherapy or patients being at different stages of treatment and in subjects who had never presented clinical manifestations but they had lived in endemic areas and migrated to nonendemic regions [8].

Moreover, several studies reported that PCR detects parasitaemia a few weeks before the appearance of clinical manifestations. The detection of asymptomatic infected humans contributes to the prevention of the sand fly infection and the transfusion-transmitted kala-azar especially for the patients that require multiple transfusions, at least in endemic areas [3,9].

Regarding canine leishmaniasis, PCR assays constitute useful tools in cases of clinically healthy dogs which harbour infection but may never develop clinical disease. As the PCR positive results indicate infection, these assays could contribute to the prevention of the importation of infected clinically healthy dogs to nonendemic areas where infection may spread via local sand fly vectors and the transmission via blood transfusion [10]. Finally, the parasite detection is crucial in case of negative results obtained by serology. This discrepancy may be attributed to the gap between infection and seroconversion, the transient presence of specific antibodies and the possibility for some infected dogs never to be seroconverted. In contrast, false positive results may be obtained due to the existence of anti-*Leishmania* antibodies for a considerable time after convalescence [11]. On the other hand, a positive PCR result in asymptomatic dogs cannot support decision-making regarding treatment as the parasite DNA may be present for a long time after the parasite has been cleared while also a single negative PCR result in a clinically suspected dog cannot rule out infection. Along with the need for PCR assays simplification, there is also a demand for standardization and optimization due to the lack of a universal PCR assay for the diagnosis of leishmaniasis [12]. Most laboratories perform "in-house" PCR assays using different primer pairs, DNA targets and PCR protocols [13].

A variety of clinical samples have been used for the detection of *Leishmania* DNA such as whole blood, buffy coat, bone marrow, lymph node, spleen, conjunctival swabs [14,15] and other biological samples such liver, lung, heart, penis, vagina, testis, semen, uterus, placenta, kidney, intestine, milk and urine [16] and more recently nasal, ear and oral swabs [17,18]. Bone marrow, lymph node, spleen and skin are the tissues presenting the highest sensitivity for the diagnosis of canine leishmaniasis [11,19]. The same holds true for the non invasive sampling techniques using conjunctival swabs [15,17]. Whole blood, buffy coat, urine and the other biological samples mentioned above have been shown to be less sensitive.

Several target sequences and different PCR protocols have been described for the detection of *Leishmania* DNA. The most frequently used amplification targets are the Kinetoplast DNA minicircle (kDNA) [20–25] and the small subunit ribosomal RNA (SSU rRNA) [26–29]. There are various gene targets which are also commonly used such as the ribosomal internal transcriped spacer (ITS) [15,30–34], the mini-exon gene (spliced leader) [32,35–40] and a repetitive genomic sequence [41,42].

It is worth mentioning that variable and sometimes conflicting results have been reported by several studies evaluating PCR using different target sequences in different host tissues. These results have been mostly obtained from asymptomatic infected hosts and they may vary depending on the sampling technique, storage method and the PCR protocol employed [1]. Some indicative studies evaluating the most frequently used PCR targets in different tissues are summarized in Table 1.

Target	PCR product size (bp)	Tissue tested	Sensitivity %	Specificity %	References
kDNA	120,297,790,792	WB,BM	68.8-100	100	[21] [22] [24] [25]
ssurRNA	358, 603	WB,BM	72.2-97	100	[27] [43][29] [28]
ITS1	300-350	BM,WB,SB,SS,DS,CS,CB,SA	68-100	100	[44] [33] [30] [32] [31]
Mini-exon	378-450	BM,WB,SB,LA,DB,GB	53.8-89.7	100	[37] [38] [35] [32]

BM: Bone marrow, WB: whole blood, SB: Skin biopsy, SS: Skin scrapings, DS: Dermal smear, SA: Skin aspirates LA: Lesion aspirates CS: Conjunctival swab, CB: Cultured biopsies, DB: Duodenal biopsy, GB: Gastric biopsy

Table 1. Evaluation of the most frequently used PCR targets in different tissues

Real time PCR (or quantitative PCR-qPCR), a molecular technique which has revolutionized the pathogen diagnosis, is considered to be the future reference method for molecular diagnosis. In recent years, qPCR assays based either on SYBR Green or TaqMan chemistries have been developed and evaluated for the detection, quantification and even species differentiation of *Leishmania spp* in a variety of clinical samples showing high sensitivity and reproducibility [45,46]. qPCR is considered to be a helpful tool for *Leishmania* diagnosis, monitoring during therapy, development of new drugs and diagnostic tools, comparison of drug efficacy or prophylactic schemes, and for epidemiological studies. Regarding diagnosis of leishmaniasis, the kinetic study of parasitemia in the immunocompromised hosts, the diagnosis of relapses and the quantification of the low parasitic load in asymptomatic patients are of great interest [47].

qPCR is highly sensitive especially at the lower parasite loads [48,49], specific and reproducible offering the ability to monitor therapy and to prevent relapses. The applications mentioned above make qPCR an attractive alternative to conventional PCR in routine diagnosis [47,49]. Some of the studies carried out so far and their findings regarding the detection threshold, sensitivity and specificity are summarized in Table 2.

Target	Tissue tested	Detection threshold	Sensitivity %	Specificity %	References
kDNA	BM, WB	0.001 p/ r			[50]
kDNA	WB	0.07 p/ r	100	83.33	[51]
kDNA	BM, WB, LN, CS, S, L, LU,K, BC	0.03 p/ r			[52]
kDNA	WB	0.004 p/ r			[53]
TRYP	BS		98.7	59.8	[54]
ITS1	WB, SB, S	0.25 p/s			[55]

BM: Bone marrow, WB: whole blood, SB: Skin biopsy, CS: Conjunctival swab, LN: Lymph node, S: Spleen, L: Liver, LU: Lung, K: Kidney, BC: Buffy coat, BS: Biopsy specimen, p/r:parasites/reaction, p/s: parasite/sample TRYP: tryparedoxin peroxidase gene

Table 2. Detection threshold, sensitivity and specificity of qPCR using various targets in different tissues

Given that PCR is restricted to well equiped laboratory settings, and that there is a need for simplification of the PCR assay and a demand for standardization and optimization [56], the described tools below may represent a good alternative for rapid and simple diagnosis of leishmaniasis in endemic areas and epidemiological studies [12,57].

Quantitative nucleic acid sequence-based amplification (QT-NASBA) has proven to be a very sensitive and specific assay in diagnostic microbiology which is based on the amplification of single-stranded RNA sequences. In fact, this technique detects RNA in a background of DNA [13]. Several QT-NASBA assays have been developed for the detection of *Leishmania* parasites including QT-NASBA combined with electro-chemiluminescence (ECL) [57,58] and QT-NASBA combined with oligochromatographic technology (OC) [12,59] for the detection of NASBA products. The QT-NASBA assays developed, are commonly based on amplification of single-stranded 18S ribosomal RNA sequences [12,57,58,60,61]. This target is considered to be highly efficient for the diagnosis of leishmaniasis as each parasite contains a large number of copies of the 18SrRNA gene [62] while also the cytoplasm is assumed to contain approximately 104 rRNA copies [62]. Moreover the target is present in all *Leishmania* species and it does not vary between different species allowing high sensitivity and quantification of all species in a similar manner [12,57,58]. However, this target shows high similarity with the 18S rRNA gene sequence of *Endotrypanum, Crithidia, Wallacein*a, and *Leptomonas* organisms which may result in false positive results especially in the case of immunocompromised patients [12]. The fact that NASBA detects RNA, makes it a molecular tool of great importance for the measurement of viable parasites. As a consequence, its application makes possible the assessment of the efficacy of drug therapies, the prediction of treatment outcome and the monitoring of the emergence of drug resistance. As it is well known, the DNA is still detected for a long time after parasite death, thus making RNA a preferable amplification target for the demonstration of parasite viability [13,56,58]. Moreover, when targeting RNA, the starting number of the template molecules is much higher resulting in increased assay sensitivity and decreased sample volume required [56]. The latter, makes also QT-NASBA a highly sensitive assay as it is able to detect very low target levels on clinical samples.

Loop-mediated isothermal amplification (LAMP), a novel method of DNA amplification under isothermal condition [63], has been developed to detect *Trypanosoma spp, Plasmodium spp, Mycobacterium spp and Filaria spp* [64]. Recently a reverse transcriptase step has been developed to specifically amplify RNA so as to amplify RNA viruses such as HIV and avian influenza viruses and to increase the assay sensitivity [65]. The recently developed LAMP seems to be a promising diagnostic tool. The results obtained from several studies are encouraging as this assay is much faster than conventional or nested PCR, it may be applied in field conditions, it shows high specificity and sensitivity [63,64,66–69].

In the context of a generalized effort for simplification of the parasite detection, assays including PCR-ELISA and PCR-OC have been developed and evaluated. Several studies reported that PCR-ELISA showed high sensitivity. In a study, PCR-ELISA in blood samples from HIV negative VL patients was evaluated and presented higher sensitivity (83.9% and 73.2%) and specificity (100% and 87.2%) than conventional PCR [70]. Other investigators have also evaluated the use of the assay in blood samples from HIV co-infected VL patients and PCR-ELISA found to be highly sensitive [23,71,72]. Basiye et al, reported that PCR-OC is highly sensitive for *Leishmania* diagnosis on blood samples from VL patients (sensitivity 96,4% and specificity 88.8%) compared to NASBA-OC which was shown to be more specific (specificity 100%) [60]. In another study the repeatability and reproducibility of the assay was studied and found to be 95.9% and 98.1% in purified nucleic acid specimens and 87.1% and 91.7% in blood specimens spiked with parasites respectively [73].

3. Species identification

The species identification is useful in areas with various sympatric *Leishmania* species such as the southern Mediterranean Basin where CL is caused by *L. major, L. tropica* or *L.infantum* and South America where CL may be caused by *L.mexicana* and *L.amazonensis* as well as the species of the subgenus *L.(Viannia)*. Regarding the areas where only one species is considered to be responsible for the disease, the species identification is an important tool for the differentiation between *Leishmania* species and lower trypanosomatids related to the monoxenous parasites of insects of the genera *Leptomonas* or *Herpetomonas* which are also considered to cause VL in Southern Europe, South America and in the Indian subcontinent. As far as it concerns the non-endemic areas, they seem to be at risk for parasite importation due to the increasing international travel and population migration [74].

In recent years, there has been great scientific interest in the development of molecular tools, based on PCR or other amplification techniques, for *Leishmania* parasites identification at species and even strain level. The molecular tools used, range from amplification and subsequent RFLP or DNA sequence analysis of multicopy targets or multigene families, including coding and non-coding regions, and PCR-fingerprinting techniques to the recently developed MLST and MLMT with different discriminatory power, sensitivity and specificity while also each one has its specific advantages and drawbacks [74]. Additionally, in most cases, the level of polymorphism found with coding or repeated non-coding PCR-amplified sequences is not refined enough to distinguish between closely related strains while application of MLST and MLMT approaches may reveal important strain polymorphisms.

PCR assays amplifying the conserved region of kinetoplast minicircle DNA or SSU rDNA have been shown to be the most sensitive, but they are able to identify *Leishmania* parasites only to the generic and/or subgeneric level [34,35,41,62]. However, the kDNA PCR-RFLP assay has been used as a molecular marker for *Leishmania* identification at strain level and found to be discriminative between closely related organisms such as *L.infantum* MON-1. In this case, PCR-RFLP of whole minicircle DNA, a highly polymorphic assay, has been applied for differentiation between recrudescence and re-infection [75,76] and for *L.infantum* strain typing [77]. However, the interpretation of the RFLP patterns is difficult as well as the comparison of the results obtained between laboratories [74,77].

The targets used for species identification include the ribosomal internal transcribed spacer (ITS) [34,78,79]; the mini-exon gene [38,39]; repetitive nuclear DNA sequences [80]; the glucose-6-phosphate dehydrogenase gene [81]; gp63 genes [82]; hsp70 genes[83,84]; cytochrome b gene [85], 7SL RNA gene sequences [86].

Other PCR-based approaches used for *Leishmania* parasites identification at strain level include the sequences of cysteine protease B (cpb) gene [87–90], the gp63 [87,91], the ITS1 [33,92–94], the mini-exon [95] and the kinetoplast minicircles [76,96–99].

The digestion of ITS1 PCR product with the restriction enzyme HaeIII can distinguish all medically relevant *Leishmania* species. However, almost identical RFLP patterns arise for the representatives of the *L. donovani* complex *(L. donovani* and *L.infantum)* or *L. braziliensis* complex *(L. braziliensis, L. guyanensis, L. panamensis, L. peruviana* etc.) with a great variety of restriction enzymes [34]. According to Schönian et al, in such a case, the sequencing of the ITS1 PCR product will allow the species differentiation [74]. Nasereddin et al developed a simple reverse line blot hybridization (RLB) assay based on ITS1 sequences, which could distinguish all Old World *Leishmania* species, even *L. donovani* from *L.infantum*. This approach was found to be highly sensitive, approximately 10- to100-fold more sensitive than ITS1 PCR while the results obtained were comparable to those found by kDNA PCR [79]. Moreover, Talmi-Frank et al, described a new application of high resolution melt (HRM) analysis of a real time PCR product from the ITS1 region in samples from human, reservoir hosts and sand flies for rapid detection, quantification and speciation of Old World *Leishmania* species. In this assay, different characteristic high resolution melt analysis patterns were exhibited by *L.major, L.tropica, L. aethiopica,* and *L.infantum* making this approach able to distinguish all Old World *Leishmania* species causing human disease, except *L. donovani* from *L.infantum* [55]. Recently, an alternative technique, PCR-fluorescent fragment length analysis (PCR-FFL), has been developed by Tomás-Pérez et al, for use in *Leishmania* while its use has been reported previously for species identification in Trypanosoma [100,101]. In this study the fluorescently tagged primers used, were designed in the rRNA fragment ITS1 and 7SL region. The amplified fragments were digested and their sizes were determined by an automated DNA sequencer. PCR-FFL was found to be accurate and more sensitive than PCR-RFLP analysis [101].

Regarding the hsp70 PCR-RFLP approach, it is considered to be useful for the *L.(Viannia)* species discrimination while its sensitivity is poor for *L.(Leishmania)* species. Diagnostic RFLP patterns for the *L.guyanensis* species complex as well as for *L. lainsoni* and *L. shawi* are produced after restriction with the enzyme HaeIII [84,102]. However, this assay was not able to discriminate between *L. braziliensis* and *L. peruviana* as well as *L. naiffi*, requiring a second restriction enzyme for the differentiation [102] while also *L. guyanensis* and *L. panamensis* both belonging to the *L. guyanensis* complex share identical RFLP pattern [83]. The discrimination of the species mentioned above is of great significance due to the fact that even if *L. braziliensis* is considered to be the main causative agent of MCL [103] other *L.(Viannia)* species are also suspected of causing MCL. Additionally, a differential response to antimonial treatment has been documented [104–106]. This assay was suggested to be applicable on clinical samples [107,108].

Montalvo et al, extended the use of the hsp70 PCR-RFLP for identification of Old World and additional New World species and improved resolution within New World species complexes [108]. Recently, they developed an adequate and flexible toolbox which consists of one improved and three new PCR approaches based on hsp70 target amplification and subsequent RFLP, able to diagnose and identify the most medically relevant New and Old World *Leishmania* species. The new PCR variants were highly sensitive and specific and they presented improved amplification efficiency in clinical samples compared to hsp70 PCR described previously by Garcia et al [84]. The choice of the most suitable PCR among the four described, depends on factors like the origin of infection, the sympatry of species, the imported versus endemic pathology, the clinical presentation and the clinical sample [109].

Fernandes et al first developed a PCR approach based on mini-exon gene [36] which was later adapted by Mauricio et al. In this study the mini-exon PCR-RFLP was compared with ITS1 PCR-RFLP. Both targets were shown to be able to identify the strains studied but mini-exon was found to be more polymorphic than ITS1 whereas neither ITS1 nor mini -exon produced as many robust groups as gp63 based restriction analyses published before [91,95]. Marfurt et al also developed a mini-exon PCR-RFLP assay [39]. The pair of primers deriving from the conserved region was able to amplify DNA from Old and New World *Leishmania* species while the diversity detected in the non transcribed spacers represented an informative phylogenetic marker. The digestion of the PCR products with one or two different restriction enzymes resulted in species-specific patterns allowing the species differentiation. Thus, they designed a mini-exon PCR-RFLP genotyping scheme, using different restriction enzymes. However, a single EaeI digest was informative enough for the speciation needed in clinical setting [39]. Furthermore, the repetitive character of this template made it highly sensitive even when applied to clinical samples [38]. On the other hand, when Bensoussan et al compared three PCR assays (kDNA,ITS1 and mini-exon used as targets) found that mini-exon presented the lowest sensitivity (53.8%) and suggested that this discrepancy may be attributed to the examination of stored clinical samples collected on filter papers instead of fresh samples, the extraction or the purification technique [110]. Rocha et al also adapted the PCR approach of Fernades et al and compared four PCR assays (kDNA and mini-exon used as targets) for the evaluation of New World *Leishmania* strains typing. Species belonging to the subgenus *Leishmania* were not amplified with the mini-exon target and the author suggested that this difference probably resulted from intraspecific variation [111]. Recently, in another study, ITS1 and mini-exon targets were compared with 18SrRNA in terms of sensitivity and discriminatory power in clinical samples, under routine laboratory settings. A new pair of primers for mini-exon target was designed due to the inability of the previous published primers to amplify the target in all clinical samples while also the protocol was slightly modified in order to achieve better diagnostic sensitivity. However, ITS1 was found to be more sensitive and practical than mini-exon. In contrast, mini-exon was again more polymorphic and revealed a great discriminatory power in *L.(Viannia)* subgenus [32].

The *L.donovani* complex is the causative agent of visceral leishmaniasis, the most severe form of the disease. The discrimination between the representatives of *L.donovani* complex, *L.infantum* and *L.donovani*, is important as they are morphologically indistinguishable while also they are associated with different epidemiology, ecology and pathology as *L.donovani* is anthroponotic and *L.infantum* is anthropozoonotic. Moreover, there are not discriminative markers to identify certain strains which status is questioned. Thus, the development of molecular tools capable of identifying diagnostic markers and allowing a better understanding of phylogenetic relationships is of great importance. In a study a PCR assay based on cysteine proteinase B (cpb) was developed which was able to differentiate between the two species. The cathepsin-1 proteases CPB which belong to the papain-like superfamily, clan CA and family C1, play an important role in the host protein destruction and evasion of the host immune response [88,112]. CPB enzymes are encoded by a tandem array located in a single locus. Mundodi et al, have compared a *L. donovani* strain and a *L.chagasi*(syn *L.infantum*) strain and revealed at least five tandemly arranged genes [113]. Hide and Banuls, used the last repeats of the cluster (cpbE for *L.infantum* and cpbF for *L.donovani*) and designed a PCR assay able to differentiate the two species by their fragment length as *L.donovani* strains were characterized by a 741-bp product and *L.infantum* strains by a 702-bp product. This PCR assay did not generate amplification for other *Leishmania* species nor trypanosomatids. Although sensitive and specific in cultured parasites, the assay is not sensitive enough for diagnosis on clinical samples [88]. The fact that the species discrimination is based on 39 bp difference in PCR product may cause problems in species identification when using normal agarose gel electrophoresis and where both species are not available for comparison. Thus, another cpb PCR assay was developed with subsequent digestion with DraIII which cuts the 741-bp amplicon of *L.donovani* into 400 and 341 bp and a PCR using a species-specific primer pair capable of amplifying a 317 bp of *L. donovani* whereas it did not amplify *L.infantum* [89]. Two cpb PCR-RFLP and one fluorogenic PCR assay for the molecular typing of *L.donovani* complex have been also developed and it was reported that the assays described were valid and informative for *Leishmania* typing in clinical samples [90,114]. Furthermore, a multilocus approach, using new and previously reported targets including cpb genes, was applied to neotropical isolates (*L.braziliensis, L.peruviana, L.guyanensis, L.lainsoni and L. amazonensis*) and was shown to be a highly robust method of distinguishing different strains [87].

Real-time PCR is considered to be a useful, sensitive, accurate and rapid tool for detection, quantification and even genetic characterization of *Leishmania* parasites. A LightCycler RT-PCR assay based on fluorescence melting curve analysis of PCR products generated from the minicircles of kDNA was developed. This assay was able to detect and differentiate four Old World *Leishmania* species (*L. major* was differentiated from *L. donovani* and from *L.tropica* and *L.infantum*) [45]. In another study, a qPCR based on glucosephosphate isomerase (GPI) gene was able to discriminate between subgenus *Viannia* and the complexes *L.mexicana, L.donovani/infantum* and *L.major* [115]. A qPCR based on glucose-6-phosphate dehydrogenase (g6pd) using either SYBR-Green or TaqMan probes has also been described. This assay was able to differentiate *L.braziliensis* from other *L. (Viannia)* species and from those of *L.(Leishmania)* [116]. Weirather et al used a set of primers and probes for serial qPCR assays based on kDNA which was able to detect and differentiate *Leishmania* species in clinical samples due to different melt temperature of the amplicon or by observing the presence or absence of some amplicons [117]. Recently, tryparedoxine peroxidase gene was used as amplification target in a qPCR assay able to identify Old-World *Leishmania* species causing CL [54]. An alternative 18S rDNA based qPCR using fluorescence resonance energy transfer probes (FRET) was able to discriminate the *L.donovani* complex, the *L.brasiliensis* complex, and species other than these based on the distinct melting temperature obtained [46]. Finally, a new qPCR assay based on FRET technology and melting curve analysis was designed based on mannose phosphate isomerase (MPI) and 6-phosphogluconate dehydrogenase (6PGD) genes which found to be highly sensitive and discriminative for the five species of *Leishmania* being evaluated (*L.braziliensis, L.panamensis, L.guyanensis, L.peruviana and L.lainsoni*) [118].

MLEE, the technique which is regarded as the 'gold standard' for the identification of *Leishmania* parasites to species and subspecific levels and for genetic diversity studies, has been widely used since its introduction [119]. MLEE detects different alleles of housekeeping genes indirectly by scoring the electrophoretic mobility of the enzymes they encode. The nucleotide differences in the genes encoding the enzymes are reflected by their mobility differences. Thus, the parasites are identified by their enzymatic profile and are grouped in taxonomic units termed zymodemes, each one of whom consists of all the strains showing exactly the same profiles for all the enzymatic systems under study. Distinct combinations of isoenzyme mobilities for up to 15 enzymes have been assigned zymodeme numbers (MON-1–MON-274) [120].

However, this molecular method presents several disadvantages including the need for mass culture of *Leishmania* parasites and large amount of protein, it is timeconsuming, labour-intensive, costly and technically demanding. It is also worth mentioning that the MLEE methods used in Europe and in South America are based on different enzyme panels and cannot be compared directly [74,93,119]. As far as it concerns its discriminatory power, it is considered to be poor due to its inability to detect nucleotide substitutions that do not change the amino acid composition and changes in the amino acid composition that does not modify the electrophoretic mobility. The discriminatory power of MLEE for classifications below species level is limited. For instance, the *L.infantum* zymodeme MON-1, the causative agent of the majority of visceral leishmaniasis cases around the Mediterranean basin and South America, has been shown to be genetically heterogeneous and polyphyletic with molecular markers presenting higher resolution level [121,122]. Moreover, other molecular studies do not always agree with the classification of *Leishmania* parasites by MLEE. For instance, the differentiation between the representatives of *L.donovani* complex, *L.donovani* and *L.infantum*, is based on only one enzymatic system (glutamate–oxaloacetate transaminase-GOT) making the species distinction poor. In fact, the zymodeme MON-30 which was regarded as *L.infantum*, has recently shown to be *L.donovani* [123,124]. Furthermore, the existence of *L.archibaldi* as a distinct species belonging to *L.donovani* complex was supported by MLEE but it was not in agreement with the results of many different molecular markers [125] while also *L.killicki* was not confirmed to be a separate species [94,126] and *L.donovani* zymodeme MON-37 was assigned to strains of different genetic background [74,120,127]. However, the codominant character of this molecular tool is advantageous as it is able to identify heterozygous profiles and thus potential hybrids while also if the proteins are highly polymeric, the distinction can be made between a heterozygous profile and a mixed infection [120].

Randomly Amplified Polymorphic DNA (RAPD), a simple process, distinct from the PCR, based in the amplification of genomic DNA with short oligonucleotides of arbitrary nucleotide sequence used as primers, has been also applied for *Leishmania spp*. The primers are designed and used for the detection of polymorphisms without relying on prior knowledge of the DNA sequence to be amplified [128]. From the advent of RAPD technique [128,129] numerous studies, only a few of them can be cited here, have been published reporting the use of RAPD as a molecular tool for *Leishmania* species identification and strain characterization. RAPD has been used for the investigation of the genomic diversity of *L.braziliensis* strains [130,131], *L.major* isolates [132], *L.donovani* complex [124,133,134] and *L.infantum* [77,121,135]. Regarding the use of RAPD in species identification, it has been applied for the differentiation between the species *L.braziliensis*, *L.mexicana*, *L.infantum*, *L.tropica*, *L.chagasi*, *L.amazonensis and L.major* [136], the identification and differentiation of Old World species at complex level [137] and recently for the characterization of clinical isolates responsible for kala-azar in India [138]. The main disadvantages of this technique are the need for parasite culture due to the use of non *Leishmania* specific primers and the poor reproducibility of the assay. Moreover, the bands of equal electrophoretic mobility may not be homologous and it is impossible to distinguish homozygous from heterozygous genotypes at specific loci because it is difficult to recognize allelic variants of randomly amplified polymorphic DNA markers in the absence of crossing data [74,120]

PCR hybridization is one of the first molecular methods for species identification and genotyping. DNA probes have been designed for *Leishmania* species identification. The most common target used for *Leishmania spp* identification is kDNA. DNA probes targeting kDNA have been applied for *L.major* [139], *L.infantum* [140], *L.aethiopica* [141], *L.mexicana* and *L.braziliensis* [142], and *L.mexicana, L.donovani* and *L.braziliensis* complexes [143]. Other specific probes developed include a cDNA probe, designed from a repetitive degenerate sequence isolated from *L.donovani*, which specifically hybridized only with isolates of the *L.donovani* complex [144] and two probes, the pDK10 and the pDK20, which were able to differentiate between the Old World *Leishmania* species belonging to *L.donovani* complex and between all Old World *Leishmania* species respectively [145,146]. DNA probes generated from mini-exon genes have also been developed [147]. Other probes developed so far include a *L.braziliensis* specific probe [148] and *L.guyanensis* specific one [149].

MLEE has been recently modified in a direct sequencing allele detection method at each locus, called MLST. Partial sequences of approximately 700 bp in size, belonging to a defined set of housekeeping genes, are directly compared; the alleles are scored as identical or not and the same allele combinations are referred as sequence types. Alternatively, data analysis by sequencing of the alleles may be implemented. This technique was first used for bacterial pathogens whereas in *Leishmania*, steps have been taken to develop a MLST system [150]. The *L. donovani* complex has been studied by 2 sets of 5 loci for genes coding for enzymes used in MLEE [151,152]. These 10 targets in combination should be a complete MLST system for application in *L. donovani* complex. These studies showed that results from MLST are in agreement with results from MLEE whereas some discrepancies were found and MLST presented higher resolution level such as a silent Single Nucleotide Polymorphism (SNP) in gpi that distinguishes between strains of *L.infantum* [151]. Moreover, SNPs resulting in amino acid changes were also found in genes coding for enzymes giving indistinguishable electrophoretic profiles such as in nh2, which has the same protein band size for all *L.donovani* complex strains. These authors reported that MLST could be applied directly to clinical samples or to small-volume cultures. Furthermore, it can be used to detect recombination indirectly and for population genetics studies [151]. Tsukayama et al investigated the intraspecific and interspecific variation in the coding sequences of four enzymes (gpi, mdh, mpi and 6pgd), used in the MLEE typing method, in order to identify SNPs able to discriminate among closely related species. The assay was applied to clinical samples and successfully identified the species of *Leishmania* responsible for the clinical disease [153]. However, the analysis did not include sufficient diversity of strains for each species [74]. Recently, in another study a combination of the previous published enzyme-coding genes (fh, g6pdh, icd, mpi and pgd) was used so as to differentiate the Chinese *Leishmania* isolates and to investigate their phylogenetic relationships [154]. MLST is likely to become the gold standard basis for taxonomy and identification of *Leishmania*.

MLMT is based on the amplification of microsatellites sequences, tandem repeats of a simple nucleotide motif, 1-6 nucleotides, which are distributed abundantly in the eukaryotic and prokaryotic genomes and may reveal important strain polymorphisms. These markers are very useful for studying genetic variation between closely related organisms. Length polymorphisms in microsatellites sequences result from gain and loss of single repeat units which can be detected after amplification with specific to their flanking regions primers. MLMT approaches developed so far for *Leishmania spp*, make use of sets of 14–20 unlinked microsatellite loci. Microsatellite loci with high discriminatory power and being suitable for characterizing closely related strains have been published for the *L.donovani* complex [155–158], *L.donovani* strains [127] *L.major* [159], *L.tropica* [126,160] and for species of the subgenus *L. (Viannia)* [161]. Moreover, as the genetic diversity of *L.infantum* strains has been the subject of intense interest, several studies used MLMT approaches for the evaluation of the genomic variation in *L.infantum* strains [122,135]. It is worth mentioning that when MLMT was compared with other molecular markers for strain typing of *L.infantum*, the results obtained with kDNA PCR-RFLP were comparable to MLMT. kDNA and MLMT presented the highest discriminatory power especially for the MON-1 strains discrimination and appeared to be the most adequate for strain fingerprinting. However, MLMT is advantageous over kDNA PCR-RFLP because of its better reproducibility and feasibility of inter-lab comparisons and the co-dominant character of the markers used, making MLMT suitable for population genetic studies [77]. MLMT is suitable for high-throughput analysis and the data obtained are reproducible and exchangeable between laboratories. Moreover, accurate, quality controlled microsatellite profiles can be stored in databases and compared between different laboratories. In contrast to MLEE, selection does not seem to act on polymorphisms in microsatellite length while also the codominant nature of these markers permits the detection of the allelic variants. MLMT can be used directly on biological samples without prior culture of the parasite. DNA extracted from specimens spotted on filter paper or glass slides or from old Giemsa stained microscope slides was successfully applied in MLMT approaches [155]. It is recommended to use a panel of 10–20 unlinked microsatellite markers in all studies for nearly every species because microsatellite sequences are prone to homoplasy. Additionally, polymorphic repeats are not conserved between different species of *Leishmania* [74,122,157].

4. Phylogenetic analysis

Phylogenetics is the study of evolutionary relationships among various groups of organisms (e.g., species or populations). Their relatedness is evaluated through morphological and molecular sequencing data. This analysis leads to a hypothesis about the evolutionary history of taxonomic groups, their phylogeny. Regarding evolution, it is considered to be a branching process. Populations are altered with time and may split into separate branches, hybridize or be eliminated. The order in which evolutionary events are assumed to have occurred is revealed and may be visualized in a phylogenetic tree.

As mentioned before, MLEE is still regarded as the reference technique for the identification of *Leishmania* species and subspecies. The data obtained from MLEE were analyzed by phenetic and cladistic techniques and led to the construction of the first phylogenetic tree of the genus *Leishmania* [162]. The latter, revealed the monophyletic origin of the genus *Leishmania* and its subdivision into two subgenera, the *L.(Leishmania)* and the *L.(Viannia)* subgenus. *L.(Leishmania)* included the Old World species and *L.mexicana* and complexes from the New World. *L. (Viannia)* subgenus was composed from the other New World species. As *Sauroleishmania* was considered to be a separate genus, the lizard species were not included in these studies. MLEE has been applied to a great variety and amount of isolates in comparison to other molecular methods in the past 25 years, resulting in the current classification system [93,162]. Phylogenetics based on different molecular methods, has confirmed the previous suggested taxonomy of the genus *Leishmania* by MLEE. However, the existence of a larger number of species has been proposed.

PCR-based methods with subsequent RFLP or DNA sequence analysis of multicopy targets or multigene families, to the recently developed MLST and MLMT, have been applied for the identification of the *Leishmania* species being responsible for the disease and for epidemiological studies in different endemic regions, as well as for taxonomic, phylogenetic, and population genetic studies. These tools except from their enhanced sensitivity they are also able to distinguish *Leishmania* parasites at species and intraspecies level. As for phylogenetic studies, the sequence analysis of single-copy gene targets is preferred while also the recombination and the different mutation rates between lineages make the use of one gene less suitable for the phylogenic analysis of the Trypanosomatidae or its subgroups[163].

Several DNA targets have been used to reveal the phylogeny of the *Leishmania* genus including single-copy genes encoding the catalytic polypeptide of DNA polymerase a (polA), the largest subunit of RNA polymerase II (rpoIILS) [164] and 7SL RNA [86], the ITS [165,166], the N-acetylglucosamine-1-phosphate transferase (NAGT) gene [167], the mitochondrial cytochrome b gene (cytb) [168], and most recently, sequences of the hsp70 subfamily [83]. Sequence analysis of these targets led to the conclusion that the subgenera L. (*Leishmania*) and L. (*Viannia*) constitute distinct monophyletic clades and that species of the Old and New World are segregated within the L. (*Leishmania*) subgenus. *Sauroleishmania* species branched off between the L.(*Leishmania*) and L.(*Viannia*) subgenera as an independent taxon suggesting that lizard *Leishmania* might be derived from mammalian parasites [164] and that they should be regarded as a subgenus of *Leishmania* rather than an independent genus [99]. However, the fact that RNA and DNA polymerase genes presented higher evolution rate in the lizard *Leishmania* than in the mammalian *Leishmania* species set into question the exact taxonomic position of lizard parasites [164].

In another study, Cupolillo et al. based on various molecular criteria, suggested the division of the genus *Leishmania* into two sections, *Euleishmania* and *Paraleishmania*. *Euleishmania* consisted of the subgenera L.(*Leishmania*), L.(*Sauroleishmania*), and L.(*Viannia*). *Paraleishmania* included L. hertigi, L.deanei, L.colombiensis, L.equatorensis, L.herreri, and strains of *Endotrypanum*. In the latter section, the parasites of hystricomorph rodents, L.hertigi and L.deanei and the remaining species that are mainly parasites of sloths were genetically different while strains of *Endotrypanum* formed a paraphyletic group [169].

More recently Fraga et al. analyzed the phylogeny of the genus *Leishmania* based on the hsp70 gene. In this study the isolates and strains used, were of different geographic origins. The resulting phylogeny supported that the monophyletic genus *Leishmania* consisted of three distinct subgenera, the L.(*Leishmania*), L.(*Viannia*), and L.(*Sauroleishmania*). The obtained phylogeny supported the following eight species: *L.donovani, L.major, L.tropica, L.mexicana, L.lainsoni, L.naiffi, L.guyanensis* and *L.braziliensis*. In some of these species, subspecies were recognized including *L.donovani infantum, L.guyanensis panamensis,* and *L.braziliensis peruvi-*

ana. The so far recognized species *L.aethiopica, L.garnhami, and L.amazonensis* did not form monophyletic clusters [83].

Several discrepancies were reported for the taxonomic status of species obtained by MLEE compared to DNA based sequences. It is worth mentioning that the existence of *L.chagasi* and *L. archibaldi* as distinct species, was not supported by any molecular analyses as *L.chagasi* cannot be distinguished from strains of *L.infantum* and should therefore be regarded as South American strains of *L.infantum* [170,171] whereas *L. archibaldi* is not a valid species [125,159]. Numerous molecular studies did not even support the monophyly of the two remaining species, *L.donovani* and *L.infantum* [83,164,168]. Therefore, it was proposed that *L.donovani* is the only species of the *L.donovani* complex [83] while *L.donovani infantum* was recognized as subspecies. Regarding other geographically defined genetic groups within *L.donovani*, it was suggested that they could be delimited. Furthermore, the status of *L.killicki* has been debated. MLEE analysis supported the classification of *L.killicki* as a separate species while other molecular methods proposed that it was identical to *L.tropica* [94,126,168]. At the same time, *L.tropica* clusters to a single branch with *L.aethiopica*, making it difficult to be distinguished by the most of the DNA-based phylogenies [83,86,168]. It was suggested that they may represent different subspecies of the species *L.tropica* which is however needed to be investigated with a larger number of strains. Another discrepancy concerns the existence of the *L.mexicana* complex species. The strains of *L.mexicana* and *L.amazonensis* species are overpresented in DNA based phylogenies while only one *L. garnhami* strain was analysed in the hsp70 trees. In the latter study, none of these species could be distinguished as a monophyletic clade and *L.mexicana* was the only recognized species [83]. These results are in agreement with previous published studies [164,172,173] whereas they are in contrast to others [86,165,168]. Thus, the *L.mexicana* complex should be investigated, including *L.venezuelensis* and *L.aristidesi* strains, in order to evaluate the species and subspecies constituting this complex. The same holds true for the *L.braziliensis* complex species. Several molecular phylogenies including hsp70, RAPD and MLEE, supported the distinction of *L.peruviana* from other strains of *L.braziliensis* [83,174] and it was recognized as a subspecies in the *L.braziliensis* complex. However, this classification was questioned by a study using monoclonal antibodies [175] and another one analyzing the microsatellite variation [161] which suggested that strains of *L.peruviana* were grouped together with strains of *L.braziliensis* from Peru and from the Acre State, a Brazilian region bordering Peru. The use of a sufficiently large number of strains from different areas of distribution is needed so as the taxonomic status of the repsesentatives of the *L.braziliensis* complex to be evaluated. Moreover, in different phylogenetic trees, strains of *L.guyanensis* and *L.panamensis* formed a monophyletic cluster which was then divided into two monophyletic subclusters. Thus, the existence of two subspecies within the species *L.guyanensis* was proposed. A possible explanation for these discrepancies reported in different studies regarding the taxonomic status of both *L.peruviana* and *L.panamensis*, is the application of different molecular markers and the analysis of different strains.

Several molecular methods including MLEE [93], PCR-RFLP of ITSrDNA [78] and PCR-RFLP and sequence analysis of the hsp70 gene [102], were also suggested the inclusion of *L.shawi* in the *L. guyanensis* group. The same applies for *L.naiffi* whereas *L.lainsoni* was confirmed to be the most divergent species inside the *L.(Viannia)* subgenus [83,102].

Noyes et al. (2002) identified a parasite isolated from human cutaneous lesions. Both stains were analysed by MLEE and found to be identical to each other and distantly related to all other *Leishmania* species. The application of other molecular methods revealed a low support for both its position basal to all *Euleishmania* and its clustering with *L.enriettii*. Thus, it was suggested that this strain may cluster with *L.(Leishmania)* or *L.(Viannia)* or form a novel clade within the *Euleishmania* either with or without *L.enriettii* [176]. Recently *Leishmania* species isolated from clinical samples from immunocompetent and immunosuppressed patients in Thailand [177,178] and a focal CL outbreak in Ghana [179] were identified and named as *L.siamensis*. Furthermore, novel *Leishmania* species, genetically indistinguishable, were isolated from kangaroos, wallaroos, and wallabies, living in captivity in the Northern Territory of Australia, a region that was considered free of *Leishmania* parasites [180]. Additionally, autochthonous cases of CL in German and Swiss horses and in a Swiss cow could not be classified neither as Old World nor New World *Leishmania* species while they were found to be most closely related to *L.siamensis* [181,182]. Finally, two new *L.(Viannia)* species were described and named *L.lindenbergi* [183] and *L.utingensis*. The last one was represented by only one sample isolated from a *Lutzomyia tuberculata* sand fly. Although the sequence analysis of single-copy gene targets has shown to be informative, the use of several independent genes displaying different evolutionary histories is preferable [184]. Such genes have applied in MLST and provided new insights on taxonomy and evolutionary history of *Leishmania*. MLST is currently considered the most powerful phylogenetic approach, it has been shown to have high discriminatory power, reproducibility and transportability of results between laboratories. Thus far, there are 10 published MLST targets available for the *L.donovani* complex [151,152], most of which are also applicable to other Old World *Leishmania* [185] and 4 targets for the sub-genus *Leishmania (Viannia)* [153]. This should form a complete MLST system applicable to *Leishmania* parasites.

5. Conclusion

Molecular methods have revolutionised the diagnosis of leishmaniasis. A variety of target sequences has been used and evaluated in different clinical samples of parasite hosts. Regarding PCR based assays, they were found to be rapid, sensitive and discriminative at species or even strain level. However the diagnosis of leishmaniasis remains a scientific challenge. There is a gap between the scientific advances, diagnostics and management of *Leishmania* infections in the field which should be decreased and an urgent need for standardization, optimization and simplification of PCR based applications. In this context, there is a generalized effort to make these assays available mainly in endemic areas around the world which will have an impact in disease control.

The great scientific interest for species identification may be attributed to its significance in prompt diagnosis and prognosis of the disease, decision making regarding treatment and control measures. Despite the abundance of the studies carried out and the molecular markers used so far, the species discrimination is still tough in several closely related species. Thus, molecular tools with high discriminatory power are currently under development, optimization and evaluation.

Many molecular tools have been used for the *Leishmania* phylogeny and the definition of its taxonomy. However, evaluation of the phylogenetic relationships of *Leishmania* species is not an easy task. Moreover, there is a need for simplification of the classification and a meaningful nomenclature of *Leishmania* genus particularly for the clinicians.

Acknowledgements

This research has been co-financed by the European Union (European Social Fund – ESF) and Greek national funds through the Operational Program "Education and Lifelong Learning" of the National Strategic Reference Framework (NSRF) - Research Funding Program: THALES. Investing in knowledge society through the European Social Fund

Author details

Constantina N. Tsokana[1], Labrini V. Athanasiou[2*], George Valiakos[1], Vassiliki Spyrou[3], Katerina Manolakou[4] and Charalambos Billinis[1]

*Address all correspondence to: lathan@vet.uth.gr

1 Department of Microbiology and Parasitology, Faculty of Veterinary Medicine, University of Thessaly, Karditsa, Greece

2 Department of Medicine, Faculty of Veterinary Medicine, University of Thessaly, Karditsa, Greece

3 Department of Animal Production, Technological Education Institute of Larissa, Greece

4 Department of Animal Husbandry and Nutrition, Faculty of Veterinary Medicine, University of Thessaly, Karditsa, Greece

References

[1] Baneth G, Aroch I. Canine leishmaniasis: a diagnostic and clinical challenge. Veterinary Journal (London, England: 1997) 2008;175:14–5.

[2] Cortes S, Rolão N, Ramada J, Campino L. PCR as a rapid and sensitive tool in the diagnosis of human and canine leishmaniasis using *Leishmania donovani* s.l.-specific kinetoplastid primers. Transactions of the Royal Society of Tropical Medicine and Hygiene 2004;98:12–7.

[3] Singh S. New developments in diagnosis of leishmaniasis. The Indian Journal of Medical Research 2006;123:311–30.

[4] De Almeida Silva L, Romero HD, Prata A, Costa RT, Nascimento E, Carvalho SFG, et al. Immunologic tests in patients after clinical cure of visceral leishmaniasis. The American Journal of Tropical Medicine and Hygiene

[5] Osman OF, Oskam L, Kroon NC, Schoone GJ, Khalil ET, El-Hassan AM, et al. Use of PCR for diagnosis of post-kala-azar dermal leishmaniasis. Journal of Clinical Microbiology 1998;36:1621–4.

[6] Osman OF, Oskam L, Zijlstra EE, el-Hassan AM, el-Naeim DA, Kager PA. Use of the polymerase chain reaction to assess the success of visceral leishmaniasis treatment. Transactions of the Royal Society of Tropical Medicine and Hygiene

[7] Schubach A, Marzochi MC, Cuzzi-Maya T, Oliveira AV, Araujo ML, Oliveira AL, et al. Cutaneous scars in American tegumentary leishmaniasis patients: a site of *Leishmania* (Viannia) braziliensis persistence and viability eleven years after antimonial therapy and clinical cure. The American Journal of Tropical Medicine and Hygiene 1998;58:824–7.

[8] Guevara P, Ramírez JL, Rojas E, Scorza JV, González N, Añez N. *Leishmania braziliensis* in blood 30 years after cure. Lancet 1993;341:1341.

[9] Martín-Sánchez J, Pineda JA, Morillas-Márquez F, García-García JA, Acedo C, Macías J. Detection of *Leishmania infantum* kinetoplast DNA in peripheral blood from asymptomatic individuals at risk for parenterally transmitted infections: relationship between polymerase chain reaction results and other *Leishmania* infection markers. The American Journal of Tropical Medicine and Hygiene 2004;70:545–8.

[10] Solano-Gallego L, Koutinas A, Miró G, Cardoso L, Pennisi MG, Ferrer L, et al. Directions for the diagnosis, clinical staging, treatment and prevention of canine leishmaniosis. Veterinary Parasitology 2009;165:1–18.

[11] Maia C, Ramada J, Cristóvão JM, Gonçalves L, Campino L. Diagnosis of canine leishmaniasis: conventional and molecular techniques using different tissues. Veterinary Journal (London, England: 1997) 2009;179:142–4.

[12] Deborggraeve S, Laurent T, Espinosa D, Van der Auwera G, Mbuchi M, Wasunna M, et al. A simplified and standardized polymerase chain reaction format for the diagnosis of leishmaniasis. The Journal of Infectious Diseases 2008;198:1565–72.

[13] Schallig HDFH, Oskam L. Molecular biological applications in the diagnosis and control of leishmaniasis and parasite identification. Tropical Medicine & International Health TM IH 2002;7:641–51.

[14] Ferreira S de A, Ituassu LT, de Melo MN, de Andrade ASR. Evaluation of the conjunctival swab for canine visceral leishmaniasis diagnosis by PCR-hybridization in Minas Gerais State, Brazil. Veterinary Parasitology 2008;152:257–63.

[15] Strauss-Ayali D, Jaffe CL, Burshtain O, Gonen L, Baneth G. Polymerase chain reaction using noninvasively obtained samples, for the detection of *Leishmania infantum* DNA in dogs. The Journal of Infectious Diseases 2004;189:1729–33.

[16] Maia C, Campino L. Methods for diagnosis of canine leishmaniasis and immune response to infection. Veterinary Parasitology 2008;158:274–87.

[17] Ferreira S de A, Almeida GG, Silva S de O, Vogas GP, Fujiwara RT, de Andrade ASR, et al. Nasal, oral and ear swabs for canine visceral leishmaniasis diagnosis: new practical approaches for detection of *Leishmania infantum* DNA. PLoS Neglected Tropical Diseases 2013;7:e2150.

[18] Lombardo G, Pennisi MG, Lupo T, Migliazzo A, Caprì A, Solano-Gallego L. Detection of *Leishmania infantum* DNA by real-time PCR in canine oral and conjunctival swabs and comparison with other diagnostic techniques. Veterinary Parasitology 2012;184:10–7.

[19] Manna L, Reale S, Vitale F, Picillo E, Pavone LM, Gravino AE. Real-time PCR assay in *Leishmania*-infected dogs treated with meglumine antimoniate and allopurinol. Veterinary Journal (London, England: 1997) 2008;177:279–82.

[20] Andresen K, Gasim S, Elhassan AM, Khalil EA, Barker DC, Theander TG, et al. Diagnosis of visceral leishmaniasis by the polymerase chain reaction using blood, bone marrow and lymph node samples from patients from the Sudan. Tropical Medicine & International Health TM IH 1997;2:440–4.

[21] Da Silva ES, Gontijo CMF, Pacheco R da S, Brazil RP. Diagnosis of human visceral leishmaniasis by PCR using blood samples spotted on filter paper.Genetics and Molecular Research GMR 2004;3:251–7.

[22] Hu XS, Yang WT, Lu HG, Yan HP, Cheng JP, Ma Y, et al. Sequencing a specific kinetoplast DNA fragment of *Leishmania donovani* for polymerase chain reaction amplification in diagnosis of leishmaniasis in bone marrow and blood samples. The Journal of Parasitology 2000;86:822–6.

[23] Martín-Sánchez J, Pineda JA, Andreu-Lopez M, Delgado J, Macías J, De La Rosa R, et al. The high sensitivity of a PCR-ELISA in the diagnosis of cutaneous and visceral leishmaniasis caused by *Leishmania infantum*. Annals of Tropical Medicine and Parasitology 2002;96:669–77.

[24] Pal S, Aggarwal G, Haldar A, Majumdar A, Majumdar HK, Duttagupta S. Diagnosis of symptomatic kala-azar by polymerase chain reaction using patient's blood. Medi-

cal Science Monitor: International Medical Journal of Experimental and Clinical Research 2004;10:MT1–5.

[25] Salotra P, Sreenivas G, Pogue GP, Lee N, Nakhasi HL, Ramesh V, et al. Development of a species-specific PCR assay for detection of *Leishmania donovani* in clinical samples from patients with kala-azar and post-kala-azar dermal leishmaniasis. Journal of Clinical Microbiology 2001;39:849–54.

[26] Cruz I, Chicharro C, Nieto J, Bailo B, Canavate C, Figueras M-C, et al. Comparison of New Diagnostic Tools for Management of Pediatric Mediterranean Visceral Leishmaniasis. Journal of Clinical Microbiology 2006;44:2343–7.

[27] Cruz I, Cañavate C, Rubio JM, Morales MA, Chicharro C, Laguna F, et al. A nested polymerase chain reaction (Ln-PCR) for diagnosing and monitoring *Leishmania infantum* infection in patients co-infected with human immunodeficiency virus. Transactions of the Royal Society of Tropical Medicine and Hygiene 2002;96 Suppl 1:S185–189.

[28] Lachaud L, Dereure J, Chabbert E, Reynes J, Mauboussin JM, Oziol E, et al. Optimized PCR using patient blood samples for diagnosis and follow-up of visceral leishmaniasis, with special reference to AIDS patients. Journal of Clinical Microbiology 2000;38:236–40.

[29] Mathis A, Deplazes P. PCR and in vitro cultivation for detection of *Leishmania* spp. in diagnostic samples from humans and dogs. Journal of Clinical Microbiology 1995;33:1145–9.

[30] Azmi K, Nasereddin A, Ereqat S, Schnur L, Schonian G, Abdeen Z. Methods incorporating a polymerase chain reaction and restriction fragment length polymorphism and their use as a "gold standard" in diagnosing Old World cutaneous leishmaniasis.Diagnostic Microbiology and Infectious Disease 2011;71:151–5.

[31] Leite RS, Ferreira S de A, Ituassu LT, de Melo MN, de Andrade ASR. PCR diagnosis of visceral leishmaniasis in asymptomatic dogs using conjunctival swab samples. Veterinary Parasitology 2010;170:201–6.

[32] Roelfsema JH, Nozari N, Herremans T, Kortbeek LM, Pinelli E. Evaluation and improvement of two PCR targets in molecular typing of clinical samples of *Leishmania* patients. Experimental Parasitology 2011;127:36–41.

[33] Rotureau B, Ravel C, Couppie P, Pratlong F, Nacher M, Dedet J-P, et al. Use of PCR-Restriction Fragment Length Polymorphism Analysis To Identify the Main New World *Leishmania* Species and Analyze Their Taxonomic Properties and Polymorphism by Application of the Assay to Clinical Samples. Journal of Clinical Microbiology 2006;44:459–67.

[34] Schönian G, Nasereddin A, Dinse N, Schweynoch C, Schallig HDF., Presber W, et al. PCR diagnosis and characterization of *Leishmania* in local and imported clinical samples.Diagnostic Microbiology and Infectious Disease 2003;47:349–58.

[35] Bensoussan E, Nasereddin A, Jonas F, Schnur LF, Jaffe CL. Comparison of PCR Assays for Diagnosis of Cutaneous Leishmaniasis. Journal of Clinical Microbiology 2006;44:1435–9.

[36] Fernandes O, Murthy VK, Kurath U, Degrave WM, Campbell DA. Mini-exon gene variation in human pathogenic *Leishmania* species. Molecular and Biochemical Parasitology 1994;66:261–71.

[37] Katakura K, Kawazu S, Naya T, Nagakura K, Ito M, Aikawa M, et al. Diagnosis of kala-azar by nested PCR based on amplification of the *Leishmania* mini-exon gene. Journal of Clinical Microbiology 1998;36:2173–7.

[38] Marfurt J, Nasereddin A, Niederwieser I, Jaffe CL, Beck H-P, Felger I. Identification and Differentiation of *Leishmania* Species in Clinical Samples by PCR Amplification of the Miniexon Sequence and Subsequent Restriction Fragment Length Polymorphism Analysis. Journal of Clinical Microbiology 2003;41:3147–53.

[39] Marfurt J, Niederwieser I, Makia ND, Beck H-P, Felger I. Diagnostic genotyping of Old and New World *Leishmania* species by PCR-RFLP.Diagnostic Microbiology and Infectious Disease 2003;46:115–24.

[40] Serin MS, Waki K, Chang K-P, Aslan G, Direkel S, Otag F, et al. Consistence of mini-exon polymerase chain reaction–restriction fragment length polymorphism and single-copy gene sequence analyses in discriminating *Leishmania* genotypes.Diagnostic Microbiology and Infectious Disease 2007;57:295–9.

[41] Lachaud L, Marchergui-Hammami S, Chabbert E, Dereure J, Dedet JP, Bastien P. Comparison of Six PCR Methods Using Peripheral Blood for Detection of Canine Visceral Leishmaniasis. Journal of Clinical Microbiology 2002;40:210–5.

[42] Minodier P, Piarroux R, Gambarelli F, Joblet C, Dumon H. Rapid identification of causative species in patients with Old World leishmaniasis. Journal of Clinical Microbiology 1997;35:2551–5.

[43] Cruz I, Chicharro C, Nieto J, Bailo B, Canavate C, Figueras M-C, et al. Comparison of New Diagnostic Tools for Management of Pediatric Mediterranean Visceral Leishmaniasis. Journal of Clinical Microbiology 2006;44:2343–7.

[44] Schönian G, Nasereddin A, Dinse N, Schweynoch C, Schallig HDF., Presber W, et al. PCR diagnosis and characterization of *Leishmania* in local and imported clinical samples.Diagnostic Microbiology and Infectious Disease 2003;47:349–58.

[45] Nicolas L, Milon G, Prina E. Rapid differentiation of Old World *Leishmania* species by LightCycler polymerase chain reaction and melting curve analysis. Journal of Microbiological Methods 2002;51:295–9.

[46] Schulz A, Mellenthin K, Schonian G, Fleischer B, Drosten C. Detection, Differentiation, and Quantitation of Pathogenic *Leishmania* Organisms by a Fluorescence Resonance Energy Transfer-Based Real-Time PCR Assay. Journal of Clinical Microbiology 2003;41:1529–35.

[47] Paiva-Cavalcanti M, Regis-da-Silva C, Gomes Y. Comparison of real-time PCR and conventional PCR for detection of *Leishmania (Leishmania infantum)* infection: a mini-review. Journal of Venomous Animals and Toxins Including Tropical Diseases 2010;16:537–42.

[48] Mary C, Faraut F, Lascombe L, Dumon H. Quantification of *Leishmania infantum* DNA by a Real-Time PCR Assay with High Sensitivity. Journal of Clinical Microbiology 2004;42:5249–55.

[49] Vitale F, Reale S, Vitale M, Petrotta E, Torina A, Caracappa S. TaqMan-based detection of *Leishmania infantum* DNA using canine samples. Annals of the New York Academy of Sciences 2004;1026:139–43.

[50] Francino O, Altet L, Sánchez-Robert E, Rodriguez A, Solano-Gallego L, Alberola J, et al. Advantages of real-time PCR assay for diagnosis and monitoring of canine leishmaniosis. Veterinary Parasitology 2006;137:214–21.

[51] De Paiva Cavalcanti M, Felinto de Brito ME, de Souza WV, de Miranda Gomes Y, Abath FGC. The development of a real-time PCR assay for the quantification of *Leishmania infantum* DNA in canine blood. Veterinary Journal (London, England: 1997) 2009;182:356–8.

[52] Galletti E, Bonilauri P, Bardasi L, Fontana MC, Ramini M, Renzi M, et al. Development of a minor groove binding probe based real-time PCR for the diagnosis and quantification of *Leishmania infantum* in dog specimens. Research in Veterinary Science 2011;91:243–5.

[53] Abbasi I, Aramin S, Hailu A, Shiferaw W, Kassahun A, Belay S, et al. Evaluation of PCR procedures for detecting and quantifying *Leishmania donovani* DNA in large numbers of dried human blood samples from a visceral leishmaniasis focus in Northern Ethiopia. BMC Infectious Diseases 2013;13:153.

[54] Khosravi S, Hejazi SH, Hashemzadeh M, Eslami G, Darani HY. Molecular diagnosis of Old World leishmaniasis: real-time PCR based on tryparedoxin peroxidase gene for the detection and identification of *Leishmania* spp. Journal of Vector Borne Diseases 2012;49:15–8.

[55] Talmi-Frank D, Nasereddin A, Schnur LF, Schönian G, Töz SO, Jaffe CL, et al. Detection and identification of old world *Leishmania* by high resolution melt analysis. PLoS Neglected Tropical Diseases 2010;4:e581.

[56] Reithinger R, Dujardin J-C. Molecular Diagnosis of Leishmaniasis: Current Status and Future Applications. Journal of Clinical Microbiology 2006;45:21–5.

[57] Van der Meide W, Guerra J, Schoone G, Farenhorst M, Coelho L, Faber W, et al. Comparison between quantitative nucleic acid sequence-based amplification, real-time reverse transcriptase PCR, and real-time PCR for quantification of *Leishmania* parasites. Journal of Clinical Microbiology 2008;46:73–8.

[58] Van der Meide WF, Schoone GJ, Faber WR, Zeegelaar JE, de Vries HJC, Ozbel Y, et al. Quantitative nucleic acid sequence-based assay as a new molecular tool for detection and quantification of *Leishmania* parasites in skin biopsy samples. Journal of Clinical Microbiology 2005;43:5560–6.

[59] Mugasa CM, Laurent T, Schoone GJ, Basiye FL, Saad AA, El Safi S, et al. Simplified molecular detection of *Leishmania* parasites in various clinical samples from patients with leishmaniasis. Parasites & Vectors 2010;3:13.

[60] Basiye FL, Mbuchi M, Magiri C, Kirigi G, Deborggraeve S, Schoone GJ, et al. Sensitivity and specificity of the *Leishmania* OligoC-TesT and NASBA-oligochromatography for diagnosis of visceral leishmaniasis in Kenya. Tropical Medicine & International Health TM IH 2010;15:806–10.

[61] Saad AA, Ahmed NG, Osman OS, Al-Basheer AA, Hamad A, Deborggraeve S, et al. Diagnostic Accuracy of the *Leishmania* OligoC-TesT and NASBA-Oligochromatography for Diagnosis of Leishmaniasis in Sudan. PLoS Neglected Tropical Diseases 2010;4:e776.

[62] Van Eys GJ, Schoone GJ, Kroon NC, Ebeling SB. Sequence analysis of small subunit ribosomal RNA genes and its use for detection and identification of *Leishmania* parasites. Molecular and Biochemical Parasitology 1992;51:133–42.

[63] Notomi T, Okayama H, Masubuchi H, Yonekawa T, Watanabe K, Amino N, et al. Loop-mediated isothermal amplification of DNA.Nucleic Acids Research 2000;28:E63.

[64] Khan MGM, Bhaskar KRH, Salam MA, Akther T, Pluschke G, Mondal D. Diagnostic accuracy of loop-mediated isothermal amplification (LAMP) for detection of *Leishmania* DNA in buffy coat from visceral leishmaniasis patients. Parasites & Vectors 2012;5:280.

[65] Adams ER, Schoone GJ, Ageed AF, Safi SE, Schallig HDFH. Development of a reverse transcriptase loop-mediated isothermal amplification (LAMP) assay for the sensitive detection of *Leishmania* parasites in clinical samples. The American Journal of Tropical Medicine and Hygiene 2010;82:591–6.

[66] Mori Y, Notomi T. Loop-mediated isothermal amplification (LAMP): a rapid, accurate, and cost-effective diagnostic method for infectious diseases. Journal of Infection and Chemotherapy: Official Journal of the Japan Society of Chemotherapy 2009;15:62–9.

[67] Nagamine K, Hase T, Notomi T. Accelerated reaction by loop-mediated isothermal amplification using loop primers. Molecular and Cellular Probes 2002;16:223–9.

[68] Takagi H, Itoh M, Islam MZ, Razzaque A, Ekram ARMS, Hashighuchi Y, et al. Sensitive, specific, and rapid detection of *Leishmania donovani* DNA by loop-mediated isothermal amplification. The American Journal of Tropical Medicine and Hygiene 2009;81:578–82.

[69] Verma S, Avishek K, Sharma V, Negi NS, Ramesh V, Salotra P. Application of loop-mediated isothermal amplification assay for the sensitive and rapid diagnosis of visceral leishmaniasis and post-kala-azar dermal leishmaniasis. Diagnostic Microbiology and Infectious Disease 2013;75:390–5.

[70] De Doncker S, Hutse V, Abdellati S, Rijal S, Singh Karki BM, Decuypere S, et al. A new PCR-ELISA for diagnosis of visceral leishmaniasis in blood of HIV-negative subjects. Transactions of the Royal Society of Tropical Medicine and Hygiene 2005;99:25–31.

[71] Costa JM, Durand R, Deniau M, Rivollet D, Izri M, Houin R, et al. PCR enzyme-linked immunosorbent assay for diagnosis of leishmaniasis in human immunodeficiency virus-infected patients. Journal of Clinical Microbiology 1996;34:1831–3.

[72] Martin-Sanchez J, Lopez-Lopez MC, Acedo-Sanchez C, Castro-Fajardo JJ, Pineda JA, Morillas-Marquez F. Diagnosis of infections with *Leishmania infantum* using PCR-ELISA. Parasitology 2001;122:607–15.

[73] Mugasa CM, Deborggraeve S, Schoone GJ, Laurent T, Leeflang MM, Ekangu RA, et al. Accordance and concordance of PCR and NASBA followed by oligochromatography for the molecular diagnosis of Trypanosoma brucei and *Leishmania*. Tropical Medicine & International Health TM IH 2010;15:800–5.

[74] SchöNian G, Kuhls K, Mauricio IL. Molecular approaches for a better understanding of the epidemiology and population genetics of *Leishmania*. Parasitology 2010;138:405–25.

[75] Morales MA, Cruz I, Rubio JM, Chicharro C, Cañavate C, Laguna F, et al. Relapses versus reinfections in patients coinfected with *Leishmania infantum* and human immunodeficiency virus type 1. The Journal of Infectious Diseases 2002;185:1533–7.

[76] Morales MA, Chicharro C, Ares M, Cañavate C, Barker DC, Alvar J. Molecular tracking of infections by *Leishmania infantum*. Transactions of the Royal Society of Tropical Medicine and Hygiene 2001;95:104–7.

[77] Botilde Y, Laurent T, Quispe Tintaya W, Chicharro C, Cañavate C, Cruz I, et al. Comparison of molecular markers for strain typing of *Leishmania infantum*.Infection, Genetics and Evolution: Journal of Molecular Epidemiology and Evolutionary Genetics in Infectious Diseases 2006;6:440–6.

[78] Cupolillo E, Grimaldi Júnior G, Momen H, Beverley SM. Intergenic region typing (IRT): a rapid molecular approach to the characterization and evolution of *Leishmania*. Molecular and Biochemical Parasitology 1995;73:145–55.

[79] Nasereddin A, Bensoussan-Hermano E, Schönian G, Baneth G, Jaffe CL. Molecular diagnosis of Old World cutaneous leishmaniasis and species identification by use of a reverse line blot hybridization assay. Journal of Clinical Microbiology 2008;46:2848–55.

[80] Piarroux R, Azaiez R, Lossi AM, Reynier P, Muscatelli F, Gambarelli F, et al. Isolation and characterization of a repetitive DNA sequence from *Leishmania infantum*: development of a visceral leishmaniasis polymerase chain reaction. The American Journal of Tropical Medicine and Hygiene 1993;49:364–9.

[81] Castilho TM, Shaw JJ, Floeter-Winter LM. New PCR assay using glucose-6-phosphate dehydrogenase for identification of *Leishmania* species. Journal of Clinical Microbiology 2003;41:540–6.

[82] Victoir K, Bañuls AL, Arevalo J, Llanos-Cuentas A, Hamers R, Noël S, et al. The gp63 gene locus, a target for genetic characterization of *Leishmania* belonging to subgenus Viannia. Parasitology 1998;117 (Pt 1):1–13.

[83] Fraga J, Montalvo AM, De Doncker S, Dujardin J-C, Van der Auwera G. Phylogeny of *Leishmania* species based on the heat-shock protein 70 gene. Infection, Genetics and Evolution 2010;10:238–45.

[84] Garcia L, Kindt A, Bermudez H, Llanos-Cuentas A, De Doncker S, Arevalo J, et al. Culture-Independent Species Typing of Neotropical *Leishmania* for Clinical Validation of a PCR-Based Assay Targeting Heat Shock Protein 70 Genes. Journal of Clinical Microbiology 2004;42:2294–7.

[85] Kato H, Uezato H, Katakura K, Calvopiña M, Marco JD, Barroso PA, et al. Detection and identification of *Leishmania* species within naturally infected sand flies in the andean areas of ecuador by a polymerase chain reaction. The American Journal of Tropical Medicine and Hygiene 2005;72:87–93.

[86] Zelazny AM, Fedorko DP, Li L, Neva FA, Fischer SH. Evaluation of 7SL RNA gene sequences for the identification of *Leishmania* spp. The American Journal of Tropical Medicine and Hygiene 2005;72:415–20.

[87] Garcia AL, Kindt A, Quispe-Tintaya KW, Bermudez H, Llanos A, Arevalo J, et al. American tegumentary leishmaniasis: antigen-gene polymorphism, taxonomy and clinical pleomorphism.Infection, Genetics and Evolution: Journal of Molecular Epidemiology and Evolutionary Genetics in Infectious Diseases 2005;5:109–16.

[88] Hide M, Bañuls A-L. Species-specific PCR assay for L. infantum/L. donovani discrimination. Acta Tropica 2006;100:241–5.

[89] Oshaghi MA, Ravasan NM, Hide M, Javadian E-A, Rassi Y, Sedaghat MM, et al. Development of species-specific PCR and PCR-restriction fragment length polymor-

phism assays for L.infantum/L.donovani discrimination. Experimental Parasitology 2009;122:61–5.

[90] Quispe-Tintaya KW, Laurent T, Decuypere S, Hide M, Bañuls A-L, De Doncker S, et al. Fluorogenic assay for molecular typing of the *Leishmania donovani* complex: taxonomic and clinical applications. The Journal of Infectious Diseases 2005;192:685–92.

[91] Mauricio IL, Gaunt MW, Stothard JR, Miles MA. Genetic typing and phylogeny of the *Leishmania donovani* complex by restriction analysis of PCR amplified gp63 intergenic regions. Parasitology 2001;122:393–403.

[92] Cupolillo E, Brahim LR, Toaldo CB, de Oliveira-Neto MP, de Brito MEF, Falqueto A, et al. Genetic Polymorphism and Molecular Epidemiology of *Leishmania (Viannia) braziliensis* from Different Hosts and Geographic Areas in Brazil. Journal of Clinical Microbiology 2003;41:3126–32.

[93] Cupolillo E, Grimaldi G Jr, Momen H. A general classification of New World *Leishmania* using numerical zymotaxonomy. The American Journal of Tropical Medicine and Hygiene 1994;50:296–311.

[94] Schönian G, Schnur L, el Fari M, Oskam L, Kolesnikov AA, Sokolowska-Köhler W, et al. Genetic heterogeneity in the species *Leishmania tropica* revealed by different PCR-based methods. Transactions of the Royal Society of Tropical Medicine and Hygiene 2001;95:217–24.

[95] Mauricio IL, Stothard JR, Miles MA. *Leishmania donovani* complex: genotyping with the ribosomal internal transcribed spacer and the mini-exon. Parasitology 2004;128:263–7.

[96] Chicharro C, Morales MA, Serra T, Ares M, Salas A, Alvar J. Molecular epidemiology of *Leishmania infantum* on the island of Majorca: a comparison of phenotypic and genotypic tools. Transactions of the Royal Society of Tropical Medicine and Hygiene 2002;96 Suppl 1:S93–99.

[97] Cortes S, Mauricio I, Almeida A, Cristovão JM, Pratlong F, Dedet JP, et al. Application of kDNA as a molecular marker to analyse *Leishmania infantum* diversity in Portugal. Parasitology International 2006;55:277–83.

[98] Laurent T, Rijal S, Yardley V, Croft S, De Doncker S, Decuypere S, et al. Epidemiological dynamics of antimonial resistance in *Leishmania donovani*: genotyping reveals a polyclonal population structure among naturally-resistant clinical isolates from Nepal.Infection, Genetics and Evolution: Journal of Molecular Epidemiology and Evolutionary Genetics in Infectious Diseases 2007;7:206–12.

[99] Noyes HA, Reyburn H, Bailey JW, Smith D. A nested-PCR-based schizodeme method for identifying *Leishmania* kinetoplast minicircle classes directly from clinical samples and its application to the study of the epidemiology of *Leishmania tropica* in Pakistan. Journal of Clinical Microbiology 1998;36:2877–81.

[100] Hamilton PB, Adams ER, Malele II, Gibson WC. A novel, high-throughput technique for species identification reveals a new species of tsetse-transmitted trypanosome related to the Trypanosoma brucei subgenus, Trypanozoon. Infection, Genetics and Evolution 2008;8:26–33.

[101] Tomas-Perez M, Fisa R, Riera C. The Use of Fluorescent Fragment Length Analysis (PCR-FFL) in the Direct Diagnosis and Identification of Cutaneous *Leishmania* Species. The American Journal of Tropical Medicine and Hygiene 2013;88:586–91.

[102] Da Silva LA, de Sousa CDS, da Graça GC, Porrozzi R, Cupolillo E. Sequence analysis and PCR-RFLP profiling of the hsp70 gene as a valuable tool for identifying *Leishmania* species associated with human leishmaniasis in Brazil.Infection, Genetics and Evolution: Journal of Molecular Epidemiology and Evolutionary Genetics in Infectious Diseases 2010;10:77–83.

[103] Lessa MM, Lessa HA, Castro TWN, Oliveira A, Scherifer A, Machado P, et al. Mucosal leishmaniasis: epidemiological and clinical aspects. Brazilian Journal of Otorhinolaryngology 2007;73:843–7.

[104] Arevalo J, Ramirez L, Adaui V, Zimic M, Tulliano G, Miranda-Verástegui C, et al. Influence of *Leishmania (Viannia)* species on the response to antimonial treatment in patients with American tegumentary leishmaniasis. The Journal of Infectious Diseases 2007;195:1846–51.

[105] Llanos-Cuentas A, Tulliano G, Araujo-Castillo R, Miranda-Verastegui C, Santamaria-Castrellon G, Ramirez L, et al. Clinical and parasite species risk factors for pentavalent antimonial treatment failure in cutaneous leishmaniasis in Peru.Clinical Infectious Diseases: An Official Publication of the Infectious Diseases Society of America 2008;46:223–31.

[106] Thomaz-Soccol V, Velez ID, Pratlong F, Agudelos S, Lanotte G, Rioux JA. Enzymatic polymorphism and phylogenetic relationships in *Leishmania* Ross, 1903 (Sarcomastigophora: Kinetoplastida): a case study in Colombia. Systematic Parasitolog 2000;46:59–68.

[107] Garcia AL, Parrado R, De Doncker S, Bermudez H, Dujardin J-C. American tegumentary leishmaniasis: direct species identification of *Leishmania* in non-invasive clinical samples. Transactions of the Royal Society of Tropical Medicine and Hygiene 2007;101:368–71.

[108] Montalvo AM, Fraga J, Monzote L, Montano I, De Doncker S, Dujardin JC, et al. Heat-shock protein 70 PCR-RFLP: a universal simple tool for *Leishmania* species discrimination in the New and Old World. Parasitology 2010;137:1159–68.

[109] Montalvo AM, Fraga J, Maes I, Dujardin J-C, Van der Auwera G. Three new sensitive and specific heat-shock protein 70 PCRs for global *Leishmania* species identification. European Journal of Clinical Microbiology & Infectious Diseases2011;31:1453–61.

[110] Bensoussan E, Nasereddin A, Jonas F, Schnur LF, Jaffe CL. Comparison of PCR assays for diagnosis of cutaneous leishmaniasis. Journal of Clinical Microbiology 2006;44:1435–9.

[111] Rocha MN, Margonari C, Presot IM, Soares RP. Evaluation of 4 polymerase chain reaction protocols for cultured *Leishmania* spp. typing. Diagnostic Microbiology and Infectious Disease 2010;68:401–9.

[112] Alexander J, Coombs GH, Mottram JC. *Leishmania mexicana* cysteine proteinase-deficient mutants have attenuated virulence for mice and potentiate a Th1 response. Journal of Immunology (Baltimore, Md.: 1950) 1950 1998;161:6794–801.

[113] Mundodi V, Somanna A, Farrell PJ, Gedamu L. Genomic organization and functional expression of differentially regulated cysteine protease genes of *Leishmania donovani* complex. Gene 2002;282:257–65.

[114] Quispe Tintaya KW, Ying X, Dedet J-P, Rijal S, De Bolle X, Dujardin J-C. Antigen genes for molecular epidemiology of leishmaniasis: polymorphism of cysteine proteinase B and surface metalloprotease glycoprotein 63 in the *Leishmania donovani* complex. The Journal of Infectious Diseases 2004;189:1035–43.

[115] Wortmann G, Hochberg L, Houng H-H, Sweeney C, Zapor M, Aronson N, et al. Rapid identification of *Leishmania* complexes by a real-time PCR assay. The American Journal of Tropical Medicine and Hygiene 2005;73:999–1004.

[116] Castilho TM, Camargo LMA, McMahon-Pratt D, Shaw JJ, Floeter-Winter LM. A real-time polymerase chain reaction assay for the identification and quantification of American *Leishmania* species on the basis of glucose-6-phosphate dehydrogenase. The American Journal of Tropical Medicine and Hygiene 2008;78:122–32.

[117] Weirather JL, Jeronimo SMB, Gautam S, Sundar S, Kang M, Kurtz MA, et al. Serial quantitative PCR assay for detection, species discrimination, and quantification of *Leishmania* spp. in human samples. Journal of Clinical Microbiology 2011;49:3892–904.

[118] Tsukayama P, Núñez JH, De Los Santos M, Soberón V, Lucas CM, Matlashewski G, et al. A FRET-based real-time PCR assay to identify the main causal agents of New World tegumentary leishmaniasis. PLoS Neglected Tropical Diseases 2013;7:e1956.

[119] Rioux JA, Lanotte G, Serres E, Pratlong F, Bastien P, Perieres J. Taxonomy of *Leishmania*. Use of isoenzymes. Suggestions for a new classification. Annales de Parasitologie Humaine et Comparée 1990;65:111–25.

[120] Bañuls A-L, Hide M, Prugnolle F. *Leishmania* and the Leishmaniases: A Parasite Genetic Update and Advances in Taxonomy, Epidemiology and Pathogenicity in Humans. Advances in Parasitology., vol. 64, Elsevier; 2007, p. 1–458.

[121] Hide M, Bañuls AL, Tibayrenc M. Genetic heterogeneity and phylogenetic status of *Leishmania (Leishmania) infantum* zymodeme MON-1: epidemiological implications. Parasitology 2001;123:425–32.

[122] Ochsenreither S, Kuhls K, Schaar M, Presber W, Schönian G. Multilocus microsatellite typing as a new tool for discrimination of *Leishmania infantum* MON-1 strains. Journal of Clinical Microbiology 2006;44:495–503.

[123] Jamjoom MB, Ashford RW, Bates PA, Chance ML, Kemp SJ, Watts PC, et al. *Leishmania donovani* is the only cause of visceral leishmaniasis in East Africa; previous descriptions of *L. infantum* and *"L. archibaldi"* from this region are a consequence of convergent evolution in the isoenzyme data. Parasitology 2004;129:399–409.

[124] Zemanová E, Jirků M, Mauricio IL, Miles MA, Lukes J. Genetic polymorphism within the *Leishmania donovani* complex: correlation with geographic origin. The American Journal of Tropical Medicine and Hygiene 2004;70:613–7.

[125] Lukes J, Mauricio IL, Schönian G, Dujardin J-C, Soteriadou K, Dedet J-P, et al. Evolutionary and geographical history of the *Leishmania donovani* complex with a revision of current taxonomy. Proceedings of the National Academy of Sciences of the United States of America 2007;104:9375–80.

[126] Schwenkenbecher JM, Wirth T, Schnur LF, Jaffe CL, Schallig H, Al-Jawabreh A, et al. Microsatellite analysis reveals genetic structure of *Leishmania tropica*. International Journal for Parasitology 2006;36:237–46.

[127] Alam MZ, Haralambous C, Kuhls K, Gouzelou E, Sgouras D, Soteriadou K, et al. The paraphyletic composition of *Leishmania donovani* zymodeme MON-37 revealed by multilocus microsatellite typing. Microbes and Infection / Institut Pasteur 2009;11:707–15.

[128] Williams JG, Kubelik AR, Livak KJ, Rafalski JA, Tingey SV. DNA polymorphisms amplified by arbitrary primers are useful as genetic markers.Nucleic Acids Research 1990;18:6531–5.

[129] Welsh J, McClelland M. Fingerprinting genomes using PCR with arbitrary primers.Nucleic Acids Research 1990;18:7213–8.

[130] Baptista C, Schubach AO, Madeira MF, Leal CA, Pires MQ, Oliveira FS, et al. *Leishmania (Viannia) braziliensis* genotypes identified in lesions of patients with atypical or typical manifestations of tegumentary leishmaniasis: Evaluation by two molecular markers. Experimental Parasitology 2009;121:317–22.

[131] Gomes RF, Macedo AM, Pena SD, Melo MN. *Leishmania (Viannia) braziliensis*: genetic relationships between strains isolated from different areas of Brazil as revealed by DNA fingerprinting and RAPD. Experimental Parasitology 1995;80:681–7.

[132] Mahmoudzadeh-Niknam H, Ajdary S, Riazi-Rad F, Mirzadegan E, Rezaeian A, Khaze V, et al. Molecular epidemiology of cutaneous leishmaniasis and heterogenei-

ty of *Leishmania major* strains in Iran: Molecular epidemiology of cutaneous leishmaniasis. Tropical Medicine & International Health 2012;17:1335–44.

[133] Hamad SH, Khalil EAG, Musa AM, Ibrahim ME, Younis BM, Elfaki MEE, et al. *Leishmania donovani*: genetic diversity of isolates from Sudan characterized by PCR-based RAPD. Experimental Parasitology 2010;125:389–93.

[134] Mauricio IL, Howard MK, Stothard JR, Miles MA. Genomic diversity in the *Leishmania donovani* complex. Parasitology 1999;119 (Pt 3):237–46.

[135] Segatto M, Ribeiro LS, Costa DL, Costa CHN, Oliveira MR de, Carvalho SFG, et al. Genetic diversity of *Leishmania infantum* field populations from Brazil. Memórias Do Instituto Oswaldo Cruz 2012;107:39–47.

[136] Martinez E, Alonso V, Quispe A, Thomas MC, Alonso R, Piero JE, et al. RAPD method useful for distinguishing *Leishmania* species: design of specific primers for *L. braziliensis*. Parasitology 2003;127:513–7.

[137] Ikram G, Dellagi K, Ismaïl RB. Random amplified polymorphic DNA technique for identification and differentiation of old world *Leishmania* species. The American Journal of Tropical Medicine and Hygiene 2002;66:152–6.

[138] Khanra S, Bandopadhyay SK, Chakraborty P, Datta S, Mondal D, Chatterjee M, et al. Characterization of the recent clinical isolates of Indian Kala-azar patients by RAPD-PCR method. Journal of Parasitic Diseases: Official Organ of the Indian Society for Parasitology 2011;35:116–22.

[139] Smith DF, Searle S, Ready PD, Gramiccia M, Ben-Ismail R. A kinetoplast DNA probe diagnostic for *Leishmania major*: sequence homologies between regions of *Leishmania* minicircles. Molecular and Biochemical Parasitology 1989;37:213–23.

[140] Gramiccia M, Smith DF, Angelici MC, Ready PD, Gradoni L. A kinetoplast DNA probe diagnostic for *Leishmania infantum*. Parasitology 1992;105 (Pt 1):29–34.

[141] Laskay T, Kiessling R, Rinke deWit TF, Wirth DF. Generation of species-specific DNA probes for *Leishmania aethiopica*. Molecular and Biochemical Parasitology 1991;44:279–86.

[142] Rodríguez N, Guzman B, Rodas A, Takiff H, Bloom BR, Convit J. Diagnosis of cutaneous leishmaniasis and species discrimination of parasites by PCR and hybridization. Journal of Clinical Microbiology 1994;32:2246–52.

[143] Brenière SF, Telleria J, Bosseno MF, Buitrago R, Bastrenta B, Cuny G, et al. Polymerase chain reaction-based identification of New World *Leishmania* species complexes by specific kDNA probes. Acta Tropica 1999;73:283–93.

[144] Howard MK, Kelly JM, Lane RP, Miles MA. A sensitive repetitive DNA probe that is specific to the *Leishmania donovani* complex and its use as an epidemiological and diagnostic reagent. Molecular and Biochemical Parasitology 1991;44:63–72.

[145] Van Eys GJ, Guizani I, Ligthart GS, Dellagi K. A nuclear DNA probe for the identification of strains within the *Leishmania donovani* complex. Experimental Parasitology 1991;72:459–63.

[146] Van Eys GJ, Schoone GJ, Ligthart GS, Alvar J, Evans DA, Terpstra WJ. Identification of "Old World" *Leishmania* by DNA recombinant probes. Molecular and Biochemical Parasitology 1989;34:53–62.

[147] Grisard EC, Steindel M, Shaw JJ, Ishikawa EA, Carvalho-Pinto CJ, Eger-Mangrich I, et al. Characterization of *Leishmania* sp. strains isolated from autochthonous cases of human cutaneous leishmaniasis in Santa Catarina State, southern Brazil. Acta Tropica 2000;74:89–93.

[148] Rodriguez N, De Lima H, Rodriguez A, Brewster S, Barker DC. Genomic DNA repeat from *Leishmania (Viannia) braziliensis* (Venezuelan strain) containing simple repeats and microsatellites. Parasitology 1997;115 (Pt 4):349–58.

[149] Rodriguez N, Rodriguez A, Cardona M, Barrios MA, McCann SH, Barker DC. *Leishmania (Viannia) guyanensis*: a new minicircle class exclusive to this specie isolated from a DNA cosmid library useful for taxonomic purposes. Experimental Parasitology 2000;94:143–9.

[150] Schönian G, Mauricio I, Gramiccia M, Cañavate C, Boelaert M, Dujardin J-C. Leishmaniases in the Mediterranean in the era of molecular epidemiology. Trends in Parasitology 2008;24:135–42.

[151] Mauricio IL, Yeo M, Baghaei M, Doto D, Pratlong F, Zemanova E, et al. Towards multilocus sequence typing of the *Leishmania donovani* complex: resolving genotypes and haplotypes for five polymorphic metabolic enzymes (ASAT, GPI, NH1, NH2, PGD).International Journal for Parasitology 2006;36:757–69.

[152] Zemanová E, Jirků M, Mauricio IL, Horák A, Miles MA, Lukeš J. The *Leishmania donovani* complex: Genotypes of five metabolic enzymes (ICD, ME, MPI, G6PDH, and FH), new targets for multilocus sequence typing.International Journal for Parasitology 2007;37:149–60.

[153] Tsukayama P, Lucas C, Bacon DJ. Typing of four genetic loci discriminates among closely related species of New World *Leishmania*. International Journal for Parasitology 2009;39:355–62.

[154] Zhang C-Y, Lu X-J, Du X-Q, Jian J, Shu L, Ma Y. Phylogenetic and Evolutionary Analysis of Chinese *Leishmania* Isolates Based on Multilocus Sequence Typing. PLoS ONE 2013;8:e63124.

[155] Alam MZ, Kovalenko DA, Kuhls K, Nasyrova RM, Ponomareva VI, Fatullaeva AA, et al. Identification of the agent causing visceral leishmaniasis in Uzbeki and Tajiki foci by analysing parasite DNA extracted from patients' Giemsa-stained tissue preparations. Parasitology 2009;136:981.

[156] Gouzelou E, Haralambous C, Amro A, Mentis A, Pratlong F, Dedet J-P, et al. Multilocus microsatellite typing (MLMT) of strains from Turkey and Cyprus reveals a novel monophyletic *L. donovani* sensu lato group. PLoS Neglected Tropical Diseases 2012;6:e1507.

[157] Jamjoom MB, Ashford RW, Bates PA, Kemp SJ, Noyes HA. Towards a standard battery of microsatellite markers for the analysis of the *Leishmania donovani* complex. Annals of Tropical Medicine and Parasitology 2002;96:265–70.

[158] Kuhls K, Keilonat L, Ochsenreither S, Schaar M, Schweynoch C, Presber W, et al. Multilocus microsatellite typing (MLMT) reveals genetically isolated populations between and within the main endemic regions of visceral leishmaniasis. Microbes and Infection 2007;9:334–43.

[159] Jamjoom MB, Ashford RW, Bates PA, Kemp SJ, Noyes HA. Polymorphic microsatellite repeats are not conserved between *Leishmania donovani* and *Leishmania major*. Molecular Ecology Notes 2002;2:104–6.

[160] Azmi K, Schnur L, Schonian G, Nasereddin A, Pratlong F, El Baidouri F, et al. Genetic, serological and biochemical characterization of *Leishmania tropica* from foci in northern Palestine and discovery of zymodeme MON-307. Parasites & Vectors 2012;5:121.

[161] Oddone R, Schweynoch C, Schönian G, de Sousa C dos S, Cupolillo E, Espinosa D, et al. Development of a multilocus microsatellite typing approach for discriminating strains of *Leishmania (Viannia)* species. Journal of Clinical Microbiology 2009;47:2818–25.

[162] Rioux JA, Lanotte G, Serres E, Pratlong F, Bastien P, Perieres J. Taxonomy of *Leishmania*. Use of isoenzymes. Suggestions for a new classification. Annales de Parasitologie Humaine et Comparée 1990;65:111–25.

[163] Schönian G, Cupolillo E, Mauricio I. Molecular Evolution and Phylogeny of *Leishmania*. In: Ponte-Sucre A, Diaz E, Padrón-Nieves M, editors. Drug Resistance in *Leishmania* Parasites,, Vienna: Springer Vienna; 2013, p. 15–44.

[164] Croan DG, Morrison DA, Ellis JT. Evolution of the genus *Leishmania* revealed by comparison of DNA and RNA polymerase gene sequences. Molecular and Biochemical Parasitology 1997;89:149–59.

[165] Berzunza-Cruz M, Cabrera N, Crippa-Rossi M, Sosa Cabrera T, Pérez-Montfort R, Becker I. Polymorphism analysis of the internal transcribed spacer and small subunit of ribosomal RNA genes of *Leishmania mexicana*. Parasitology Research 2002;88:918–25.

[166] Dávila AM, Momen H. Internal-transcribed-spacer (ITS) sequences used to explore phylogenetic relationships within *Leishmania*. Annals of Tropical Medicine and Parasitology 2000;94:651–4.

[167] Waki K, Dutta S, Ray D, Kolli BK, Akman L, Kawazu S-I, et al. Transmembrane molecules for phylogenetic analyses of pathogenic protists: *Leishmania*-specific informative sites in hydrophilic loops of trans- endoplasmic reticulum N-acetylglucosamine-1-phosphate transferase. Eukaryotic Cell 2007;6:198–210.

[168] Asato Y, Oshiro M, Myint CK, Yamamoto Y, Kato H, Marco JD, et al. Phylogenic analysis of the genus *Leishmania* by cytochrome b gene sequencing. Experimental Parasitology 2009;121:352–61.

[169] Cupolillo E, Medina-Acosta E, Noyes H, Momen H, Grimaldi G Jr. A revised classification for *Leishmania* and *Endotrypanum*. Parasitology Today (Personal Ed.) 2000;16:142–4.

[170] Kuhls K, Alam MZ, Cupolillo E, Ferreira GEM, Mauricio IL, Oddone R, et al. Comparative microsatellite typing of new world *Leishmania infantum* reveals low heterogeneity among populations and its recent old world origin. PLoS Neglected Tropical Diseases 2011;5:e1155.

[171] Maurício IL, Stothard JR, Miles MA. The strange case of *Leishmania chagasi*. Parasitology Today (Personal Ed.) 2000;16:188–9.

[172] Spanakos G, Piperaki E-T, Menounos PG, Tegos N, Flemetakis A, Vakalis NC. Detection and species identification of Old World *Leishmania* in clinical samples using a PCR-based method. Transactions of the Royal Society of Tropical Medicine and Hygiene 2008;102:46–53.

[173] Yurchenko VY, Lukes J, Jirku M, Zeledón R, Maslov DA. Leptomonas costaricensis sp. n. (Kinetoplastea: Trypanosomatidae), a member of the novel phylogenetic group of insect trypanosomatids closely related to the genus *Leishmania*. Parasitology 2006;133:537–46.

[174] Banũls AL, Hide M, Tibayrenc M. Molecular epidemiology and evolutionary genetics of Leischmania parasites.International Journal for Parasitology 1999;29:1137–47.

[175] Grimaldi G Jr, Tesh RB. Leishmaniases of the New World: current concepts and implications for future research. Clinical Microbiology Reviews 1993;6:230–50.

[176] Noyes H, Pratlong F, Chance M, Ellis J, Lanotte G, Dedet JP. A previously unclassified trypanosomatid responsible for human cutaneous lesions in Martinique (French West Indies) is the most divergent member of the genus *Leishmania* sp. Parasitology 2002;124:17–24.

[177] Suankratay C, Suwanpimolkul G, Wilde H, Siriyasatien P. Autochthonous visceral leishmaniasis in a human immunodeficiency virus (HIV)-infected patient: the first in thailand and review of the literature. The American Journal of Tropical Medicine and Hygiene 2010;82:4–8.

[178] Sukmee T, Siripattanapipong S, Mungthin M, Worapong J, Rangsin R, Samung Y, et al. A suspected new species of *Leishmania*, the causative agent of visceral leishmaniasis in a Thai patient.International Journal for Parasitology 2008;38:617–22.

[179] Villinski JT, Klena JD, Abbassy M, Hoel DF, Puplampu N, Mechta S, et al. Evidence for a new species of *Leishmania* associated with a focal disease outbreak in Ghana.Diagnostic Microbiology and Infectious Disease 2008;60:323–7.

[180] Rose K, Curtis J, Baldwin T, Mathis A, Kumar B, Sakthianandeswaren A, et al. Cutaneous leishmaniasis in red kangaroos: isolation and characterisation of the causative organisms.International Journal for Parasitology 2004;34:655–64.

[181] Lobsiger L, Müller N, Schweizer T, Frey CF, Wiederkehr D, Zumkehr B, et al. An autochthonous case of cutaneous bovine leishmaniasis in Switzerland. Veterinary Parasitology 2010;169:408–14.

[182] Müller N, Welle M, Lobsiger L, Stoffel MH, Boghenbor KK, Hilbe M, et al. Occurrence of *Leishmania* sp. in cutaneous lesions of horses in Central Europe. Veterinary Parasitology 2009;166:346–51.

[183] Silveira FT, Ishikawa EAY, De Souza AAA, Lainson R. An outbreak of cutaneous leishmaniasis among soldiers in Belém, Pará State, Brazil, caused by *Leishmania (Viannia) lindenbergi* n. sp. A new leishmanial parasite of man in the Amazon region. Parasite (Paris, France) 2002;9:43–50.

[184] Simpson AGB, Stevens JR, Lukeš J. The evolution and diversity of kinetoplastid flagellates. Trends in Parasitology 2006;22:168–74.

[185] Miles MA, Llewellyn MS, Lewis MD, Yeo M, Baleela R, Fitzpatrick S, et al. The molecular epidemiology and phylogeography of *Trypanosoma cruzi* and parallel research on *Leishmania*: looking back and to the future. Parasitology 2009;136:1509–28.

Molecular Tools for Understanding Eco-Epidemiology, Diversity and Pathogenesis of *Leishmania* Parasites

Souheila Guerbouj, Imen Mkada–Driss and
Ikram Guizani

1. Introduction

Protozoan parasites of the genus *Leishmania* are responsible of a large variety of clinical manifestations ranging from self-healing cutaneous forms (CL), through mucocutaneous lesions (MCL), to lethal if untreated visceral disease (VL). Nevertheless, there is no absolute correlation between a particular clinical form and a causative species [1]. For instance, parasites of the *L. donovani* complex are generally responsible for VL cases in the Old and New World but can also cause CL. Another example is the *L. tropica* species, which causes a CL form but its association to VL cases was occasionally reported [2]. Identification of *Leishmania* parasites is a central issue to patients' management and to control. Leishmaniases have a worldwide distribution but only absent in the poles regions, and in Australia where in spite of presence of the parasites in Kangourous no human cases were described. According to the WHO, 350 million people are at risk, with a prevalence of 12 million and more than 98 countries affected [3]. More than twenty species are responsible for leishmaniasis in humans. However, *Leishmania* species present very similar morphologies in their flagellated, promastigote forms and their intracellular, amastigote forms which renders necessary the use of molecular or biochemical assays for their identification and characterization (see for review [4]).

The current identification and classification of *Leishmania* is still based on isoenzyme typing, using multilocus enzyme electrophoresis (MLEE) (reviewed in [5]). This approach has been widely used for the identification of *Leishmania*, but several limitations were reported. Most importantly, differences in electrophoretic profiles were shown to be due to heterozygosity at a single nucleotide position [6–8]. Molecular studies showed also that zymodemes included distinct DNA genotypes [7,9]. Consequently, other molecular studies do not always agree with the classification of *Leishmania* by MLEE. The other limitations of MLEE are that it requires bulk cultures of parasites, it is time-consuming, and it can be performed only in specialized laboratories. Therefore, alternative DNA based tools and assays are increasingly developed and used for effective investigation and characterization of the parasites.

Indeed, the diversity of *Leishmania* species, their vectors and their reservoir hosts is a main feature of leishmaniasis, so consequently the transmission cycles are very much dependent on the environment and are very prone to changes. So not only parasite identification is needed to establish etiology of the disease and understand the pathogeny, but knowledge of parasite diversity and its population structure is also needed for a better understanding of eco-epidemiology and its changing trends. For this purpose, molecular tools have been developed to allow differentiation of *Leishmania* parasites at species and strain levels within environmental or patients' samples.

Molecular tools are based mainly on the amplification and subsequent restriction fragment length polymorphism (PCR-RFLP) of several targets including repeated gene families and coding and non-coding regions, or the sequence analysis of the products. Recently multilocus sequence typing (MLST) and multilocus microsatellite typing (MLMT) were also developed for *Leishmania* DNA typing. Each of these molecular markers or tools has its specific discriminatory power, advantages and drawbacks.

2. Parasite identification

2.1. Differentiation at the genus level

This is based on the amplification of the kinetoplast minicircle DNA (kDNA, about 10000 copies per cell) or the variable sequences of the small subunit ribosomal DNA genes (SSU rDNA, 40–200 copies per cell) [10–13].

kDNA and SSU rDNA primers were initially designed for Trypanosomatids including *Leishmania, Sauroleishmania, Crithidia* and Trypanosomes. They allow identification of *Leishmania* parasites only at the generic and/ or subgeneric level. Both targets have also been used for the development of real-time PCR assays in order to determine parasite burden in clinical samples [14,15].

2.2. Differentiation at the species level

The ability to distinguish between *Leishmania* species is crucial for a correct diagnosis of the disease as well as for making decisions regarding treatment and control measures. This is especially useful in areas where several *Leishmania* species co-exist.

Numerous PCR approaches have been published based on different coding and non-coding regions in the *Leishmania* genome. Different targets have been used, including the ribosomal internal transcribed spacer (ITS) [12,16,17], the mini-exon genes [18,19], gp63 genes [20,21], hsp70 genes [22–24] and cysteine proteinase B gene sequences (cpB) [25,26].

2.2.1. Randomly amplified polymorphic DNA (RAPD) and anonymous markers

Randomly amplified polymorphic DNA (RAPD) technique is based on the PCR amplification of DNA fragments using only one short primer that was arbitrarily defined and thus could be applied to any organism without a prior knowledge on the genome [27]. Such primers correspond to decamers having 60-70 % GC content and no self-complementary ends, thus the number of primers that could be used is virtually unlimited. Only in few occasions, two primers were used for *Leishmania* DNA analysis [28]; primers longer than 10 mers like universal primers used in cloning technologies have been used in some instances [29–32]. A list of selected primers used for *Leishmania* characterization is reported on Table 1. The RAPD technique generates monomorphic or polymorphic banding patterns, analyzed upon electrophoresis on agarose gels (or other supports) like DNA fingerprints. Given the fact that in comparison studies absence of bands does not reflect absence of corresponding DNA fragment in the compared DNA [33,34], the analysis is based only on Jaccard (or equivalent) distance or Similarity index [33] that only takes into account the presence of bands. RAPD reaction is very sensitive to reaction conditions even when variations are minor. Relaxed conditions and particularly low annealing temperature underlie DNA amplification but concentration or batch (quality) of DNA, reaction component, additives, brand of DNA polymerase, thermocyclers impact size range, complexity and reproducibility of the amplification profiles [33,35]. Molecular mechanisms underlying *Leishmania* DNA amplification was proposed to be based mainly on DNA mutations occurring on potential priming sites, that seem to be in regions enriched for short repeated motives [34].

Potential of RAPD and a selection of 28 primers was assessed for the discrimination between members of the *Leishmania Viannia* sub-genus which have overlapping geographical distribution in Latin America and that were difficult to distinguish by the conventional PCR using the primers then available. The authors have identified primers able to distinguish the 4 species (*L. braziliensis, L. guyanensis, L. panamensis* and *L. peruviana*) in a pair wise way. They also addressed the reliability of the technique by developing a statistical measure of the variation range of Jaccard coefficient when comparing the parasites [33].

Primer	Nucleotide sequence 5'-3'	References	Primer	Nucleotide sequence 5'-3'	References
OPA-01	CAGGCCCTTC	[30,34,36,43,44]	OPR-16	CTCTGCGCGT	[38]
H4 (OPA-02)	TGCCGAGCTG	[31,41,46]	OPR-20	ACGGCAAGGA	[38]
C4 (OPA-04)	AATCGGGCTG	[41]	OPU-15	ACGGGCCAGT	[38]
A5, P8, (OPA-05)	AGGGGTCTTG	[31,38,41,48]	OPU-16	CTGCGCTGGA	[38]
A4, (OPA-07)	GAAACGGGTG	[30,31,36,41,43]	OPU-02	CTGAGGTCTC	[43]
OPA-08	GTGACGTAGG	[28,30,31,33]	ILO 509	TGGTCAGTGA	[42]
OPA-09	GGGTAACGCC	[31]	ILO 526	GCCGTCCGA	[42]
OPA-10	GTGATCGCAG	[28,30,31,36,38,43, 48]	ILO 872	CCCGCCATCT	[42]
A12 (OPA-12)	TCGGCGATAG	[41]	ILO875	GTCCGTGAGC	[41,42]

Primer	Nucleotide sequence 5'-3'	References	Primer	Nucleotide sequence 5'-3'	References
A15 (OPA-15)	TTCCGAACCC	[41]	ILO 876	GGGACGTCTC	[42]
D10 (OPA-20)	GTTGCGATCC	[41]	ILO 878	GTCGCGGAG	[42]
D8 (OPA-16)	AGCCAGCGAA	[41]	A5, C5	CTCACGTAGG	[39,41]
OPB-01	GTTTCGCTCC	[30]	C6	CTGATCGCAG	[41]
C (OPB-04)	GGACTGGAGT	[28,33,43,44]	L2	CGGACGTCGC	[41]
B5 (OPB-05)	TGCGCCCTTC	[41]	H1	CGCGCCCGCT	[39,41]
B6 (OPB-06)	TGCTCTGCCC	[41]	L15996	CTCCACCATTAGCACCC AAAGC	[29,32]
OPB-07	GGTGACGCAG	[30,41]	λg11R	TTGACACCAGACCAACT GGTAAT	[29,32]
OPB-08	GTCCACACGG	[38,41]	M13a, M13	GTAAAACGACGGCCAG T	[30,33]
OPB-09	TGGGGGACTC	[30,33]	M13-40 F/ M13 (−40) a	GTTTTCCCAGTCACGAC	[29,30,32]
OPB-10	CTGCTGGGAC	[43,44]	M13/pUC	CGCCAGGGTTTTCCCAG TCACGA	[31]
OPB-12	CCTTGACGCA	[30,41]	P53-1	ACGACAGGGCTGGTTG CCCA	[32]
OPB-13	TTCCCCCGCT	[33,41]	PLiD2-9	CAAAAGTCCCCACCAA TCCC	[42]
OPB-15	GGAGGGTGTT	[30,43]	QG1	CCATTAGCACCCAAAG CAGACCTCACCCTGTGG AGC	[29,32]
A (OPB-18)	CCACAGCAGT	[28,30,33]	TA150	ATGCGATGAGTGGTTG AG	[41,42]
OPF-01	ACGGATCCTG	[38]	TA610	TCAACCGATTACAAACC A	[42]
OPF-10	GGAAGCTTGG	[43,44]	UMS	GGGGTTGGTGTA	[31,46]
OPF-13	GGCTGCAGAA	[38,43]	37	TGGATCCGGAATTTCGG CTTCACTAC	[42]
OPN-13	AGCGTCACTC	[38]	198	GCAGGACTGC	[41]
OPN-20	GGTGCTCCGT	[38]	233	CTATGCGCGC	[35]
OPR-13	GGACGACAAG	[38]	283	CGGCCACCGT	[35,48]
OPR-14	CAGGATTCCC	[38]	3301	TCGTAGCCAA	[30,33]
OPR-15	GGACAACGAG	[38,43,44]			

Name and sequence of the primers are reported on the table as described in the references. However, for the purpose of this work all the sequences were compared to lists provided by Operon Technologies (OP); primers thus identified are reported within brackets. Primers presenting discrepancies were not reported.

Table 1. Selection of primers used in RAPD analyses of *Leishmania* parasites generating polymorphic patterns.

We have used the RAPD technique to identify and discriminate Old World species using 57 strains from different hosts, countries and reservoirs. Six random primers were tested from which 3 allowed to distinguish *L. aethiopica, L. arabica, L. donovani, L. major, L. tropica and L. turanica* species. We have analyzed the RAPD profiles considering criteria of consistent presence of amplified bands at the same electrophoretic presence for strains/ isolates of the same species, and the discrimination between parasites belonging to different species. This constitutes a simpler way to results interpretation that emphasizes on presence of consistently amplified and discriminative bands within a profile to overcome lack of reliability of RAPD [36]. RAPD also allowed differentiating Old World *Leishmania* species from the often co-sympatric *Sauroleishmania* parasites [30,36].

Random amplification of polymorphic DNA has been also used alone or with other techniques to confirm taxonomic status of parasites, for instance putative natural hybrids such as *L. braziliensis/L. panamensis* hybrids isolated in Nicaragua [33] or *L. braziliensis* and *L. panamensis/ guyanensis* in Ecuador [37]. In another example, genetic analysis of *Leishmania* parasites in Ecuador with MLEE and RAPD questioned the separation of *L. panamensis* and *L. guyanensis* as distinct taxa as these tools failed to generate clearly distinct clusters of parasites [38].

The RAPD technique was also used to investigate genetic diversity within *Leishmania* species or complexes in diverse settings. Causal agents of visceral leishmaniasis belong to the *L. donovani* complex, which includes the species *L. donovani, L. infantum, L. chagasi* and *L. archibaldi* [39]; however, taxonomy within this complex is controversial considering for instance *L. infantum* as forming its own complex [40]. The RAPD technique has been used to investigate intraspecific diversity of the *L. donovani* complex, using an initial set of 43 random primers [41]. Like in other studies [36,42], some primers differentiated the *L. donovani* complex from the other Old World taxa. Seven distinguished within the complex, differentiating in the tested panel of DNAs, Mediterranean *L. infantum* from the other parasites of the complex. Strikingly, none of the primers distinguished *L. donovani, L. infantum* and *L. archibaldi* taxa. Geographical clustering was observed with 2 strong Indian and East African *L. donovani* groups and a third Mediterranean *L. infantum* group in support to a previous study using RAPD in addition to other DNA tools [39]. Distribution of other *L. infantum* in the dendrogram also supports the paraphyly of *L. infantum* [41].

L. infantum zymodeme MON-1 has a worldwide distribution and is responsible mainly for a form of VL. RAPD analysis contributed to describe heterogeneity within this zymodeme and to demonstrate its polyphyletic nature [43]. The RAPD technique also highlighted geographical structures of *L. infantum* in diverse settings. In [42] they have shown that 17 (out of 18) primers tested on 33 strains isolated from diverse hosts in various Spanish regions generated highly polymorphic RAPD patterns that grouped the parasites into two main clusters that included parasites from central–western region in one side and from eastern Spain in the other. This study in addition illustrated intra-zymodemic diversity and lack of correlation with the MLEE analysis conducted on these strains, the clinical or host origin of the parasites. In another example, 53 *L. infantum* isolates from VL cases and dogs originating from different endemic regions in Brazil were analyzed with 5 RAPD primers (also used in [43]), MLMT and SSR-PCR. RAPD analysis was shown to be the most appropriate to illustrate genetic diversity of the parasites. Interestingly, in spite of the homogenous genetic background the polymorphisms observed demonstrated correlation with geographical origin [44].

In Corte Pedra, North Eastern Brazil, *L. braziliensis* is causing different American Tegumentary Leishmaniasis (ATL) forms. Forty-five *L. braziliensis* strains isolated from patients having different ATL forms were shown to generate with 3 primers and 4 protocols, RAPD patterns having overall more than 80% fingerprint identity classifying the parasites into 5 clades. Significant distribution frequency of the different clinical forms along the clades was observed. The authors thus concluded on the suitability of the RAPD analysis of parasite strains' variability in Corte Pedra and that in such a spatially limited population geographical isolation precludes geographic sequestration as the mechanism for the observed genetic structures. In addition they assumed that infection with some *L. braziliensis* genotypes could be accompanied with different pathogenic mechanisms [28]. Other studies investigating *L. braziliensis* diversity in Brazil with other primers also highlighted contrasted diversity extent of parasites isolated from cutaneous leishmaniasis according to the transmission areas; parasites from Mato Grosso [32] or from Para [29] states were more diverse than the ones in Minas Gerais. These authors proposed that eco-epidemiology of the parasites in relation to environmental and geographical differences could explain in part such diversity patterns. Genetic diversity using intergenic region typing (ITSrDNA PCR-RFLP) and MLEE of *L. braziliensis* from diverse hosts and geographical origins in Brazil also illustrated occurrence of geographical clusters of parasites exerting different levels of variability; association of *L. braziliensis* to specific transmission cycles likely reflecting adaptation of different parasite clones to the vector (and diversity of) species involved in the transmission has been inferred [45].

The RAPD technique has also been used to investigate epidemiology of leishmaniases, characterizing clinical or field isolates in diverse settings. For instance, in India the increasing reports on drug resistance of the VL patients and the implication of *L. tropica* as a causal agent of VL, also hypothesized to be a potential reason for drug unresponsiveness [2], has prompted investigations of the causal agents of VL using various DNA tools. A first study for example characterized by MLEE and 8 RAPD primers 15 clinical isolates collected over 20 years from the eastern part of India from confirmed VL patients; this sample study comprised 1 PKDL and 6 antimony unresponsive cases. All parasites proved to be *L. donovani* [31]. Another study investigated with the same primers 9 other parasites isolated over the period 2006-2010 from hospital clinics in Kolkata from confirmed VL and a PKDL cases; one parasite was similar to *L. tropica* while the others were very close to *L. donovani* [46]. The association of *L. tropica* with the disease was further confirmed in another study using ITS, ITS1 and HP70 based assays [47]. In Iran, where cutaneous leishmaniasis is highly endemic, MLEE and kDNA were used to identify species of 565 parasites obtained from confirmed CL patients from the different provinces of the country during the 2002–2008 period [48]; this study associated *L. major* mainly to rural transmission and *L. tropica* to urban settings. RAPD using 3 primers allowed describing extensive genetic heterogeneity of a random selection of 65 *L. major* strains across the different transmission area and within the same foci.

In addition, RAPD technique constitutes a powerful alternative to the identification of PCR targets and markers. RAPD markers have been exploited for the design of species or complex specific PCR assays like for instance a PCR that only amplifies DNA of parasites of the *L. donovani* complex [34] or another that amplifies exclusively *L. braziliensis* [49]. Such markers proved to be highly informative as probes or as PCR targets [34].

Randomly amplified polymorphic DNA products were used to develop markers that were targeted to develop typing strategies. For example, RAPD products that were amplified consistently across tested DNAs with a combination of 2 primers have been selected and sequenced partially to design marker specific PCR primers. The resulting PCR products were then screened for single stranded conformation polymorphisms (SSCP) and subsequently confirmed by sequence analysis [50]. This sequence confirmed amplified region analysis (SCAR) approach was used to differentiate 29 *L. donovani* strains from Sudan, Kenya, India and China using 8 different markers. The study identified 19 unique multilocus genotypes and a correlation between genotypes and geographical origin; SCAR markers were considered as co-dominant for their ability to detect all possible allele combinations in a diploid organism and as a representative random sample of neutral genetic variation in natural populations thus constituting appropriate tools for population studies [50].

Alternatively, with the objective to identify markers and develop simple assays for the discrimination of viscerotropic parasites encountered in Africa, we have screened 5 Operon kits (100 primers) for reproducible profiles and a selection of 28 primers was then used to screen for DNA markers within a panel of viscerotropic parasites from different countries in Africa and India [51]. These primers organized the parasites according to their geographical origin in a similar way to other studies using RAPD or other types of tools [39,41]. Some of the differentially amplified RAPD bands obtained in our study were cloned and sequenced; their analysis with bioinformatics tools and comparison to their respective genomic sites in *L. infantum*, *L. donovani* and *L. major* genomes highlighted the markers' association with simple sequence repeats and microsatellites in non coding regions [51]. A selection of such markers in *L. archibaldi* was used to develop simple PCR assays differentiating viscerotropic parasites, some of which in a country–specific way [52].

Randomly amplified polymorphic DNA is highly suitable for analysis of cultured *Leishmania* promastigotes but of limited interest for analysis of patients or zoonotic samples due to sample contamination with host DNA. Its use could be however contemplated to characterize promastigotes at the isolation step given the technique does not require large amounts of DNA (20 ng or less). Another generally admitted drawback is the lack of reproducibility generated by complex reactions occurring under the relaxed reaction conditions, therefore inter-laboratory or inter-study comparison using the same primers appear difficult to achieve. Options to overcome this drawback were the prior selection of primers of interest, or the use of defined criteria for analysis as for example relying only on consistently observed bands within RAPD patterns to assign the parasites to taxonomic groups [36] or using statistical tools to assess significance of the range of distances evaluated [33]. Use of well–standardized protocols may also help overcoming such a drawback. Although simple and having potential for detecting variation where other techniques fail, other drawbacks of this technique could be that bands of equal electrophoretic mobility may not be homologous [34]; identification of allelic variants is also not possible in *Leishmania*. Yet, RAPD constitutes a powerful tool for the identification of markers and the design of PCR based assays [34, 49–52]. Diverse RAPD *Leishmania* studies reached conclusions that were confirmed by other tools or alternative studies making the RAPD approach still valuable.

2.2.2. Gp63 PCR-RFLP and sequencing analyses

Gp63 genes encode for the major metalloprotease of *Leishmania*, which is the most abundant surface glycoprotein found in promastigote and amastigote forms of the parasite. GP63 protein is encoded by a cluster of tandemly repeated genes, and has been identified as a virulence factor in several *Leishmania* species. Several groups have studied the potential of gp63 as a species discriminatory tool in *Leishmania*. Amplification of gp63 genes coupled with restriction analysis (PCR-RFLP) was applied to a large number of isolates belonging to 4 species of the subgenus *Viannia*, namely *L. (V.) braziliensis, L. (V.) peruviana, L. (V.) guyanensis* and *L. (V.) lainsoni* and allowed discrimination of all the species tested [20] (Table2).

Target	Primers sequences (5'–3')	Product size (bp)	Discrimination by		Refs
			PCR-RFLP	Seq.	
	(F) Pia1: ACGAGGTCAGCTCCACTCC	100	-	-	[11,13]
	(R) Pia2: CTGCAACGCCTGTGTCTACG		-	-	
	(F) Pia3: CGGCTTCGCACCATGCGGTG	260	-	-	
	(R) Pia4: ACATCCCTGCCCACATACGC		-	-	
kDNA	(F) K13A : GTGGGGGAGGGGCGTTCT	120			
	(R) K13B: ATTTTACACCAACCCCCAGTT				
	(F) RV1: CTTTTCTGGTCCCGCGGGTAGG	145			
	(R) RV2: CCACCTGGCCTATTTTACACCA				
SSU rDNA	(F) R221: GGTTCCTTTCCTGATTTACG	603	+	+	[10]
	(R) R332: GGCCGGTAAAGGCCGAATAG				
	(F) TDM1: GTCTCCACCGCAGACCTCACGGA	1300	+	-	[20]
	(R) TDM2: TGATGTAGCTGCCATTCACGAAG				
	(F) SG1: GTCTCCACCGAGGACCTCACCGA	1300	+	-	
Gp63	(R) SG2: TGATGTAGCCGCCCTCCTCGAAG				[21]
	(F) PDD1: TCGGTGAGGTCCTCGGTGGAGAC	1700	+	-	
	(R) PDD2: CTTCGAGGAGGGCGGCTACATCA				
	(F) C9F: GGCTCCCGACGTGAGTTA	1750	+	-	
	(R) C1R: GGGCCCGGGCGACAGCAGCGATGACTG				[58]

	(F) C10F: GGGAAGCTTACGTACAGCGTGCAGGTG	1600, 2000 and 4500	+	-	
	(R) C1R: GGGCCCGGGCGACAGCAGCGATGACTG				
ITS	(F) LITSV: ACACTCAGGTCTGTAAAC	1040 or	+	+	[64,65,69]
	(R) LITSR: CTGGATCATTTTCCGATG	950–1100	+	+	
ITS1	(F) IR1: GCTGTAGGTGAACCTGCAGCAGCTGGATCATT	1000–1200	+	-	[16]
	(R) IR2: GCGGGTAGTCCI'GCCAAACACTCAGGTCTG				
	(F) LITSR: CTGGATCATTTTCCGATG	300–350	+	+	[12,13,61,65,82]
	(R) L5.8S: TGATACCACTTATCGCACTT				
ITS2	(F) LGITSF2: GCATGCCATATTCTCAGTGTC	372–450	-	+	[63]
	(R) LGITSR2: GGCCAACGCGAAGTTGAATTC				
	(F) L5.8SR: AAGTGCG-ATAAGTGGTA	720	-	+	[65]
	(R) LITSV: ACACTCAGGTCTGTAAAC				
ITS1and part of ITS2	(F) LITS-MG: ATG CCC AAC GCG AAG TTG	800	-	+	[69]
	(R) LITSR: CTGGATCATTTTCCGATG				
Hsp70	PCR-G : (F) HSP70sen: GACGGTGCCTGCCTACTTCAA	1422	+	-	[22,72]
	(R) HSP70ant: CCGCCCATGCTCTGGTACATC				
	PCR-F : (F) F25: GGACGCCGGCACGATTKCT	1286	+	-	
	(R) R1310: CCTGGTTGTTGTTCAGCCACTC				
	PCR-N : (F) F25: GGACGCCGGCACGATTKCT	593	+	-	[73–75]
	(R) R617: CGAAGAAGTCCGATACGAGGGA				
	PCR-C : (F) F251: GACAACCGCCTCGTCACGTTC	741	+	-	
	(R) R991: GTCGAACGTCACCTCGATCTGC				
	(F) HSP70sen: GACGGTGCCTGCCTACTTCAA	1422	-	+	
	(R) HSP70ant: CCGCCCATGCTCTGGTACATC				
	(F) HSP70-F335 CACGCTGTCGTCCGCGACG	113	-	+	
	(R) HSP70-R429 AACAGGTCGCCGCACAGCTCC				
	(F) HSP70-2F CTGAACAAGAGCATCAACCC	170	-	+	[23]
	(R) HSP70-2R CTTGATCAGCGCCGTCATCAC				
	(F) HSP70-F893 GTTCGACCTGTCCGGCATCC	130	-	+	
	(R) HSP70-R1005 GTGATCTGGTTGCGCTTGCC				
	PCR-F : (F) HSP70-F25: GGACGCCGGCACGATTKCT	1286	-	+	
	(R) HSP70-R1310: CCTGGTTGTTGTTCAGCCACTC				
	PCR-T : (F) HSP70-6F GTGCACGACGTGGTGCTGGTG	766	-	+	[76]
	(R) HSP70-R1310: CCTGGTTGTTGTTCAGCCACTC				
	PCR-N : (F) HSP70-F25: GGACGCCGGCACGATTKCT	593	-	+	
	(R) HSP70-R617 CGAAGAAGTCCGATACGAGGGA				

3'UTR : (F) 70-IR-D: CCAAGGTCGAGGAGGTCGACTA (R) 70-IR-M: ACGGGTAGGGGGAGGAAAGA	516–733	-	+	[77]

Mini-exon					
	(F) Fme: TATTGGTATGCGAAACTTCCG (R) Rme: GAAACTGATACTTATATAGCG	220–443	+	+	[19,13,78]
	(F) FME2: ACTTCCGGAACCTGTCTTCC (*Leishmania* subgenus) or ACTTCCGGGACCCGTCTTCC (*Viannia* subgenus) (R) ME2R: CAGAAACTGATACTTATATAGCGTTA	220–443	+	+	[82]

Cysteine protease B					
	intragenic region : (F) CPBFOR: CGAACTTCGAGCGCAACCT (R) CPBREV: CAGCCCAGGACCAAAGCAA	1079	+	-	[83,84]
	Intergenic region : (F) PIGS1A: CCTCATTGCTTTGGTCCTGG (R) PIGS2B: GGCGTGCCCACGTATATCGC	1600	+	-	
	cpbEF: (F) CGTGACGCCGGTGAAGAAT (R) CGTGCACTCGGCCGTCTT	702–741	-	-	[25,85]
	cpbEF: (F) CGTGACGCCGGTGAAGAAT (R) CGTGCACTCGGCCGTCTT	702–741	+	+	[26]
	Leishmania cpb: (F) LmcpbUNIF: ACGGTCTTAGCGTGCGAGTTGTG (R) LmcpbUNIR: CAAGGAGGTCCCCTCACGCG	1440	-	+	[85]
	L. major cpb (variant 1): (F) LmcpbUNIF: ACGGTCTTAGCGTGCGAGTTGTG (R) LmcpbR: TCGTGCAGCACATGTCGCTTG	1176	-	+	
	L. infantum cpb: (F) cpbEF For: CGTGACGCCGGTGAAGAAT (R) L. inf Rev: CGTTTCGTTGCTCGGGATCAT	325	-	-	
	L. tropica cpb: (F) LmcpbUNIF: ACGGTCTTAGCGTGCGAGTTGTG (R) Ltro Rev: ACAGGGCCGTCAGCCCGTGGC	600	-	-	
	L. infantum cpb: (F) infcpbE: GTCTTACCAGAGCGGAGTGCTACT (R) Inf2.1: ATAACCAGCCATTCGGTTTTG	278	-	-	[86]
	L. donovani cpb: (F) cpbF2.1: GCGGCGTGATGACCAGC (R) Do2.1: CAATAACCAGCCATTCGTTTTTA	309	-	-	
	(F) MATRAE2: GGCGATGGTGGAGCAGATGATCT		-	-	

(R) Ma4.1: CGGTTCTCGTAGCACACTTGTTG	99 (*L. major*)		
(R) Tr4.1: CTCCCCCGTTCGGAT	100 (*L. tropica*)		
(R) Ae2.1: AGTACGTGCACATCAGCACATGGG	154 (*L. aethiopica*)		
(F) V5F: GGTGATGTGCCCGAGTGCA (R) V10R: CGTGCACATCAGCACATGGG	564	-	-
(F) CpbF: GTGCGTGCGGGTCGTGC (R) CpbR: AAAGCCCCGGACCAAAGCA	735	-	-	[87]

(F): Forward primer; (R): Reverse primer; Seq.: sequence analysis; Refs: references

Table 2. Overview of DNA targets, primers sequences, product sizes and the technique used to achieve discrimination of *Leishmania* taxa.

Gp63 PCR-RFLP tool was also used to characterize isolates representative of the *L. donovani* complex (*L. infantum, L. donovani, L. archibaldi* and *L. chagasi*), with special attention to Mediterranean *L. infantum* from different geographical origins, in addition to representative strains of Old World *Leishmania* (*L. major, L. tropica* and *L. aethiopica*) [21] (Table2). This allowed discrimination of the 4 species of the *L. donovani* complex, which were quite distinct from the outgroup. Within *L. infantum*, the parasites were found to be polymorphic showing a geographical structuring [21]. Sequences of the gp63 genes were explored in 33 strains of the *L. donovani* complex having different origins and zymodemes, in addition to reference strains of other Old World species [53]. Evolution of the gp63 multigene family was inferred to be under the influence of a mosaic or fragmental gene conversion mechanism. The sequences clustered according to the species, showing a concerted evolution of the different gene classes. Phylogenetic analyses confirmed the genetic diversity of the *L. donovani* complex, which showed that gp63 genes could provide the basis for rapid and reliable genotyping of strains in this complex [53].

Furthermore, still using gp63 coding sequences PCR-RFLP evaluated intra-specific polymorphism of *L. infantum* isolates in Tunisia [54]. In total, 22 *L. infantum* isolates responsible of visceral (14 isolates) and cutaneous (8 isolates) forms of leishmaniasis in Tunisia were analysed, in addition to reference isolates, representative of Old World complexes. The *Sal*I, *Hinc*II, *Bal*I and *Bsi*EI restriction enzymes were used in this intragenic gp63 PCR-RFLP analysis. Results showed profiles that allowed distinction of *L. infantum* from the other species belonging to the *L. donovani* complex (*L. donovani, L. archibaldi* and *L. chagasi*) but also from the Old World species *L. major, L. tropica* and *L. aethiopica*. Besides, polymorphic patterns were observed among *L. infantum* isolates that tend to be correlated to the clinical presentation of the disease; the phenetic analysis using a UPGMA clustering method (Phylip package) grouped all VL isolates together while most of the CL parasites clustered in a separate branch. Good bootstrapping values supported the clusters [54].

The gp63 PCR-RFLP method was applied to characterise parasites contained within the lesions of patients having cutaneous leishmaniasis, originating from areas in central Tunisia, known to be free of CL. This analysis confirmed assignment of the parasites to the *L. infantum* species, thus demonstrating the occurrence/emergence of sporadic cutaneous leishmaniasis (SCL) due to *L. infantum* in central Tunisia [55].

The gp63 PCR associated to RFLP analysis was also used to characterise transmitted *Leishmania* in Sudan. Patients that presented with uncommon cutaneous leishmaniasis, including one case with a *L. tropica* like-lesion, were confirmed, using this tool, to be infected by *L. major* [56]. In another study, *Leishmania* parasites from Sudanese patients having cutaneous ulcers were analyzed by gp63 PCR-RFLP and shown to belong to the *L. donovani* species [56]. This work allowed concluding that, in addition to *L. major*, *L. donovani* species can also be a major cause of CL in Sudan [57].

Another PCR-RFLP analysis of the gp63 intergenic region was also developed and tested on the *L. donovani* complex [58]. The markers generated robust and congruent phylogenies, identifying 5 genetic clusters within *L. donovani* complex. Furthermore, clusters strongly correlated with isoenzyme typing and some with geographical origin, which may be important for epidemiological and clinical studies [58].

Although the gp63 PCR RFLP technique has been successfully used for *Leishmania* discrimination at the species and strains levels, it presents several disadvantages. The fragment patterns obtained are sometimes vey complex and can be difficult to analyze and compare between laboratories. Also, partial restriction needs to be carefully evaluated as a potential source of artefacts. This technique depends therefore, on careful standardization and is recommended for comparative studies involving few strains rather than for large-scale epidemiological studies. Given the size of the sequences amplified (1.3Kb for the intragenic PCR) and the number of (GC rich) copies, the PCR assay requires good quality DNA and additives like DMSO [21] and thus a careful establishment step.

2.2.3. ITS1 PCR–RFLP and ITS2 targets

Ribosomal RNA (rRNA) genes are highly repetitive and conserved sequences. The ITS1 region is the sequence in between the 18S rRNA and 5.8S rRNA genes. It has enough conservation to serve as a PCR target but sufficient polymorphisms to facilitate species typing. ITS1 PCR has been developed in combination with an RFLP analysis (Table2) with different restriction enzymes (*Alu*I, *Bst*UI, *Eco*RI, *Fsp*I, *Hae*III, *Hha*I, *Rsa*I, *Sau*3AI, *Sph*I and *Taq*I) [16]; *Hae*III is the mostly used restriction enzyme used for species identification. Indeed, ITS1 PCR–RFLP using *Hae*III is the most widely used assay for direct detection and identification of *Leishmania* species in the Old World.

It has been applied for the distinction of sympatric species, especially in the Mediterranean region [59,60]. However, representatives of the *L. donovani* complex (*L. donovani* and *L. infantum*) and also of the *L. braziliensis* complex (*L. braziliensis*, *L. guyanensis*, *L. panamensis*, *L. peruviana*) cannot be distinguished by this approach, even using a great variety of restriction enzymes [12]. This limitation can however be bypassed by sequencing of the ITS1 PCR product thus allowing for a clear separation of these species and also assignment of different strains [61].

Recently, real-time PCR product from the ITS1 region has been used in a high-resolution melt (HRM) analysis in order to identify and quantify Old World *Leishmania* species [62]. High resolution melt analysis is a molecular technique that uses a fluorescent intercalating dye to measure the rate of double stranded DNA dissociation consequent to an increase of temperature. The observed melting curve is characteristic of a particular DNA and depends on its sequence length, GC content, complementarity, and nearest neighbour thermodynamics. The dye is incorporated during the amplification; the DNA dissociation measures occur at the end of the PCR, which is performed in a dedicated thermocycler. The results are computerized and analyzed through a graphic output. When tested on 300 samples from human cases, reservoir hosts and sand flies, this approach distinguished all Old World *Leishmania* species causing human disease, except *L. donovani* from *L. infantum* [62].

The ITS2 region is located in between the 5.8S rRNA and LSU rRNA genes. It has been studied and found to be adequate for species identification. Indeed, generic PCR primers (LGITSF2/LGITSR2) were designed to amplify this fragment from *Leishmania* spp. associated with human infection, using reference isolates [63] (Table 2). Substantial differences in the ITS2 region amplified by these primers followed by sequencing analysis, allowed detection of and discrimination among *Leishmania* species from the Old and New World [63]. The ITS2 PCR followed by DNA sequence analysis approach was validated on clinical specimens, which allowed identification of a total of 8 *Leishmania* species (*L. (V.) braziliensis*, *L. (V.) guyanensis*, *L. (V.) panamensis*, *L. (L.) mexicana*, *L. aethiopica*, *L. major*, *L. tropica* and the *L. donovani* complex) among 159 patients corresponding to U.S. civilians that had travel and immigration history to leishmaniasis endemic countries [63].

The ITS1 and ITS2 region have also been used to assess intra-specific DNA polymorphisms among *L. donovani* isolates from different geographical origins [64,65] (Table 2). Single-stranded conformation polymorphism (SSCP), and sequencing of the ITS regions were applied to clinical samples of *L. donovani* from Sudan and one from Kenya, one from India and one from China. Intra-specific variation in SSCP banding patterns was clearly observed in the ITS1 region and gave five different SSCP profiles; 3 profiles were detected among Sudan isolates and 2 ITS1-SSCP profiles were observed among the samples from Kenya, India, and China [65]. This corroborates the results of a previous study in which 11 polymorphic ITS1-SSCP patterns were identified among 63 clinical samples of *L. donovani* from eastern Sudan [64]. On the other hand, no variation was observed in the ITS2 region among the 63 studied cases from Sudan [64] and the study that analyzed the ITS2 locus among 23 Sudanese samples, showed again the same ITS2 SSCP pattern, with the exception of 1 isolate that had a different one [65].

When the species *L. tropica* was studied using ITS1 amplification and SSCP analysis, 14 SSCP profiles within 29 strains from different Old World geographical areas were found [66,67]. The *L. major* species was also investigated for DNA polymorphisms using ITS1 and ITS2 PCR amplification followed by SSCP analysis and sequencing [68]. Results revealed in total five genotypic variants among *L. major* isolates from Iran [68].

Recently, authors from Iran used primers LITSR and LITSV to amplify whole ITS region and found a double banded electrophoretic pattern in *L. tropica* species, while a sharp single band was observed for *L. infantum* and *L. major* isolates [69]. In order to explain how this two-band pattern occur in *L. tropica,* an *in silico* analysis of ITS sequences was conducted and showed the existence of two groups of sequences that differ by a 100bp gap, indicating existence of at least two alleles for ITS in ribosomal DNA. Thus, a specific reverse primer was developed (LITS-MG, Table 2) in order to amplify, with LITSR, sequences located just before the gap, which included ITS1 5.8S and a part of the ITS2 sequence. Amplification using LITS-MG/ LITSR primer set, followed by sequencing, allowed discriminating *L. tropica* from *L. infantum* or *L. major* [69].

Although PCR-RFLP of the ITS1 spacer is the most widely used assay for direct detection and identification of *Leishmania* species in the Old World, it has some limitations. Despite that all medically relevant *Leishmania* species can be distinguished by digesting the ITS1 PCR product with *Hae*III restriction enzyme, representatives of the *L. donovani* complex (*L. donovani* and *L. infantum*) or *L. braziliensis* complex (*L. braziliensis, L. guyanensis, L. panamensis* and *L. peruviana*) have almost identical RFLP patterns with a great variety of restriction enzymes and cannot be resolved further by this approach [12]. This problem can, however be solved partially by sequencing the ITS1 PCR product. Use of a highly resolutive agarose or SSCP analysis may be needed to resolve differences between some species or to investigate intra-specific polymorphism, respectively. ITS2 region has also served for species identification but the drawback of this approach is the need for DNA sequencing analysis. Sequencing or SSCP analysis may not be available in most laboratories in areas of endemicity.

2.2.4. hsp70 PCR–RFLP and sequencing

The 70kDa heat-shock proteins (HSP70) are encoded by genes that are highly conserved across prokaryotes and eukaryotes both in sequence and function. They have great importance as molecular chaperones in protein folding and transport [70]. Genes encoding cytoplasmic HSP70s were among the first kinetoplastid genes that were cloned and characterized because of their conserved nature [71]. HSP70 protein and its encoding gene have been widely used for phylogenetic and taxonomic studies of different parasites, including *Leishmania*.

The PCR-RFLP approach targeting hsp70 sequences has proven to be most useful for the differentiation between South American *Leishmania* species from the subgenus *Viannia* (Table2). Using the restriction enzyme *Hae*III to digest the amplified product, the produced RFLP patterns allowed discrimination between *L. guyanensis* species complex as well as for *L. lainsoni* and *L. shawi* [22,24]. However, *L. braziliensis* and *L. peruviana,* both belonging to the *L. braziliensis* complex, as well as *L. naiffi* showed an identical *Hae*III RFLP pattern. They can be distinguished by using other restriction endonucleases like *Mbo*I and *Bst*UI [24]. The Hsp70 PCR-RFLP approach was extended for identification of Old World and additional New World species with an improved resolution within species complexes; in total 139 strains from 14 species were studied using *Hae*III, *Bcc*I, *Rsa*I, *Mlu*I, and *Bsa*HI restriction enzymes [72]. Two subsequent digestions of the PCR products identified the species *L. infantum* and *L. donovani* (*Hae*III and *Mlu*I), *L. tropica* and *L. aethiopica* (*Hae*III and *Bsa*HI), *L. braziliensis* and *L. peruviana* (*Hae*III and *Rsa*I), *L. guyanensis* and *L. panamensis* (*Hae*III and *Bcc*I); the first digestion using *Hae*III discriminates among the broad groups while the additional ones discriminate within these groups; the species *L. major, L. lainsoni* and *L. naiffi* had specific patterns with *Hae*III restriction enzyme, without need to use an additional digestion [72]. However, it was not possible to differentiate between the species *L. mexicana, L. amazonensis*, and *L. garnhami* [72].

In order to improve the sensitivity and specificity of the previously reported hsp70 PCR, alternative PCR primers and RFLPs were used [73] (Table2). Thus, three new PCR primer sets (PCR-F, PCR-N, and PCR-C) and their corresponding restriction scheme (RFLP-F, RFLP-N, and RFLP-C) were tested. The detection limit of the new PCRs was between 0.05 and 0.5 parasite genomes; they amplified clinical samples more efficiently, and were *Leishmania* specific. A specific discriminative power was found for each new RFLP analysis: in general species from the Old World (*L. major, L. tropica, L. aethiopica, L. donovani, L. infantum*) and from the New World (*L. infantum, L. lainsoni, L. peruviana, L. guyanensis, L. panamensis*) were well differentiated [73]. Discrimination of *L. guyanensis* and *L. panamensis* species, both belonging to the *L. guyanensis* complex is important for epidemiological purposes and has also consequences for the prognosis of the disease, since MCL, which is principally associated with *L. braziliensis*, can also be caused by other *L. (Viannia)* suspected species. Recently, an updated hsp70PCR RFLP protocol for RFLP-F and RFLP-N designed in [73] was published, with new restriction enzymes [74]. These new enzymes showed reduced cost and allowed better separation of some New World (sub)species [74].

Relevance of the hsp70 PCR-RFLP approach [72–74] is illustrated by a study that applied it on 89 clinical samples from a total of 73 Peruvian patients with either cutaneous or mucocutaneous leishmaniasis. The new PCRs were tested on tissue samples, lesion biopsies, aspirates, and scrapings. They showed an improved sensitivity both for genus detection and species typing and identified the species *L. braziliensis, L. peruviana* and *L. guyanensis* [75].

In addition to PCR-RFLP analysis, the hsp70 gene was also used in sequencing. Indeed, the 1380bp fragment of the coding region commonly used in RFLP analysis was sequenced in 43 isolates from different geographic origins for studying evolutionary relationships [23]. Fifty-two hsp70 sequences representing 17 species commonly causing leishmaniasis both in the New and Old World were analyzed. The authors found that the genus *Leishmania* formed a monophyletic group with three distinct subgenera *L. (Leishmania), L. (Viannia)*, and *L. (Sauroleishmania)*. The obtained phylogeny supported the eight species *L. (L.) donovani, L. (L.) major, L. (L.) tropica, L. (L.) mexicana, L. (V.) lainsoni, L. (V.) naiffi, L. (V.) guyanensis* and *L. (V.) braziliensis*. In some of the species, subspecies *L. (L.) donovani infantum, L. (V.) guyanensis panamensis*, and *L. (V.) braziliensis peruviana* were recognized [23]. Recently, sequencing of the hsp70 gene was useful for *Leishmania* species determination within clinical samples, overcoming need for parasite isolation [76]. The results obtained were in great agreement with those from multilocus enzyme electrophoresis [76].

The 3'-untranslated region (UTR) of hsp70-type I gene constitutes an alternative target for sequence analysis [77]. These authors who used it to analyse 24 strains representing 11 *Leishmania* species, found a remarkable degree of sequence conservation in this region, even between species of the subgenera *Leishmania* and *Viannia*. In addition, the presence of many microsatellites was a common feature of the 3'-UTR of HSP70-I genes in the *Leishmania* genus. Global sequence alignments and resulting dendrograms demonstrated usefulness of this particular region of hsp70 genes for species (or species complex) typing, improving the discrimination capacity of phylogenetic trees based on hsp70 coding sequences in case of some species (*L. donovani/L. infantum; L. tropica* and *L. aethiopica; L. braziliensis/L. peruviana; L. guyanensis/L. panamensis*) [77].

Using hsp70 gene in PCR followed by RFLP or sequence analysis presents many advantages. It is easily comparable across all *Leishmania* species worldwide and discriminates all relevant species in both subgenera *L. (Leishmania)* and *L. (Viannia)*. In addition, the approach has been optimized for direct amplification from clinical samples. However, systematic sequencing of the hsp70 gene for *Leishmania* identification purposes represents the major disadvantage of this approach, since this technique needs high-resource settings. For this, it was stated, "this method is especially suited for use in non-endemic infectious disease clinics dealing with relatively few cases on an annual basis, for which no fast high throughput diagnostic tests are needed" [76].

2.2.5. Mini-exon PCR-RFLP

The mini-exon genes are involved in the trans-splicing process of nuclear mRNA in kineto-plastid protozoa and are present as 100 to 200 tandemly repeated copies per nuclear genome. Mini-exon genes contain a highly conserved exon of 39 bp with a moderately variable transcribed intron region (55 to 101 bp) and a highly variable non-transcribed spacer sequence (51 to 341 bp). These genes were extensively used as a PCR target to identify and discriminate Old and New World *Leishmania* species [19,78]. This PCR assay amplified all the miniexon sequences in a single reaction (Table2). In addition, size variability of the amplification products allowed preliminary discrimination between the major complexes (Old and New World *Leishmania,* and New World *Viannia* complexes). After enzymatic restriction of the PCR product with *Hae*III or *Eae*I, a characteristic RFLP pattern is produced that depends on size variations in the polymorphic spacer regions as well as mutations in the recognition sites of the restriction enzymes. *Eae*I profiles were shown to be more informative than *Hae*III and allowed to distinguish between the most important Old World species, *L. major, L. tropica, L. aethiopica, L. infantum* and *L. donovani* [19,78]. However, with *Hae*III, species belonging to the *L. braziliensis* complex (*L. braziliensis* and *L. peruviana*) and to the *L. guyanensis* complex (*L. guyanensis* and *L. panamensis*) could be discriminated [19].

This genotyping method was successfully applied to naturally infected clinical samples for the differentiation of New and Old World *Leishmania* species and showed a high sensitivity and a robust and reliable species differentiation power [79]. Several other research groups have applied mini-exon PCR-RFLP method for identification and characterisation of *Leishmania* species, using various types of samples from different countries. In [80], they have analyzed microcapillary cultivated isolates from cutaneous and visceral cases in Turkey and identified the species *L. infantum* and *L. tropica* in CL cases, and *L. infantum* in VL ones. In Nepal, bone marrow aspirates from VL patients were analyzed by mini-exon PCR-RFLP and the parasites have been shown similar to the standard Indian strain of *L. donovani* and different from the Kenyan strain [81].

Recently, mini-exon PCR-RFLP was compared to the ITS1 PCR RFLP approach on a set of reference strains [82]. The ITS1 PCR proved to be slightly more sensitive and more practical than the mini-exon. Analysis using the ITS1 digested with *Hae*III allowed to distinguish most species but an additional digestion with *Cfo*I may be helpful in case of *L. mexicana*. However, using the mini-exon, sequencing was found to be the most practical approach as the mini-exon sequences add information since they are more polymorphic than the ITS1 sequences [82]. Therefore, the mini-exon genes were used for typing the species that belong to the *L. Viannia* subgenus, also known as *L. braziliensis* complex, which cannot be distinguished with the ITS1 [82].

2.2.6. Cysteine protease B (cpb) based PCR and PCR RFLP

Cpb genes are multicopy genes that encode for cathepsin L-like cysteine proteinase B (cpb), a major antigen of *Leishmania* parasites.

PCR RFLP assays targeting cpb genes and their non-coding inter-genic sequences were also developed and applied for characterization of strains from the *L. donovani* complex [83] (Table2). The following enzymes were used for intra-genic cpb PCR-RFLP: *Hinf*I, *Taa*I, *Hae*III, *Cfr*I, *Hpa*II, and *Sdu*I, and for inter-genic cpb PCR-RFLP: *Eam*1104I, *Nsp*I, *Hae*III, *Acy*I, and *Hae*II [83]. The discriminatory power of this assay was compared with that of PCR-RFLP analysis of the gp63 gene, and multilocus enzyme electrophoresis (MLEE). Restriction patterns of the cpb locus were polymorphic, but less so than gp63 patterns and presented differences with MLEE, supporting a different classification of parasites. The applicability of the developed cpb PCR RFLP approach also allowed direct genotyping of parasites in bone marrow aspirates and blood samples obtained from VL patients in Nepal [83]. This cpb PCR RFLP approach, in addition to a gp63 PCR-RFLP analysis, were applied to study 59 isolates of the *L. infantum* species obtained from different regions in Algeria, originating from various clinical forms and hosts, and assigned to different zymodemes [84]. Among the four analyzed zymodemes, 15 different genotypes were obtained. Also, cpb polymorphism showed two interesting trends: a possible relationship with the cutaneous origin of the isolates and an association with a West-East cline [84].

Different species–specific PCR assays were developed using these genes as target. PCR assays discriminating *L. donovani* from *L. infantum* were developed [25,26]. An *L. donovani* species-specific PCR primer pair amplifies a 317bp at the 3' end of cpb gene of *L. donovani* whereas it does not generate an amplicon for *L. infantum* [26]. Another PCR that was developed based on cysteine protease B genes differentiates *L. infantum* from *L. donovani* by their fragment length: a 741bp product (cpbF) characterized *L. donovani* strains, and a 702bp product (cpbE) *L. infantum* strains [25]. This primer pair more recently was tested, in addition to a newly designed one (cpbEF For/L.inf Rev, Table2), on 10 Tunisian *L. infantum* isolates. The amplification showed size polymorphism of cpbEF genes with either a 702bp or a 741bp product, even though the species *L. donovani* has never been described in Tunisia and the Mediterranean region [85].

Five species-specific PCR tests that can discriminate each of the Old World species: *L. infantum*, *L. donovani*, *L. tropica*, *L. aethiopica*, and *L. major* in cultured parasite isolates were also developed [86] (Table2). All the PCRs are based on the species-specific amplification of the cpb genes as each primer pair amplifies only one of the different cpb copies present in a particular species. In addition, the authors established the adaptation of 2 of these assays for oligochromatography detection, which is a rapid dipstick test for visualization of specific amplified *L. infantum* and *L. donovani* products. They concluded to the value of these assays for the identification of parasites *in vitro* but the assays were not shown sensitive enough to identify *Leishmania* parasites within clinical samples [86].

However, upon sequencing of the cpb- coding region in clinical isolates of *L. aethiopica*, specific PCR primers (V5F/V10R) were developed to differentiate this species from *L. tropica*, *L. major*, *L. donovani* and *L. infantum* by direct PCR (Table2). This cpb PCR proved to be sensitive enough to detect *L. aethiopica* from biopsy samples [87].

Recently, primers developed in [25] were used and new ones were designed, to set up three species-specific PCR assays based on the amplification of different copies and parts of the cpb genes (Table2) [85]. They allowed amplification of 1176bp, 600bp and 325bp fragments, thus discriminating between Old World Tunisian *L. major*, *L. tropica* and *L. infantum* species, respectively [85].

Multi-copy cpb genes have been recently used to develop a species–specific *L. infantum* LAMP assay (Loop-Mediated Isothermal reaction) for the diagnosis of canine leishmaniasis in Tunisia [88]. This isothermal nucleic acid amplification technique uses intrinsic properties of the enzyme (*Bst* DNA polymerase) for auto-strand displacement DNA synthesis to amplify large amounts of DNA within 30–60 minutes. The amplification reaction that is conducted at only one temperature does not require a thermocycler and takes profit of the intricate design of a set of six specific primers [89]. LAMP has emerged as a powerful tool for diagnostics and has been successfully developed for several protozoan parasitic diseases including leishmaniasis [90]. Use of cpb genes in the LAMP assay successfully allowed to detect the *L. infantum* DNA with a specific amplification, as no cross reaction was seen, with *L. major*, *L. tropica*, *L. turanica*, *L. aethiopica*, *L. tarentolae*, *L. gerbilli*, *Trypanosoma cruzi*, or human genomic DNA. In addition, LAMP assay showed a higher sensitivity when compared to conventional cpb based PCRs [88].

Cpb coding sequence and UTR targets have a proven and good potential to characterize or identify *Leishmania* species. Their antigenic nature makes them interesting to describe epidemiological features in some areas. However in spite of being multi-copy targets, sensitivity of their detection seem to be limited likely due to sequence variations underlying the primers used.

2.2.7. Cytochrome gene sequencing

Cytochromes are involved in the electron transport process of the mitochondrial respiratory chain. They are considered one of the most useful genes for taxonomy given their slow evolution rate. They were used for discrimination of *Leishmania* parasites as well as for exploring their phylogenetic relationships. Cytochrome oxidase II gene has been first analyzed for sequence variation in 22 *Leishmania* isolates representative of the *L. donovani* complex from different geographical origins [91]. Phylogenetic analysis produced maximum parsimony, neighbor joining and maximum likelihood trees that were congruent and showed two clades corresponding to the species *L. donovani* and *L. infantum*. Furthermore, the molecular haplotypes were concordant, in general, with the isoenzyme data of the complex [91]. Interestingly, *L. donovani* isolates from Sudan were shown to possess the most ancestral cytochrome oxidase II sequence with a single haplotype that was very close to that of *L. major* [91]. The data provided in this work allowed an approximate dating of the origin of the *L. donovani* complex to a period contemporary to or predating the spread of modern humans out of Africa [91].

Cytochrome b (*Cyt b*) gene has also been used to determine the nucleotide sequence from 13 human-infecting *Leishmania* species from the New and Old Worlds [92]. The phylogenetic relationships based on this gene, showed good agreement with the classification of Lainson & Shaw [93] except for the inclusion of *L. major* in the *L. tropica* complex and the placement of *L. tarentolae* in another genus [92]. The same group has further applied this method to other *Leishmania* species to construct a new phylogenic tree [94]. A total of 30 *Leishmania* and *Endotrypanum* WHO reference strains were analyzed. The phylogenic tree obtained showed mainly the exclusion of *L. major* from the *L. tropica* complex, the placement of *L. tarentolae* in the genus and location of *L. turanica* and *L. arabica* far from human pathogenic *Leishmania* strains [94].

Since that, *Cyt b* gene have been sequenced in several studies and was shown to be able to identify the *Leishmania* species, in Pakistan [95,96], in Colombia [97] and in China [98]. Furthermore, results of *Cyt b* gene sequencing of 69 cutaneous leishmaniasis cases in Pakistan showed that only *L. tropica* was found in highland areas and only *L. major* in lowland areas [96]. Importantly, among *L. major* samples analyzed, three types of *Cyt b* polymorphism were found, including 45 cases of type I, six of type II and one of type III [96]. The authors reported for the first time on the presence of polymorphisms in *L. major* (types I, II and III) based on species identification using *Cyt b* gene sequencing from clinical samples [96].

This target is a slow evolving DNA molecule and is thus considered as a good marker for phylogeny. Being located on the mitochondrial maxicercle, the copy number constitutes another advantage. Given demonstration of natural genetic exchange experimentally [99] and naturally [100], these targets known to have a monoparental transmission (also confirmed for *Leishmania*) could be ideal for genetic exchange analyses.

2.2.8. Other molecular tools

Several other molecular tools have also been used for identification and characterization of *Leishmania*. These include quantitative PCR, AFLP, LAMP assay and others.

In recent years, quantitative PCR methods based either on SYBR Green or TaqMan technology have been set up for the quantification of *Leishmania* in different types of biopsies from mice, dogs and also from human peripheral blood, targeting either single-copy or multi-copy sequences with high sensitivity and reproducibility [101–104]. In particular, quantitative real time PCR assays (qPCR) were developed to detect and rapidly differentiate *Leishmania* species and also to quantify parasites within clinical samples. Primers used recognized kinetoplast minicircle [105,106] and ribosomal DNA [107].

Amplified fragment length polymorphism (AFLP) has also been developed for *Leishmania* typing [108]. This technique essentially probes the entire genome at random, without prior sequence knowledge. Thus, it is ideally suited as a screening tool for molecular markers linked with biological and clinical traits. It is a PCR-based technique that uses restriction enzymes to digest DNA, followed by ligation of adapters to the ends of the restriction fragments, which will be then amplified using specific primers. The amplified fragments are separated and visualised on denaturing polyacrylamide gels, through autoradiography or fluorescence methodologies or using automated capillary sequencing instruments. AFLP was adapted to the *Leishmania* genome and validated on a panel of samples from the *L. donovani* complex. Results were highly congruent with previous analyses using multiple other molecular tests [109]. AFLPs are particularly useful for assessing genetic variation and genome mapping over other existing molecular techniques (reviewed in [110]).

Assays using alternative amplification technologies such as quantitative nucleic acid sequence-based amplification (QT-NASBA) based on amplification of 18S RNA or Loop mediated isothermal amplification (LAMP) targeting rRNA, kinetoplast DNA or a multigenic family were also tested on *Leishmania* infected samples. QT-NASBA yielded a sensitivity of 97.5% and a specificity of 100% when tested on skin biopsy samples from Old and New World CL patients [111]. A generic loop mediated isothermal amplification (LAMP) of reverse transcribed 18SRNA had a 83% sensitivity on blood samples of VL patients from Sudan and 98% sensitivity on skin biopsies of CL patients from Suriname [90]. An *L. donovani* specific LAMP was developed targeting kinetoplast minicircle DNA that had 80% sensitivity on 10 blood samples of VL patients from Bengladesh [112]. This assay evaluated on a larger number of patients (N=75) and 101 negative controls had 90% sensitivity and 100% specificity; these performances were found comparable to a nested PCR assay tested on the same samples [113]. An *L. infantum* specific LAMP assay, targeting the cysteine protease B multi copy gene was also recently developed [88]. This tool applied on detection of dog infection in Tunisia had a sensitivity of 54% and a specificity of 80%, a better performance than the one obtained with a Cpb PCR assay [88]. LAMP assays constitute promising tools for rapid and sensitive detection of *Leishmania* DNA, however for discrimination of *Leishmania* species and strains other tools may appear superior at this stage. Their main advantage remains the rapid delivery of results and the minimal equipment requirement.

3. Strain typing

3.1. Multilocus sequence typing (MLST)

Multilocus sequence typing (MLST) refers to analysis based on the DNA sequence of multiple gene targets. It is based on the comparison of partial sequences (usually 700 bp) of a defined set of housekeeping genes. Similarly to MLEE, alleles are scored as identical or not, regardless of how many different polymorphic loci they have. Strains sharing the same allele combinations for the set of genes tested are referred to as sequence types. MLST is able to detect co-dominant single nucleotide polymorphisms (SNP) and although indels can complicate the analysis, they are extremely rare in protein-coding genes.

The first *Leishmania* complex that has been studied with MLST is the *L. donovani* complex. Two sets of 5 loci corresponding to genes coding for enzymes used in MLEE were studied: one set with asat, gpi, nh1, nh2 and pgd and the other one with icd, me, mpi, g6pdh, and fh [7,8]. Results were found to be largely in agreement with the results from MLEE although some key discrepancies were found and increased resolution was obtained. Thus silent SNPs were found that provide further resolution, such as a single SNP in gpi that distinguishes between strains of *L. infantum* [7]. However, SNPs responsible for amino acid changes were also found in genes coding for enzymes giving indistinguishable electrophoretic profiles, mainly in nh2, which had the same protein band for all *L. donovani* complex strains. MLST study contributed to better understanding of *L. donovani* complex phylogeny and taxonomical position of the species *L. infantum* and *L. donovani* [114]. It was a strong argument to question the position of *L. archibaldi* as a species [6] and existence of MLEE defined *L. infantum* in Sudan [8]. It also highlighted potential occurrence of genetic exchange among circulating parasites in East Africa [7,8].

MLST using 6 gene targets that are not associated with MLEE analysis (inorganic pyrophosphatase, spermidine synthase 1, hypoxanthine-guanine phosphoribosyl transferase, mitogen-activated protein kinase, RNA polymerase II largest sub-unit and adenylate kinase 2) have been used to characterize suspected *L. major/L. infantum* hybrids and representative co-endemic strains in Portugal [115]. Sequence analyses confirmed MLEE hybrid profiles and hybrid status with occurrence of heterozygous positions in the target genes that so far were not studied for their diversity within *Leishmania* species. In a more recent work, 2 of these genes and 5 others (Elongation initiation factor 2 alpha subunit, zinc binding dehydrogenase-like protein, translation initiation factor alpha subunit, nucleoside hydrolase-like protein and a hypothetical protein located on chromosome 31) were analyzed on a panel of 222 strains representative of 10 different species in 43 countries in Eurasia and Africa, corresponding to 110 zymodemes with the objective to study the genetic diversity of the genus *Leishmania*, improving our knowledge on the genetic structure and genomic evolution mechanisms of this genus [116]. Seven genetically robust clusters were obtained that overlapped with most of the biochemical taxonomy groups: clusters I, III, IV, V and VI included strains belonging to the MLEE-based species *L. aethiopica*, *L. arabica*, *L. turanica*, *L. gerbilli* and *L. major*, respectively and cluster II included the *L. tropica* and *L. killicki* strains; with the exception of the species that cause forms of visceral leishmaniasis (cluster VII that comprised strains from *L. donovani*, *L. infantum* and *L. archibaldi*) in line with the concept of species complex suggested for this group. No observations were made of interspecific recombination or genetic exchange between the different species but these strains were selected for the study as not resulting from a likely genetic exchange [116]. It is anticipated to observe more informative studies increasing the number of markers or the strains circulating within selected endemic areas notably that co-sympatry of multiple parasite species is a well-established feature in many endemic areas.

In the New World, four housekeeping genes (glucose-6-phosphate dehydrogenase (G6PD), 6-phosphogluconate dehydrogenase (6PGD), mannose phosphate isomerase (MPI) and isocitrate dehydrogenase (ICD)) were sequenced from 96 *Leishmania* (*Viannia*) strains that were chosen to be representative of the zymodeme and geographical species diversity of this subgenus, in South America, and in particular Brazil, in order to assess their discriminatory typing capacity and refine phylogeny of the *L.* (*Viannia*) species [117]. A large number of haplotypes were detected for each marker. Maximum parsimony-based haplotype networks showed separated clusters in each network, corresponding to strains of different species, congruent with the MLEE identification. Besides, NeighborNet formed by the concatenated sequences confirmed species-specific clusters. This analysis also suggested recombination occurring in *L. braziliensis* and *L. guyanensis*. However, using phylogenetic analysis, the species *L. lainsoni* and *L. naiffi* were shown to be the most divergent species and placed the *L. shawi* species in the *L. guyanensis* cluster, not as a distinct species. The authors also found the *L. braziliensis* strains to correspond to one widely geographically distributed clonal complex in Brazil and another restricted to one endemic area, in a region bordering Peru [117].

The main advantage of MLST is the possibility of generating genus-wide phylogenies, since MLST markers are co-dominant and are amenable for population and phylogenetic analyses. Also, given the high quality of sequence data, results can be easily compared between laboratories. Compared to MLEE, MLST does not necessarily require sterile culture of parasites. In addition, simultaneous typing of reference strains and sequencing can be done commercially without in-house specialized equipment. For those reasons, MLST is likely to become the gold standard basis for taxonomy and thus identification of *Leishmania*. One expected drawback could be the inherent limit of detection of nucleotide allelic diversity associated to direct sequencing of PCR products, which could be overcome by more lengthy analyses like cloning of parasites or PCR products. One consequence of this drawback is that MLST should not be considered as typing tool but an analysis tool. Another application could be diagnosis as recently new species-specific genetic polymorphisms were identified in the genes that confer the phenotypic variations in the MLEE assay [118]. Indeed, sequencing of the MPI and 6PGD genes was sufficient to differentiate among closely related species causing New World leishmaniasis, in Peru. The same group took advantage of these polymorphisms and designed a new real-time PCR assay based on FRET (fluorescence resonance energy transfer) technology and melting curve analysis using SYBR green. The assay was highly sensitive and correctly identified each of the five main species that cause tegumentary leishmaniasis in the New World, directly from clinical samples [119].

3.2. Multilocus microsatellite typing (MLMT)

Microsatellites are repeated motives of 1–6 nucleotide(s), which present allelic length variation. They mutate fast, therefore, 10–20 independent markers have to be analyzed for each strain owing to homoplasy. Microsatellite sequence variation results from the gain and loss of repeat units, which can easily be detected after amplification with specific primers annealing to their flanking regions. Then length polymorphisms are detected using PAGE, MetaPhor agarose gel electrophoresis or, preferably, automated capillary sequencers. A multilocus microsatellite profile is compiled for each sample from the fragment length measured for the microsatellite markers analyzed.

During the last years, microsatellite-based approaches have been developed for strain typing within the genus *Leishmania* to overcome the lack of discriminatory power of MLEE and other molecular tools. So far, microsatellite loci with high discriminatory power and suitable for characterizing closely related strains have been published for the *L. donovani/L. infantum* complex [120–122], *L. major* [123,124], *L. tropica* [125] and for species of the subgenus *L. (Viannia)* [126–128].

3.2.1. Subgenus L. Leishmania

3.2.1.1. L. donovani complex

Within the *L. donovani* complex, a set of 15 microsatellite markers have been applied to type strains of *L. donovani* and *L. infantum* isolated from the main endemic regions for VL (India, East Africa, Mediterranean region, Asia and South America) [129]. Six principal genetically distinct populations were identified: 2 populations of *L. infantum* from the Mediterranean area and South America comprising the MON-1 and non-MON-1 strains, respectively; 2 populations of *L. donovani* from Sudan and Ethiopia; 1 of *L. donovani* MON-2 from India; and 1 consisting of strains of *L. donovani* (MON-36, 37 and 38) from Kenya and India. These results corroborated the fragmentary data published in numerous studies using other genetic markers. Interestingly, the highest microsatellite diversity was observed for *L. infantum* from the Mediterranean basin and the lowest for *L. donovani* from India. Using 34 additional microsatellite sequences, analysis showed the homogeneity of *L. donovani* from the Indian subcontinent [130].

Different genetic groups of strains of *L. infantum* were also observed when strains from Algeria, Tunisia, the Palestinian Authority and Israel were subjected to MLMT. Microsatellite typing of strains belonging to zymodemes MON-1, MON-24 and MON-80 identified 3 different populations in Algeria and in Tunisia [131,132]. The MON-1 strains were assigned to 2 different populations one of which contained only local strains and the other local and European strains of MON-1. The non-MON-1 strains were always separated from the MON-1 ones. Gene flow was detected between the two MON-1 populations and the local MON-1 and the non-MON-1 populations, respectively [131,132]. *L. infantum* Israeli and Palestinian strains obtained from infected dogs and human cases showed 2 main populations genetically different from European populations, one of which is sub-divided in geographically distributed sub populations [133].

In Spain, *L. infantum* strains from a rural leishmaniasis-endemic area, from which 94 were obtained from dogs, 15 from sand flies, and 1 from a human visceral case, were MLMT studied [134]. Results showed existence of 17 genotypes that were detected using 10 microsatellite markers belonging to 3 different targets. They also showed the heterogeneous distribution of *L. infantum* species in hosts living in sympatric conditions.

Analysis of *L. infantum* strains having a New World origin by MLMT indicated that these strains were more similar to MON-1 and non-MON-1 sub-populations of *L. infantum* from southwest Europe, than to any other Old World sub-population [135] thus indicating that the parasite has been recently imported multiple times to the New World from southwest Europe.

Within the *L. donovani* complex, *L. donovani*, *L. infantum* and *L. archibaldi* strains from Sudan were studied by MLMT technique [6]. The authors found one single monophyletic *L. donovani* clade and argued that the isoenzyme differentiation of *L. donovani* and *L. infantum* in East Africa was misleading and that *L. archibaldi* is an invalid taxon [6].

Analysis of *L. donovani* strains from India, Bangladesh, Sri Lanka and Nepal showed that in Sri Lanka the causative agent of CL is most closely related to parasites causing VL in India [136] and that genetically homogeneous strains are circulating in the Indian subcontinent [130]. On the other hand, *L. donovani* strains belonging to the MON-37 zymodeme and originating from different geographical origins (India, Sri Lanka, Middle East, Cyprus and East Africa) were MLMT analyzed [9]. Zymodeme MON-37 was found to be paraphyletic, representing different genetic groups corresponding to their geographical origin and strains from Cyprus were clearly different from all others and could be autochthonous [9].

3.2.1.2. L. tropica

MLMT technique was also applied for *L. tropica* strain typing. Indeed, 117 strains from Asia and Africa were used and revealed 10 genetic groups, which were largely correlated to the geographical origin of the strains [125]. Different genetic groups were shown to co-exist in strains from the Middle East and Morocco. However, the authors postulated that recent spread of new genotypes has occurred recently in the Middle East and suspected an African origin of the *L. tropica* species [125].

3.2.1.3. L. major

Concerning *L. major*, 106 strains from Central Asia, Africa and the Middle East were analyzed using MLMT, based on 10 different microsatellite markers [124]. The study showed three main populations corresponding to the three geographical regions studied that were further subdivided into 2 sub-populations. Interestingly, the African and Middle Eastern populations seemed to be more genetically diversified than the Central Asian population [124].

3.2.2. Subgenus L. Viannia

Within the New World *L. Viannia* subgenus, the first MLMT studied species were *L. braziliensis* and *L. peruviana*. Fifty- nine analyzed Peruvian strains showed emergence of multiple *L. braziliensis/L. peruviana* hybrids [137]. Then, 124 *L. braziliensis* strains from Peru and Bolivia were investigated for their genetic polymorphism at 12 microsatellite loci [127,138]. A substantial genetic diversity with high levels of inbreeding, inconsistent with a strictly clonal reproduction was shown. Besides, a large genetic heterogeneity between populations within countries was described, which evidenced a strong population structure at a microgeographic scale [138].

In another study, polymorphisms of 30 strains of *L. braziliensis*, 21 strains of *L. guyanensis*, and 2 strains of *L. peruviana* from Brazil, Paraguay and Peru were analyzed at 15 independent microsatellite loci [128]. All strains except two *L. guyanensis* had individual MLMT types. In addition, three main clades were found, that consisted of one population of strains of *L.*

guyanensis only, another one with strains of *L. braziliensis* from Paraguay and Brazil, and the last one with strains of *L. braziliensis* and *L. peruviana* [128].

Recently, 28 strains of the main species of the *L. guyanensis* complex (*L. guyanensis* and *L. panamensis*), collected in Ecuador and Peru were investigated in an MLMT study, with 12 microsatellite markers [139]. An important heterozygote deficit was observed in these populations, similar to the previously reported results in *L. braziliensis* complex [138]. They further showed genetic polymorphism and geographical differentiation on the *L. guyanensis* complex [139].

All together, these studies confirmed that microsatellite markers constitute good tools for typing and population genetic studies of *Leishmania*. Their additional advantage resides in the possibility of their use directly in biological material without culturing of parasites [130,140]. Moreover, accurate, quality controlled microsatellite profiles could be stored in databases and compared between different laboratories.

4. *Leishmania* parasite evolution, genetics and genome analyses – Consequences and prospects

For many years *Leishmania* parasites have been considered to replicate clonally, without genetic exchange. Indeed, Tibayrenc proposed that clonal evolution in micropathogens be defined as restrained recombination on an evolutionary scale, with genetic exchange scarce enough to not break the prevalent pattern of clonal population structure (Reviewed in [141,142]). The two main manifestations of clonal evolution are strong linkage disequilibrium (LD) and wide-spread genetic clustering ("near-clading"). These authors hypothesized that this pattern is not mainly due to natural selection, but would originate chiefly from in-built genetic properties of pathogens, that would allow like for other microorganisms (viruses, bacteria, protozoan parasites) to keep a balance between clonality and recombination, which would help escape from recombinational load. This way, to face evolutionary challenges, pathogens would be equipped with "clonality/sexuality machinery" that would function as alternative allelic systems [141,142]. However, an accumulation of molecular evidence indicates that there are inter-specific [115,137,143–146] and intra-specific [132,138] hybrids among natural populations. Genetic exchange was finally demonstrated experimentally in 2009 [99]. In fact, double drug resistant *Leishmania* major hybrids were produced by co-infecting *Phlebotomus duboscqi* (a natural *L. major* vector) sand flies with two strains carrying different drug resistance markers. The nuclear genotypes were consistent with a Mendelian transmission leading to a heterozygous first generation progeny [99]. The anticipated continuity of these studies was to co-infect sand flies with transgenic *Leishmania* carrying two different markers that are fluorescent, in an attempt to visualize the recombination events microscopically [147]. In 2011, for the first time, using a fluorescent protein detection system to observe yellow hybrid promastigotes in *Phlebotomus perniciosus* and *Lutzomyia longipalpis* midguts, *L. donovani* hybrids were observed, 2 days post bloodmeal, and the morphological stages involved were found to be short procyclic promastigotes [100]. However, the parasites could not be recovered and propagated to confirm their hybrid genotypes [100]. Recently, the analysis of the mating competency of *L. major* strains have been expanded to include pairwise matings of multiple isolates bearing independent drug markers [148]. Also, the timing of the appearance of hybrids and their developmental stage associations within both natural (*Phlebotomus duboscqi*) and unnatural (*Lutzomyia longipalpis*) sand fly vectors was followed. Genotype analysis of a large number of progeny clones showed a chromosomal inheritance of both parental alleles at 4–6 unlinked nuclear loci, consistent with a meiotic process, and a uniparental inheritance of kinetoplast DNA [148]. A low frequency of nuclear loci showed only one parental allele, suggesting loss of heterozygosity, most likely arising from aneuploidy, which is common in *Leishmania*. In the natural vector, when comparing the timing of hybrid formation and the presence of developmental stages, the authors suggested that nectomonad promastigotes are the most likely mating competent forms, with hybrids emerging before the first appearance of metacyclic promastigotes [148].

MLMT analysis showed that recombination events are much more frequent in *Leishmania* than previously thought. Indeed, MLMT analysis of Bolivian and Peruvian *L. braziliensis* showed frequent sexual crosses of individuals from the same strain (inbreeding) [138]. The substantial heterozygote deficiency and extreme inbreeding found in this study is not consistent with a strictly clonal reproduction. The authors came to the conclusion that *Leishmania* parasites may alternate between clonal and sexual modes of reproduction, occurring most probably in the vector [138]. Sexual fusion may frequently take place between genetically related parasites or even within the same strain with occasional recombination events between individuals of different genotypes.

Also, *L. braziliensis*/*L. peruviana* hybrids were found to be quite common in a Peruvian focus where both species can occur sympatrically [137]. In the Old World, natural *L. infantum*/*L. major* hybrids were experimentally transmitted by *Ph. papatasi*, usually only competent to transmit *L. major* [149]. This suggests that hybrids may circulate using this sand fly vector and spread into new foci throughout the broad range of *Ph. papatasi* distribution.

The fact that *Leishmania* can undergo genetic exchange is potentially of profound epidemiological significance since this could facilitate the emergence and spread of new genotypes and phenotypic traits. Also, hybrid offspring might show a strong selective advantage relative to the parental strains. In [149], the authors have shown that natural hybrids could have enhanced transmission potential and a positively affected fitness.

New high-throughput sequencing technologies have opened the door for population genome analyses and genome-wide association studies. Genome of the *L. major* species was the first to be fully sequenced [150] followed by *L. infantum* and *L. braziliensis* [151]. Comparison of the three genomes revealed conservation of synteny and identified only 200 genes having a differential distribution between the three species. Such genes may encode for proteins implicated in host-pathogen interactions and parasite survival in the macrophage [151]. The species *L. mexicana* and *L. donovani* were subsequently sequenced [152,153] and the reference genomes for *L. major*, *L. infantum*, and *L. braziliensis* were refined [152]. This has allowed the identification of a remarkably low number of genes or paralog groups unique to each of the species *L. mexicana*, *L. major*, *L. infantum*, and *L. braziliensis* (2, 14, 19, and 67, respectively). Besides, *L. major* and *L. infantum* were found to have a surprisingly low number of predicted heterozygous SNPs compared with *L. braziliensis* and *L. mexicana*. Chromosome copy number also varied significantly between species, with nine supernumerary chromosomes in *L. infantum*, four in *L. mexicana*, two in *L. braziliensis*, and one in *L. major*. The authors also showed that gene duplication events occur more frequently on disomic chromosomes [152]. In addition to sequencing of an *L. donovani* reference genome, a recent study also included sequence analysis of a set of 16 related clinical lines, isolated from VL patients in Nepal and India, which also differ in their *in vitro* drug response [153]. Sequence comparisons with other *Leishmania* species and analysis of single-nucleotide diversity showed evidence of selection acting on different surface- and transport-related genes, including genes associated with drug resistance. Extensive variation in chromosome copy number between the analyzed lines was also shown. In association to drug resistance, they also showed structural variation, including gene dosage and copy number variation of a circular episome, present in all lines [153].

Genomic research on *Leishmania* is taking promising directions, mainly upon sequencing of the main pathogenic species [150–153] and also the non pathogenic *L. tarentolae* [154] which will enable to answer key questions on population genetics and ultimately unravel many important aspects related to drug resistance and virulence, which are especially relevant for control of the disease.

Novel genomics technologies are expected to bring more powerful tools to characterize the pathogens and particularly the infectious stages of *Leishmania* parasites. It will be particularly useful to fully characterize the parasites within the lesions/hosts in their microenvironment. While so far expression profiling relied mainly on microarray analysis which revealed only a limited number of differentially expressed genes across developmental stages [155], or species [156]. RNA sequencing technology seems very promising to highlight transcriptional events that are associated to parasite life cycle, infection or pathology. Previous studies have demonstrated a correlation between gene expression and gene copy number [157,158]. It was further hypothesized that "Increased gene copy number due to chromosome amplification may contribute to alterations in gene expression in response to environmental conditions in the host, providing a genetic basis for disease tropism" [152]. Other studies have also suggested that *Leishmania* parasites do not respond dynamically to host immune pressure, and that any influence of varying transcript levels on virulence and pathogenicity of the different *Leishmania* species is likely to result from the differential expression of conserved genes between species and/or the expression of a small number of genes that are differentially distributed between species [159].

Genome-wide multilocus genotyping in malaria research through novel sequencing technologies has allowed the identification of almost 47000 single nucleotide polymorphisms (SNPs) across the *Plasmodium* genome [160]. This allowed development of microarray–based platforms for screening more than 3000 SNPs that were successfully applied for population genetic analyses and genome-wide association studies in *P. falciparum* [161,162]. Similar studies still need to be developed for *Leishmania*.

5. Conclusion

Epidemiological, taxonomic and population genetic studies of *Leishmania* require good sampling methods and appropriate molecular markers that allow discrimination at different levels. Answering key epidemiological questions requires new or improved tools that allow discrimination of *Leishmania* parasites at different levels. The MLEE, considered as gold standard technique, needs cultured parasites and lacks discriminatory power. PCR assays are likely to replace isoenzyme analysis since they enable direct detection and identification of different *Leishmania* species in human and animal samples and also in infected sand flies. Many of the PCR assays described in the literature have proven useful in numerous field studies. However, they still need to be standardized and validated as diagnostic PCR assays and comparisons of the sensitivity and specificity parameters of the different approaches need also validation under routine conditions. In general, more than one assay is necessary to obtain fully satisfactory analysis of field samples. Given emergence context and changing eco-epidemiological trends, multiple tools will be needed to fully investigate the transmitted parasites.

At the strain level differentiation, MLMT has potential for being a gold standard, because on its principle it is expected to be reproducible and brings possibility of data storage and exchange. However, microsatellite markers are largely species-specific in *Leishmania* and different marker sets have to be used according to species. Such databases do not exist yet and data generation will need standardization. It may also require access to automated sequencers and good knowledge of population genetics programs. On the other hand MLST appears potentially as more powerful for phylogenetic and evolutionary studies although less discriminatory than MLMT. It is most probably this technique that will advantageously replace MLEE in the future. Some results showed that the same targets could be used across the *Leishmania* genus, which will enable comparisons of distances between the species but also of the degree of genetic diversity within species [163]. Here also it will require access to automated sequencers and adequate analytical programs. Cost of both approaches are relatively high and inherent limitations will be most likely overcome by the next generation sequencing approaches expected to gain momentum in a near future. *Leishmania* population genomics still needs to be developed and made accessible to researchers in disease endemic countries to best achieve its public health potential.

Parasite knowledge is so far built on strains obtained *in vitro*. Increasing interest in *Leishmania* parasite analyses will likely identify novel genotypes or organisms, a challenge for our current knowledge on parasite taxonomy and assays to identify and characterize parasites. Improving ways to enhance knowledge on parasites within samples remains a priority.

In spite of the increasing potential of sophisticated technologies and techniques, some disease endemic areas still need simple assays for eco-epidemiological investigations or diagnosis as well as capacity building in this highly relevant area to disease control.

Acknowledgements

Research on *Leishmania* Molecular diagnostics in our laboratory has received support from the Ministry of Higher Education and Scientific Research and Technology in Tunisia (BSP46, LR00SP04 & LR11IPT04) and from different international programs: EU–Avicenne (CT920013), STD3 (CT930253), INCO-DC (CT970256); TDR–RSG (ID890266), TDR–RTG (920781), TDR–PAG (A30380); MERC–NIAID–NIH (NO1AI45183); IAEA (TUN06–12; CRP15111); CRDF (TN1–7009–TP–09); AUF (PCSI 6319PS011).

Author details

Souheila Guerbouj, Imen Mkada–Driss and Ikram Guizani

Laboratoire d'Epidemiologie et d'Ecologie Parasitaire / Epidémiologie Moléculaire et Pathologie Expérimentale Appliquée (*Leishmania* Genomics and Genetics Program), Institut Pasteur de Tunis, Université Tunis el Manar, Tunisia

The number of references for this review has been restricted by space restraints. The authors apologize to the authors whose work was not cited in this review.

References

[1] Lainson R, Shaw JJ. New World leishmaniasis–the neotropical Leishmania species. In: Cox FEG, Kreier JP, Wakelin D, editors. Topley & Wilson's *Microbiology and Microbial Infections*. London: Arnold; 1998.

[2] Sacks DL, Kenney RT, Kreutzer RD, Jaffe CL, Gupta AK, Sharma MC, *et al.* Indian kala-azar caused by *Leishmania tropica*. *Lancet*. 1995 Apr 15;345(8955):959-61.

[3] Alvar J, Vélez ID, Bern C, Herrero M, Desjeux P, Cano J, et al.; WHO Leishmaniasis Control Team. Leishmaniasis worldwide and global estimates of its incidence. *PLoS One*. 2012;7(5):e35671.

[4] Guizani I, Mukhtar M, Alvar J, Ben Abderrazak S, Shaw J. (2011) Leishmaniases. In: Nriagu JO, editor. *Encyclopedia of Environmental Health*, volume 3, pp. 453–480. Burlington: Elsevier; 2011.

[5] Schönian G, Mauricio I, Gramiccia M, Cañavate C, Boelaert M, Dujardin JC. Leishmaniases in the Mediterranean in the era of molecular epidemiology. *Trends Parasitol*. 2008 Mar;24(3):135-42.

[6] Jamjoom MB, Ashford RW, Bates PA, Chance ML, Kemp SJ, Watts PC, *et al.* Leishmania donovani is the only cause of visceral leishmaniaisis in East Africa; previous de-

scriptions of L. infantum and "L. archibaldi" from this region are a consequence of convergent evolution in the isoenzyme data. *Parasitology*. 2004 Oct;129(Pt 4):399-409.

[7]   Mauricio IL, Yeo M, Baghaei M, Doto D, Pratlong F, Zemanova E, *et al.* Towards multilocus sequence typing of the Leishmania donovani complex: resolving genotypes and haplotypes for five polymorphic metabolic enzymes (ASAT, GPI, NH1, NH2, PGD). *Int J Parasitol*. 2006 Jun;36(7):757-69.

[8]   Zemanová E, Jirků M, Mauricio IL, Horák A, Miles MA, Lukes J. The Leishmania donovani complex: genotypes of five metabolic enzymes (ICD, ME, MPI, G6PDH, and FH), new targets for multilocus sequence typing. *Int J Parasitol*. 2007 Feb;37(2):149-60.

[9]   Alam MZ, Haralambous C, Kuhls K, Gouzelou E, Sgouras D, Soteriadou K, *et al.* The paraphyletic composition of Leishmania donovani zymodeme MON-37 revealed by multilocus microsatellite typing. *Microbes Infect*. 2009 May-Jun;11(6-7):707-15.

[10] Van Eys GJ, Schoone GJ, Kroon NC, Ebeling SB. Sequence analysis of small subunit ribosomal RNA genes and its use for detection and identification of Leishmania parasites. *Mol Biochem Parasitol*. 1992 Mar;51(1):133-42.

[11] Lachaud L, Marchergui-Hammami S, Chabbert E, Dereure J, Dedet JP, Bastien P. Comparison of six PCR methods using peripheral blood for detection of canine visceral leishmaniasis. *J Clin Microbiol*. 2002 Jan;40(1):210-5.

[12] Schönian G, Nasereddin A, Dinse N, Schweynoch C, Schallig HD, Presber W, *et al.* PCR diagnosis and characterization of Leishmania in local and imported clinical samples. *Diagn Microbiol Infect Dis*. 2003 Sep;47(1):349-58.

[13] Bensoussan E, Nasereddin A, Jonas F, Schnur LF, Jaffe CL. Comparison of PCR assays for diagnosis of cutaneous leishmaniasis. *J Clin Microbiol*. 2006 Apr;44(4):1435-9.

[14] Nicolas L, Prina E, Lang T, Milon G. Real-time PCR for detection and quantitation of leishmania in mouse tissues. *J Clin Microbiol*. 2002 May;40(5):1666-9.

[15] Schulz A, Mellenthin K, Schönian G, Fleischer B, Drosten C. Detection, differentiation, and quantitation of pathogenic leishmania organisms by a fluorescence resonance energy transfer-based real-time PCR assay. *J Clin Microbiol*. 2003 Apr;41(4): 1529-35.

[16] Cupolillo E, Grimaldi Júnior G, Momen H, Beverley SM. Intergenic region typing (IRT): a rapid molecular approach to the characterization and evolution of Leishmania. *Mol Biochem Parasitol*. 1995 Jul;73(1-2):145-55.

[17] Nasereddin A, Bensoussan-Hermano E, Schönian G, Baneth G, Jaffe CL. Molecular diagnosis and species identification of Old World cutaneous leishmaniasis using a reverse line blot hybridization assay. *J Clin Microbiol*. 2008 Sep;46(9):2848-55.

[18] Harris E, Kropp G, Belli A, Rodriguez B, Agabian N. Single-step multiplex PCRassay for characterization of NewWorld Leishmania complexes. *J Clin Microbiol*. 1998 Jul; 36(7):1989-95.

[19] Marfurt J, Niederwieser I, Makia ND, Beck HP, Felger I. Diagnostic genotyping of Old and New World Leishmania species by PCR-RFLP. *Diagn Microbiol Infect Dis*. 2003 Jun;46(2):115-24.

[20] Victoir K, Bañuls AL, Arevalo J, Llanos-Cuentas A, Hamers R, Noël S, *et al*. The gp63 gene locus, a target for genetic characterization of Leishmania belonging to subgenus Viannia. *Parasitology*. 1998 Jul;117(Pt 1):1-13.

[21] Guerbouj S, Victoir K, Guizani I, Seridi N, Nuwayri-Salti N, Belkaid M, *et al*. Gp63 gene polymorphism and population structure of Leishmania donovani complex: influence of the host selection pressure? *Parasitology*. 2001 Jan;122(Pt 1):25-35.

[22] Garcia L, Kindt A, Bermudez H, Llanos-Cuentas A, De Doncker S, Arevalo J, *et al*. Culture-independent species typing of neotropical Leishmania for clinical validation of a PCR-based assay targeting heat shock protein 70 genes. *J Clin Microbiol*. 2004 May;42(5):2294-7.

[23] Fraga J, Montalvo AM, De Doncker S, Dujardin JC, Van der Auwera G. Phylogeny of Leishmania species based on the heat-shock protein 70 gene. *Infect Genet Evol*. 2010 Mar;10(2):238-45.

[24] Da Silva LA, de Sousa Cdos S, da Graça GC, Porrozzi R, Cupolillo E. Sequence analysis and PCR-RFLP profiling of the hsp70 gene as a valuable tool for identifying Leishmania species associated with human leishmaniasis in Brazil. *Infect Genet Evol*. 2010 Jan;10(1):77-83.

[25] Hide M, Bañuls AL. Species-specific PCR assay for L. infantum/L. donovani discrimination. *Acta Trop*. 2006 Dec;100(3):241-5.

[26] Oshaghi MA, Ravasan NM, Hide M, Javadian EA, Rassi Y, Sedaghat MM, *et al*. Development of species-specific PCR and PCR-restriction fragment length polymorphism assays for L.infantum/L. donovani discrimination. *Exp Parasitol*. 2009 May; 122(1):61-5.

[27] Williams JG, Kubelik AR, Livak KJ, Rafalski JA, Tingey SV. DNA polymorphisms amplified by arbitrary primers are useful as genetic markers. *Nucleic Acids Res*. 1990 Nov 25;18(22):6531-5.

[28] Schriefer AL, Góes-Neto A, Guimarães LH, Carvalho LP, Almeida RP, *et al*. Multiclonal Leishmania braziliensis population structure and its clinical implication in a region of endemicity for American tegumentary leishmaniasis. *Infect Immun*. 2004 Jan; 72(1):508-14.

[29] Gomes RF, Macedo AM, Pena SD, Melo MN. Leishmania (Viannia) braziliensis: genetic relationships between strains isolated from different areas of Brazil as revealed by DNA fingerprinting and RAPD. *Exp Parasitol*. 1995 Jun;80(4):681-7.

[30] Motazedian H, Noyes H, Maingon R. Leishmania and Sauroleishmania: the use of random amplified polymorphic DNA for the identification of parasites from vertebrates and invertebrates. *Exp Parasitol*. 1996 Jun;83(1):150-4.

[31] Manna M, Majumder HK, Sundar S, Bhaduri AN. The molecular characterization of clinical isolates from Indian Kala-azar patients by MLEE and RAPD-PCR. *Med Sci Monit*. 2005 Jul;11(7):BR220-7.

[32] Carvalho Mde L, de Andrade AS, Fontes CJ, Hueb M, de Oliveira Silva S, Melo MN. Leishmania (Viannia) braziliensis is the prevalent species infecting patients with tegumentary leishmaniasis from Mato Grosso State, Brazil. *Acta Trop*. 2006 Jul;98(3): 277-85.

[33] Noyes HA, Belli AA, Maingon R. Appraisal of various random amplified polymorphic DNA-polymerase chain reaction primers for Leishmania identification. *Am J Trop Med Hyg*. 1996 Jul;55(1):98-105.

[34] Hanafi R, Barhoumi M, Ali SB, Guizani I. Molecular analyses of Old World Leishmania RAPD markers and development of a PCR assay selective for parasites of the L. donovani species Complex. *Exp Parasitol*. 2001 Jun;98(2):90-9.

[35] Diakou A, Dovas CI. Optimization of random-amplified polymorphic DNA producing amplicons up to 8500 bp and revealing intraspecies polymorphism in Leishmania infantum isolates. *Anal Biochem*. 2001 Jan 15;288(2):195-200.

[36] Guizani I, Dellagi K, Ismaïl RB. Random amplified polymorphic DNA technique for identification and differentiation of Old World Leishmania species. *Am J Trop Med Hyg*. 2002 Feb;66(2):152-6.

[37] Bañuls AL, Guerrini F, Le Pont F, Barrera C, Espinel I, Guderian R, *et al.* Evidence for hybridization by multilocus enzyme electrophoresis and random amplified polymorphic DNA between Leishmania braziliensis and Leishmania panamemsis/ guyanensis in Ecuador. *J Eukaryot Microbiol*. 1997 Sep-Oct;44(5):408-11.

[38] Bañuls AL, Jonquieres R, Guerrini F, Le Pont F, Barrera C, Espinel I, *et al.* Genetic analysis of Leishmania parasites in Ecuador : are Leishmania (Viannia) panamensis and Leishmania (V.) guyanensis distinct taxa ? *Am J Trop Med Hyg*. 1999 Nov;61(5): 838-45.

[39] Mauricio IL, Howard MK, Stothard JR, Miles MA. Genomic diversity in the Leishmania donovani complex. *Parasitology*. 1999 Sep;119 (Pt 3):237-46.

[40] Rioux JA, Lanotte G, Serres E, Pratlong F, Bastien P, Perieres J. Taxonomy of Leishmania. Use of isoenzymes. Suggestions for a new classification. *Ann Parasitol Hum Comp*. 1990;65(3):111-25.

[41] Zemanová E, Jirků M, Mauricio IL, Miles MA, Lukes J. Genetic polymorphism within the Leishmania donovani complex: correlation with geographic origin. *Am J Trop Med Hyg*. 2004 Jun;70(6):613-7.

[42] Toledo A, Martín-Sánchez J, Pesson B, Sanchiz-Marín C, Morillas-Márquez F. Genetic variability within the species Leishmania infantum by RAPD. A lack of correlation with zymodeme structure. *Mol Biochem Parasitol*. 2002 Feb;119(2):257-64.

[43] Hide M, Bañuls AL, Tibayrenc M. Genetic heterogeneity and phylogenetic status of Leishmania (Leishmania) infantum zymodeme MON-1: epidemiological implications. *Parasitology*. 2001 Nov;123(Pt 5):425-32.

[44] Segatto M, Ribeiro LS, Costa DL, Costa CH, Oliveira MR, Carvalho SF, *et al*. Genetic diversity of Leishmania infantum field populations from Brazil. *Mem Inst Oswaldo Cruz*. 2012 Feb;107(1):39-47.

[45] Cupolillo E, Brahim LR, Toaldo CB, de Oliveira-Neto MP, de Brito ME, Falqueto A, *et al*. Genetic polymorphism and molecular epidemiology of Leishmania (Viannia) braziliensis from different hosts and geographic areas in Brazil. *J Clin Microbiol*. 2003 Jul; 41(7):3126-32.

[46] Khanra S, Bandopadhyay SK, Chakraborty P, Datta S, Mondal D, Chatterjee M, *et al*. Characterization of the recent clinical isolates of Indian Kala-azar patients by RAPD-PCR method. *J Parasit Dis*. 2011 Oct;35(2):116-22.

[47] Khanra S, Datta S, Mondal D, Saha P, Bandopadhyay SK, Roy S, *et al*. RFLPs of ITS, ITS1 and hsp70 amplicons and sequencing of ITS1 of recent clinical isolates of Kala-azar from India and Bangladesh confirms the association of L. tropica with the disease. *Acta Trop*. 2012 Dec;124(3):229-34.

[48] Mahmoudzadeh-Niknam H, Ajdary S, Riazi-Rad F, Mirzadegan E, Rezaeian A, Khaze V, *et al*. Molecular epidemiology of cutaneous leishmaniasis and heterogeneity of Leishmania major strains in Iran. *Trop Med Int Health*. 2012 Nov;17(11):1335-44.

[49] Martinez E, Alonso V, Quispe A, Thomas MC, Alonso R, Piñero JE, González AC, Ortega A, Valladares B. RAPD method useful for distinguishing Leishmania species: design of specific primers for L. braziliensis. *Parasitology*. 2003 Dec;127(Pt 6):513-7.

[50] Lewin S, Schönian G, El Tai N, Oskam L, Bastien P, Presber W. Strain typing in Leishmania donovani by using sequence-confirmed amplified region analysis. *Int J Parasitol*. 2002 Sep;32(10):1267-76.

[51] Mkada-Driss I, Lahmadi R, Chakroun AS, Talbi C, Elamin EM, Cupollilo E, *et al*. Screening and characterization of RAPD polymorphic markers in viscerotropic Leishmania parasites. In preparation.

[52] Mkada-Driss I, Talbi C, Elamin EM, Lahmadi R, Bakhiet S, Fathallah-Mili A, *et al*. Simple DNA assays for molecular epidemiology of visceral leishmaniasis in Africa:

development and evaluation of species and countries specific PCR assays. In preparation.

[53]   Mauricio IL, Gaunt MW, Stothard JR, Miles MA. Glycoprotein 63 (gp63) genes show gene conversion and reveal the evolution of Old World Leishmania. *Int J Parasitol.* 2007 Apr;37(5):565-76.

[54]   Guerbouj S, Chamekh L, Jlassi M, Jbir R, Guizani I. Genetic polymorphism of Tunisian Leishmania infantum species by restriction analysis of PCR amplified gp63 and PSA2 coding genes. Personal communication.

[55]   BenSaid M, Guerbouj S, Saghrouni F, Fathallah-Mili A, Guizani I. Occurrence of Leishmania infantum cutaneous leishmaniasis in central Tunisia. *Trans R Soc Trop Med Hyg.* 2006 Jun;100(6):521-6.

[56]   Elamin EM, Guerbouj S, Musa AM, Guizani I, Khalil EA, Mukhtar MM, *et al.* Uncommon clinical presentations of cutaneous leishmaniasis in Sudan. *Trans R Soc Trop Med Hyg.* 2005 Nov;99(11):803-8.

[57]   Elamin EM, Guizani I, Guerbouj S, Gramiccia M, El Hassan AM, Di Muccio T, *et al.* Identification of Leishmania donovani as a cause of cutaneous leishmaniasis in Sudan. *Trans R Soc Trop Med Hyg.* 2008 Jan;102(1):54-7.

[58]   Mauricio IL, Gaunt MW, Stothard JR, Miles MA. Genetic typing and phylogeny of the Leishmania donovani complex by restriction analysis of PCR amplified gp63 intergenic regions. *Parasitology.* 2001 Apr;122(Pt 4):393-403.

[59]   Al-Jawabreh A, Schnur LF, Nasereddin A, Schwenkenbecher JM, Abdeen Z, Barghuthy F, *et al.* The recent emergence of Leishmania tropica in Jericho (A'riha) and its environs, a classical focus of L. major. *Trop Med Int Health.* 2004 Jul;9(7):812-6.

[60]   Rhajaoui M, Nasereddin A, Fellah H, Azmi K, Amarir F, Al-Jawabreh A, *et al.* New clinico-epidemiologic profile of cutaneous leishmaniasis, Morocco. *Emerg Infect Dis.* 2007 Sep;13(9):1358-60.

[61]   Kuhls K, Mauricio IL, Pratlong F, Presber W, Schönian G. Analysis of ribosomal DNA internal transcribed spacer sequences of the Leishmania donovani complex. *Microbes Infect.* 2005 Aug-Sep;7(11-12):1224-34.

[62]   Talmi-Frank D, Nasereddin A, Schnur LF, Schönian G, Töz SO, Jaffe CL, *et al.* Detection and identification of Old World Leishmania by high resolution melt analysis. *PLoS Negl Trop Dis.* 2010 Jan 12;4(1):e581.

[63]   De Almeida ME, Steurer FJ, Koru O, Herwaldt BL, Pieniazek NJ, da Silva AJ. Identification of Leishmania spp. by molecular amplification and DNA sequencing analysis of a fragment of rRNA internal transcribed spacer 2. *J Clin Microbiol.* 2011 Sep;49(9): 3143-9.

[64]   El Tai NO, Osman OF, el Fari M, Presber W, Schönian G. Genetic heterogeneity of ribosomal internal transcribed spacer in clinical samples of Leishmania donovani

spotted on filter paper as revealed by single-strand conformation polymorphisms and sequencing. *Trans R Soc Trop Med Hyg.* 2000 Sep-Oct;94(5):575-9.

[65] El Tai NO, El Fari M, Mauricio I, Miles MA, Oskam L, El Safi SH, *et al.* Leishmania donovani: intra-specific polymorphisms of Sudanese isolates revealed by PCR-based analyses and DNA sequencing. *Exp Parasitol.* 2001 Jan;97(1):35-44.

[66] Schönian G, Schnur L, el Fari M, Oskam L, Kolesnikov AA, Sokolowska-Köhler W, *et al.* Genetic heterogeneity in the species Leishmania tropica revealed by different PCR-based methods. *Trans R Soc Trop Med Hyg.* 2001 Mar-Apr;95(2):217-24.

[67] Schönian G, El Fari M, Lewin S, Schweynoch C, Presber W. Molecular epidemiology and population genetics in Leishmania. *Med Microbiol Immunol.* 2001 Nov;190(1-2): 61-3.

[68] Tashakori M, Kuhls K, Al-Jawabreh A, Mauricio IL, Schönian G, Farajnia S, *et al.* Leishmania major: genetic heterogeneity of Iranian isolates by single-strand conformation polymorphism and sequence analysis of ribosomal DNA internal transcribed spacer. *Acta Trop.* 2006 Apr;98(1):52-8.

[69] Ghatee M, Sharifi I, Mirhendi H, Kanannejad Z, Hatam G. Investigation of Double-Band Electrophoretic Pattern of ITS-rDNA Region in Iranian Isolates of Leishmania tropica. *Iran J Parasitol.* 2013 Apr;8(2):264-72.

[70] Hartl FU, Hayer-Hartl M. Molecular chaperones in the cytosol: from nascent chain to folded protein. *Science.* 2002 Mar 8;295(5561):1852-8.

[71] Folgueira C, Requena JM. A postgenomic view of the heat shock proteins in kinetoplastids. *FEMS Microbiol Rev.* 2007 Jul;31(4):359-77.

[72] Montalvo AM, Fraga J, Monzote L, Montano I, De Doncker S, Dujardin JC, *et al.* Heat-shock protein 70 PCR-RFLP: a universal simple tool for *Leishmania* species discrimination in the New and Old World. *Parasitology.* 2010 Jul;137(8):1159-68.

[73] Montalvo AM, Fraga J, Maes I, Dujardin JC, Van der Auwera G. Three new sensitive and specific heat-shock protein 70 PCRs for global *Leishmania* species identification. *Eur J Clin Microbiol Infect Dis.* 2012 Jul;31(7):1453-61.

[74] Fraga J, Montalvo AM, Maes L, Dujardin JC, Van der Auwera G. HindII and SduI digests of heat-shock protein 70 PCR for *Leishmania* typing. *Diagn Microbiol Infect Dis.* 2013 Nov;77(3):245-7.

[75] Fraga J, Veland N, Montalvo AM, Praet N, Boggild AK, Valencia BM, *et al.* Accurate and rapid species typing from cutaneous and mucocutaneous leishmaniasis lesions of the New World. *Diagn Microbiol Infect Dis.* 2012 Oct;74(2):142-50.

[76] Van der Auwera G, Maes I, De Doncker S, Ravel C, Cnops L, Van Esbroeck M, *et al.* Heat-shock protein 70 gene sequencing for *Leishmania* species typing in European tropical infectious disease clinics. *Euro Surveill.* 2013 Jul 25;18(30):20543.

[77] Requena JM, Chicharro C, García L, Parrado R, Puerta CJ, Cañavate C. Sequence analysis of the 3'-untranslated region of HSP70 (type I) genes in the genus *Leishmania*: its usefulness as a molecular marker for species identification. *Parasit Vectors*. 2012 Apr 28;5:87.

[78] Serin MS, Waki K, Chang KP, Aslan G, Direkel S, Otag F, *et al.* Consistence of miniexon polymerase chain reaction–restriction fragment length polymorphism and single-copy gene sequence analyses in discriminating Leishmania genotypes. *Diagn Microbiol Infect Dis*. 2007 Mar;57(3):295-9.

[79] Marfurt J, Nasereddin A, Niederwieser I, Jaffe CL, Beck HP, Felger I. Identification and differentiation of Leishmania species in clinical samples by PCR amplification of the miniexon sequence and subsequent restriction fragment length polymorphism analysis. *J Clin Microbiol*. 2003 Jul;41(7):3147-53.

[80] Serin MS, Daglioglu K, Bagirova M, Allahverdiyev A, Uzun S, Vural Z, *et al.* Rapid diagnosis and genotyping of Leishmania isolates from cutaneous and visceral leishmaniasis by microcapillary cultivation and polymerase chain reaction-restriction fragment length polymorphism of miniexon region. *Diagn Microbiol Infect Dis*. 2005 Nov;53(3):209-14.

[81] Pandey K, Yanagi T, Pandey BD, Mallik AK, Sherchand JB, Kanbara H. Characterization of Leishmania isolates from Nepalese patients with visceral leishmaniasis. *Parasitol Res*. 2007 May;100(6):1361-9.

[82] Roelfsema JH, Nozari N, Herremans T, Kortbeek LM, Pinelli E. Evaluation and improvement of two PCR targets in molecular typing of clinical samples of Leishmania patients. *Exp Parasitol*. 2011 Jan;127(1):36-41.

[83] Quispe Tintaya KW, Ying X, Dedet JP, Rijal S, De Bolle X, Dujardin JC. Antigen genes for molecular epidemiology of leishmaniasis: polymorphism of cysteine proteinase B and surface metalloprotease glycoprotein 63 in the Leishmania donovani complex. *J Infect Dis*. 2004 Mar 15;189(6):1035-43.

[84] Seridi N, Belkaid M, Quispe-Tintaya W, Zidane C, Dujardin JC. Application of PCR-RFLP for the exploration of the molecular diversity of Leishmania infantum in Algeria. *Trans R Soc Trop Med Hyg*. 2008 Jun;102(6):556-63.

[85] Chaouch M, Fathallah-Mili A, Driss M, Lahmadi R, Ayari C, Guizani I, *et al.* Identification of Tunisian Leishmania spp. by PCR amplification of cysteine proteinase B (cpb) genes and phylogenetic analysis. *Acta Trop*. 2013 Mar;125(3):357-65.

[86] Laurent T, Van der Auwera G, Hide M, Mertens P, Quispe-Tintaya W, Deborggraeve S, *et al.* Identification of Old World Leishmania spp. by specific polymerase chain reaction amplification of cysteine proteinase B genes and rapid dipstick detection. *Diagn Microbiol Infect Dis*. 2009 Feb;63(2):173-81.

[87] Kuru T, Janusz N, Gadisa E, Gedamu L, Aseffa A. Leishmania aethiopica: development of specific and sensitive PCR diagnostic test. *Exp Parasitol*. 2011 Aug;128(4): 391-5.

[88] Chaouch M, Mhadhbi M, Adams ER, Schoone GJ, Limam S, Gharbi Z, *et al*. Development and evaluation of a loop-mediated isothermal amplification assay for rapid detection of Leishmania infantum in canine leishmaniasis based on cysteine protease B genes. *Vet Parasitol*. 2013 Nov 15;198(1-2):78-84.

[89] Notomi T, Okayama H, Masubuchi H, Yonekawa T, Watanabe K, Amino N, *et al*. Loop-mediated isothermal amplification of DNA. *Nucleic Acids Res*. 2000 Jun 15;28(12):E63.

[90] Adams ER, Schoone GJ, Ageed AF, Safi SE, Schallig HD. Development of a reverse transcriptase loopo-mediated isothermal amplification (LAMP) assay for the sensitive detection of Leishmania parasites in clinical samples. *Am J Trop Med Hyg*. 2010 Apr;82(4):591-6.

[91] Ibrahim ME, Barker DC. The origin and evolution of the Leishmania donovani complex as inferred from a mitochondrial cytochrome oxidase II gene sequence. *Infect Genet Evol*. 2001 Jul;1(1):61-8.

[92] Luyo-Acero GE, Uezato H, Oshiro M, Takei K, Kariya K, Katakura K, *et al*. Sequence variation of the cytochrome b gene of various human infecting members of the genus Leishmania and their phylogeny. *Parasitology*. 2004 May;128(Pt 5):483-91.

[93] Lainson R, Shaw JJ. Evolution, classification and geographical distribution. In: Peters W, Killick-Kendrick R, editors. The Leishmaniasis in Biology and Medicine. Vol. I *Biology and Epidemiology*. Orlando, USA: Orlando Academic Press; 1987.

[94] Asato Y, Oshiro M, Myint CK, Yamamoto Y, Kato H, Marco JD, *et al*. Phylogenic analysis of the genus Leishmania by cytochrome b gene sequencing. *Exp Parasitol*. 2009 Apr;121(4):352-61.

[95] Marco JD, Bhutto AM, Soomro FR, Baloch JH, Barroso PA, Kato H, *et al*. Multilocus enzyme electrophoresis and cytochrome B gene sequencing-based identification of Leishmania isolates from different foci of cutaneous leishmaniasis in Pakistan. *Am J Trop Med Hyg*. 2006 Aug;75(2):261-6.

[96] Myint CK, Asato Y, Yamamoto Y, Kato H, Bhutto AM, Soomro FR, *et al*. Polymorphisms of cytochrome b gene in Leishmania parasites and their relation to types of cutaneous leishmaniasis lesions in Pakistan. *J Dermatol*. 2008 Feb;35(2):76-85.

[97] Martínez LP, Rebollo JA, Luna AL, Cochero S, Bejarano EE. Molecular identification of the parasites causing cutaneous leishmaniasis on the Caribbean coast of Colombia. *Parasitol Res*. 2010 Feb;106(3):647-52.

[98] Yang BB, Chen DL, Chen JP, Liao L, Hu XS, Xu JN. Analysis of kinetoplast cytochrome b gene of 16 Leishmania isolates from different foci of China: different spe-

cies of Leishmania in China and their phylogenetic inference. *Parasit Vectors*. 2013 Feb 5;6:32.

[99]   Akopyants NS, Kimblin N, Secundino N, Patrick R, Peters N, Lawyer P, *et al.* Demonstration of genetic exchange during cyclical development of Leishmania in the sand fly vector. *Science* 2009 Apr 10;324(5924):265-8.

[100] Sadlova J, Yeo M, Seblova V, Lewis MD, Mauricio I, Volf P, *et al.* Visualisation of Leishmania donovani fluorescent hybrids during early stage development in the sand fly vector. *PLoS One*. 2011;6(5):e19851.

[101] Lombardo G, Pennisi MG, Lupo T, Migliazzo A, Caprì A, Solano-Gallego L. Detection of Leishmania infantum DNA by real-time PCR in canine oral and conjunctival swabs and comparison with other diagnostic techniques. *Vet Parasitol*. 2012 Feb 28;184(1):10-7.

[102] Da Silva RN, Amorim AC, Brandão RM, de Andrade HM, Yokoo M, Ribeiro ML, *et al.* Real-time PCR in clinical practice: a powerful tool for evaluating Leishmania chagasi loads in naturally infected dogs. *Ann Trop Med Parasitol*. 2010 Mar;104(2):137-43.

[103] De Paiva Cavalcanti M, Felinto de Brito ME, de Souza WV, de Miranda Gomes Y, Abath FG. The development of a real-time PCR assay for the quantification of Leishmania infantum DNA in canine blood. *Vet J*. 2009 Nov;182(2):356-8.

[104] Antinori S, Calattini S, Piolini R, Longhi E, Bestetti G, Cascio A, *et al.* Is real-time polymerase chain reaction (PCR) more useful than a conventional PCR for the clinical management of leishmaniasis? *Am J Trop Med Hyg*. 2009 Jul;81(1):46-51.

[105] Weirather JL, Jeronimo SM, Gautam S, Sundar S, Kang M, Kurtz MA, *et al.* Serial quantitative PCR assay for detection, species discrimination, and quantification of Leishmania spp. in human samples. *J Clin Microbiol*. 2011 Nov;49(11):3892-904.

[106] Jara M, Adaui V, Valencia BM, Martinez D, Alba M, Castrillon C, *et al.* Real-time PCR assay for detection and quantification of Leishmania (Viannia) organisms in skin and mucosal lesions: exploratory study of parasite load and clinical parameters. *J Clin Microbiol*. 2013 Jun;51(6):1826-33.

[107] De Paiva Cavalcanti M, Dantas-Torres F, da Cunha Gonçalves de Albuquerque S, Silva de Morais RC, de Brito ME, Otranto D, *et al.* Quantitative real time PCR assays for the detection of Leishmania (Viannia) braziliensis in animals and humans. *Mol Cell Probes*. 2013 Jun-Aug;27(3-4):122-8.

[108] Kumar A, Boggula VR, Misra P, Sundar S, Shasany AK, Dube A. Amplified fragment length polymorphism (AFLP) analysis is useful for distinguishing Leishmania species of visceral and cutaneous forms. *Acta Trop*. 2010 Feb;113(2):202-6.

[109] Odiwuor S, Vuylsteke M, De Doncker S, Maes I, Mbuchi M, Dujardin JC, *et al.* Leishmania AFLP: paving the way towards improved molecular assays and markers of diversity. *Infect Genet Evol*. 2011 Jul;11(5):960-7.

[110] Kumar A, Misra P, Dube A. Amplified fragment length polymorphism: an adept technique for genome mapping, genetic differentiation, and intraspecific variation in protozoan parasites. *Parasitol Res*. 2013 Feb;112(2):457-66.

[111] Van der Meide WF, Schoone GJ, Faber WR, Zeegelaar JE, de Vries HJ, Ozbel Y, *et al.* Quantitative nucleic acid sequence-based assay as a new molecular tool for detection and quantification of Leishmania parasites in skin biopsy samples. *J Clin Microbiol*. 2005 Nov;43(11):5560-6.

[112] Takagi H, Itoh M, Islam MZ, Razzaque A, Ekram AR, Hashighuchi Y, *et al.* Sensitive, specific, and rapid detection of Leishmania donovani DNA by loop-mediated isothermal amplification. *Am J Trop Med Hyg*. 2009 Oct;81(4):578-82.

[113] Khan MG, Bhaskar KR, Salam MA, Akther T, Pluschke G, Mondal D. Diagnostic accuracy of loop-mediated isothermal amplification (LAMP) for detection of Leishmania DNA in buffy coat from visceral leishmaniasis patients. *Parasit Vectors*. 2012 Dec 3;5:280.

[114] Lukes J, Mauricio IL, Schönian G, Dujardin JC, Soteriadou K, Dedet JP, *et al.* Evolutionary and geographical history of the Leishmania donovani complex with a revision of current taxonomy. *Proc Natl Acad Sci U S A*. 2007 May 29;104(22):9375-80.

[115] Ravel C, Cortes S, Pratlong F, Morio F, Dedet JP, Campino L. First report of genetic hybrids between two very divergent Leishmania species: Leishmania infantum and Leishmania major. *Int J Parasitol*. 2006 Nov;36(13):1383-8.

[116] El Baidouri F, Diancourt L, Berry V, Chevenet F, Pratlong F, Marty P, *et al.* Genetic structure and evolution of the Leishmania genus in Africa and Eurasia: what does MLSA tell us. *PLoS Negl Trop Dis*. 2013 Jun 13;7(6):e2255.

[117] Boité MC, Mauricio IL, Miles MA, Cupolillo E. New insights on taxonomy, phylogeny and population genetics of Leishmania (Viannia) parasites based on multilocus sequence analysis. *PLoS Negl Trop Dis*. 2012;6(11):e1888.

[118] Tsukayama P, Lucas C, Bacon DJ. Typing of four genetic loci discriminates among closely related species of New World Leishmania. *Int J Parasitol*. 2009 Feb;39(3): 355-62.

[119] Tsukayama P, Núñez JH, De Los Santos M, Soberón V, Lucas CM, Matlashewski G, *et al.* A FRET-based real-time PCR assay to identify the main causal agents of New World tegumentary leishmaniasis. *PLoS Negl Trop Dis*. 2013;7(1):e1956.

[120] Bulle B, Millon L, Bart JM, Gállego M, Gambarelli F, Portús M, *et al.* Practical approach for typing strains of Leishmania infantum by microsatellite analysis. *J Clin Microbiol*. 2002 Sep;40(9):3391-7.

[121] Jamjoom MB, Ashford RW, Bates PA, Kemp SJ, Noyes HA. Towards a standard battery of microsatellite markers for the analysis of the Leishmania donovani complex. *Ann Trop Med Parasitol*. 2002 Apr;96(3):265-70.

[122] Ochsenreither S, Kuhls K, Schaar M, Presber W, Schönian G. Multilocus microsatellite typing as a new tool for discrimination of Leishmania infantum MON-1 strains. *J Clin Microbiol*. 2006 Feb;44(2):495-503.

[123] Jamjoom MB, Ashford RW, Bates PA, Kemp SJ, Noyes HA. Polymorphic microsatellite repeats are not conserved between Leishmania donovani and Leishmania major. *Molecular Ecology Notes*. 2002 June;2(2):104–6.

[124] Al-Jawabreh A, Diezmann S, Müller M, Wirth T, Schnur LF, Strelkova MV, *et al*. Identification of geographically distributed subpopulations of Leishmania (Leishmania) major by microsatellite analysis. *BMC Evol Biol*. 2008 Jun 24;8:183.

[125] Schwenkenbecher JM, Wirth T, Schnur LF, Jaffe CL, Schallig H, Al-Jawabreh A, *et al*. Microsatellite analysis reveals genetic structure of Leishmania tropica. *Int J Parasitol*. 2006 Feb;36(2):237-46.

[126] Russell R, Iribar MP, Lambson B, Brewster S, Blackwell JM, Dye C, *et al*. Intra and inter-specific microsatellite variation in the Leishmania subgenus Viannia. *Mol Biochem Parasitol*. 1999 Sep 20;103(1):71-7.

[127] Rougeron V, Waleckx E, Hide M, DE Meeûs T, Arevalo J, Llanos-Cuentas A, *et al*. PERMANENT GENETIC RESOURCES: A set of 12 microsatellite loci for genetic studies of Leishmania braziliensis. *Mol Ecol Resour*. 2008 Mar;8(2):351-3.

[128] Oddone R, Schweynoch C, Schönian G, de Sousa Cdos S, Cupolillo E, Espinosa D, *et al*. Development of a multilocus microsatellite typing approach for discriminating strains of Leishmania (Viannia) species. *J Clin Microbiol*. 2009 Sep;47(9):2818-25.

[129] Kuhls K, Keilonat L, Ochsenreither S, Schaar M, Schweynoch C, Presber W, *et al*. Multilocus microsatellite typing (MLMT) reveals genetically isolated populations between and within the main endemic regions of visceral leishmaniasis. *Microbes Infect*. 2007 Mar;9(3):334-43.

[130] Alam MZ, Kuhls K, Schweynoch C, Sundar S, Rijal S, Shamsuzzaman AK, *et al*. Multilocus microsatellite typing (MLMT) reveals genetic homogeneity of Leishmania donovani strains in the Indian subcontinent. *Infect Genet Evol*. 2009 Jan;9(1):24-31.

[131] Seridi N, Amro A, Kuhls K, Belkaid M, Zidane C, Al-Jawabreh A, *et al*. Genetic polymorphism of Algerian Leishmania infantum strains revealed by multilocus microsatellite analysis. *Microbes Infect*. 2008 Oct;10(12-13):1309-15.

[132] Chargui N, Amro A, Haouas N, Schönian G, Babba H, Schmidt S, *et al*. Population structure of Tunisian Leishmania infantum and evidence for the existence of hybrids and gene flow between genetically different populations. *Int J Parasitol*. 2009 Jun; 39(7):801-11.

[133] Amro A, Schönian G, Al-Sharabati MB, Azmi K, Nasereddin A, Abdeen Z, *et al*. Population genetics of Leishmania infantum in Israel and the Palestinian Authority through microsatellite analysis. *Microbes Infect*. 2009 Apr;11(4):484-92.

[134] Montoya L, Gállego M, Gavignet B, Piarroux R, Rioux JA, Portús M, *et al.* Application of microsatellite genotyping to the study of a restricted Leishmania infantum focus: different genotype compositions in isolates from dogs and sand flies. *Am J Trop Med Hyg.* 2007 May;76(5):888-95.

[135] Kuhls K, Alam MZ, Cupolillo E, Ferreira GE, Mauricio IL, Oddone R, *et al.* Comparative microsatellite typing of new world leishmania infantum reveals low heterogeneity among populations and its recent old world origin. *PLoS Negl Trop Dis.* 2011 Jun; 5(6):e1155.

[136] Siriwardana HV, Noyes HA, Beeching NJ, Chance ML, Karunaweera ND, Bates PA. Leishmania donovani and cutaneous leishmaniasis, Sri Lanka. *Emerg Infect Dis.* 2007 Mar;13(3):476-8.

[137] Nolder D, Roncal N, Davies CR, Llanos-Cuentas A, Miles MA. Multiple hybrid genotypes of Leishmania (Viannia) in a focus of mucocutaneous leishmaniasis. *Am J Trop Med Hyg.* 2007 Mar;76(3):573-8.

[138] Rougeron V, De Meeûs T, Hide M, Waleckx E, Bermudez H, Arevalo J, *et al.* Extreme inbreeding in Leishmania braziliensis. *Proc Natl Acad Sci U S A.* 2009 Jun 23;106(25): 10224-9.

[139] Rougeron V, De Meeûs T, Hide M, Waleckx E, Dereure J, Arevalo J, *et al.* A battery of 12 microsatellite markers for genetic analysis of the Leishmania (Viannia) guyanensis complex. *Parasitology.* 2010 Nov;137(13):1879-84.

[140] Alam MZ, Kovalenko DA, Kuhls K, Nasyrova RM, Ponomareva VI, Fatullaeva AA, *et al.* Identification of the agent causing visceral leishmaniasis in Uzbeki and Tajiki foci by analysing parasite DNA extracted from patients' Giemsa-stained tissue preparations. *Parasitology.* 2009 Aug;136(9):981-6.

[141] Tibayrenc M, Ayala FJ. Reproductive clonality of pathogens: a perspective on pathogenic viruses, bacteria, fungi, and parasitic protozoa. *Proc Natl Acad Sci U S A.* 2012 Nov 27;109(48):E3305-13.

[142] Tibayrenc M, Ayala FJ. How clonal are Trypanosoma and Leishmania? *Trends Parasitol.* 2013 Jun;29(6):264-9.

[143] Delgado O, Cupolillo E, Bonfante-Garrido R, Silva S, Belfort E, Grimaldi Júnior G, *et al.* Cutaneous leishmaniasis in Venezuela caused by infection with a new hybrid between Leishmania (Viannia) braziliensis and L. (V.) guyanensis. *Mem Inst Oswaldo Cruz.* 1997 Sep-Oct;92(5):581-2.

[144] Dujardin JC, Banuls AL, Llanos-Cuentas A, Alvarez E, DeDoncker S, Jacquet D, *et al.* Putative Leishmania hybrids in the Eastern Andean valley of Huanuco, Peru. *Acta Trop.* 1995 Aug;59(4):293-307.

[145]   Belli AA, Miles MA, Kelly JM. A putative Leishmania panamensis/Leishmania brazil-
        iensis hybrid is a causative agent of human cutaneous leishmaniasis in Nicaragua.
        Parasitology. 1994 Nov;109 (Pt 4):435-42.

[146]   Kelly JM, Law JM, Chapman CJ, Van Eys GJ, Evans DA. Evidence of genetic recombi-
        nation in Leishmania. *Mol Biochem Parasitol.* 1991 Jun;46(2):253-63.

[147]   Miles MA, Yeo M, Mauricio IL. Genetics. Leishmania exploit sex. *Science.* 2009 Apr
        10;324(5924):187-9.

[148]   Inbar E, Akopyants NS, Charmoy M, Romano A, Lawyer P, Elnaiem DE, *et al.* The
        mating competence of geographically diverse Leishmania major strains in their natu-
        ral and unnatural sand fly vectors. *PLoS Genet.* 2013 Jul;9(7):e1003672.

[149]   Volf P, Benkova I, Myskova J, Sadlova J, Campino L, Ravel C. Increased transmission
        potential of Leishmania major/Leishmania infantum hybrids. *Int J Parasitol.* 2007
        May;37(6):589-93.

[150]   Ivens AC, Peacock CS, Worthey EA, Murphy L, Aggarwal G, Berriman M, *et al.* The
        genome of the kinetoplastid parasite, Leishmania major. *Science.* 2005 Jul
        15;309(5733):436-42.

[151]   Peacock CS, Seeger K, Harris D, Murphy L, Ruiz JC, Quail MA, *et al.* Comparative
        genomic analysis of three Leishmania species that cause diverse human disease. *Nat
        Genet.* 2007 Jul;39(7):839-47.

[152]   Rogers MB, Hilley JD, Dickens NJ, Wilkes J, Bates PA, Depledge DP, *et al.* Chromo-
        some and gene copy number variation allow major structural change between spe-
        cies and strains of Leishmania. *Genome Res.* 2011 Dec;21(12):2129-42.

[153]   Downing T, Imamura H, Decuypere S, Clark TG, Coombs GH, Cotton JA, *et al.*
        Whole genome sequencing of multiple Leishmania donovani clinical isolates pro-
        vides insights into population structure and mechanisms of drug resistance. *Genome
        Res.* 2011 Dec;21(12):2143-56.

[154]   Raymond F, Boisvert S, Roy G, Ritt JF, Légaré D, Isnard A, *et al.* Genome sequencing
        of the lizard parasite Leishmania tarentolae reveals loss of genes associated to the in-
        tracellular stage of human pathogenic species. *Nucleic Acids Res.* 2012 Feb;40(3):
        1131-47.

[155]   Srividya G, Duncan R, Sharma P, Raju BV, Nakhasi HL, Salotra P. Transcriptome
        analysis during the process of in vitro differentiation of Leishmania donovani using
        genomic microarrays. *Parasitology.* 2007 Oct;134(Pt 11):1527-39.

[156]   Rochette A, Raymond F, Ubeda JM, Smith M, Messier N, Boisvert S, *et al.* Genome-
        wide gene expression profiling analysis of Leishmania major and Leishmania infan-
        tum developmental stages reveals substantial differences between the two species.
        BMC Genomics. 2008 May 29;9:255.

[157] Ubeda JM, Légaré D, Raymond F, Ouameur AA, Boisvert S, Rigault P, *et al*. Modulation of gene expression in drug resistant Leishmania is associated with gene amplification, gene deletion and chromosome aneuploidy. *Genome Biol*. 2008;9(7):R115.

[158] Leprohon P, Légaré D, Raymond F, Madore E, Hardiman G, Corbeil J, *et al*. Gene expression modulation is associated with gene amplification, supernumerary chromosomes and chromosome loss in antimony-resistant Leishmania infantum. *Nucleic Acids Res*. 2009 Apr;37(5):1387-99.

[159] Depledge DP, Evans KJ, Ivens AC, Aziz N, Maroof A, Kaye PM, *et al*. Comparative expression profiling of Leishmania: modulation in gene expression between species and in different host genetic backgrounds. *PLoS Negl Trop Dis*. 2009 Jul 7;3(7):e476.

[160] Volkman SK, Sabeti PC, DeCaprio D, Neafsey DE, Schaffner SF, Milner DA Jr, *et al*. A genome-wide map of diversity in Plasmodium falciparum. *Nat Genet*. 2007 Jan;39(1): 113-9.

[161] Neafsey DE, Schaffner SF, Volkman SK, Park D, Montgomery P, Milner DA Jr, *et al*. Genome-wide SNP genotyping highlights the role of natural selection in Plasmodium falciparum population divergence. *Genome Biol*. 2008;9(12):R171.

[162] Mu J, Myers RA, Jiang H, Liu S, Ricklefs S, Waisberg M, *et al*. Plasmodium falciparum genome-wide scans for positive selection, recombination hot spots and resistance to antimalarial drugs. *Nat Genet*. 2010 Mar;42(3):268-71.

[163] Miles MA, Llewellyn MS, Lewis MD, Yeo M, Baleela R, Fitzpatrick S, *et al*. The molecular epidemiology and phylogeography of Trypanosoma cruzi and parallel research on Leishmania: looking back and to the future. *Parasitology*. 2009 Oct;136(12): 1509-28.

Permissions

List of Contributors

Miroslava Avila-García, Javier Mancilla, Enrique Segura-Cervantes and Norma Galindo-Sevilla
National Institute for Perinatology, Department of Infectious Diseases and Perinatal Immunology, Mexico City, Mexico

Luiz Alberto Alves Mota
Faculty of Medical Sciences, Universidade de Pernambuco, Brasil
ENT service, Hospital Universitário Oswaldo Cruz, Brasil

Roberta Correia Ribeiro Ferreira de Miranda
Faculty of Medical Sciences, Universidade de Pernambuco, Brasil

João Carlos Araujo Carreira
Núcleo IOC- Jacarepaguá/Fundação Oswaldo Cruz, Rio de Janeiro, Brazil

Mônica de Avelar Figueiredo Mafra Magalhães
Laboratório de Geoprocessamento, Fundação Oswaldo Cruz, Rio de Janeiro, Brazil

Alba Valéria Machado da Silva
Laboratório de Bioquímica de Proteínas e Peptídeos, Fundação Oswaldo Cruz, Rio de Janeiro, Brazil

Aldo Eloizo Job, Alexandre Fioravante de Siqueira, Caroline Silva Danna, Felipe Silva Bellucci, Flávio Camargo Cabrera and Leandra Ernst Kerche Silva
Department of Physics, Chemistry and Biology, Univ Estadual Paulista, Presidente Prudente, Sao Paulo, Brazil

Elizabeth F. Rangel, Simone M. da Costa and Bruno M. Carvalho
Oswaldo Cruz Institute, FIOCRUZ, Rio de Janeiro, Brazil

Roqueline A.G.M.F. Aversi-Ferreira
Department of Anatomy, Howard University, Washington, DC, USA
LABINECOP, Federal University of Tocantins, Palmas, state of Tocantins, Brazil
Graduate Program in Animal Biology, University of Brasilia, Brasilia, DF, Brazil

Jucimária Dantas Galvão, Sylla Figueredo da Silva and Ediana Vasconcelos da Silva
LABINECOP, Federal University of Tocantins, Palmas, state of Tocantins, Brazil
Graduate Program in Health Sciences, Federal University of Tocantins, Palmas, state of Tocantins, Brazil

Giovanna Felipe Cavalcante
LABINECOP, Federal University of Tocantins, Palmas, state of Tocantins, Brazil

Naina Bhatia-Dey
Department of Anatomy, Howard University, Washington, DC, USA

Tales Alexandre Aversi-Ferreira
Department of Anatomy, Howard University, Washington, DC, USA
LABINECOP, Federal University of Tocantins, Palmas, state of Tocantins, Brazil
Graduate Program in Health Sciences, Federal University of Tocantins, Palmas, state of Tocantins, Brazil

Ana B. Caballero
School of Chemistry, University of Birmingham, Birmingham, United Kingdom

Juan M. Salas
Department of Inorganic Chemistry, School of Sciences, University of Granada, Granada, Spain

Manuel Sánchez-Moreno
Department of Parasitology, School of Sciences, University of Granada, Granada, Spain

Constantina N. Tsokana, George Valiakos and Charalambos Billinis
Department of Microbiology and Parasitology, Faculty of Veterinary Medicine, University of Thessaly, Karditsa, Greece

Labrini V. Athanasiou
Department of Medicine, Faculty of Veterinary Medicine, University of Thessaly, Karditsa, Greece

Vassiliki Spyrou
Department of Animal Production, Technological Education Institute of Larissa, Greece

Katerina Manolakou
Department of Animal Husbandry and Nutrition, Faculty of Veterinary Medicine, University of Thessaly, Karditsa, Greece

Souheila Guerbouj, Imen Mkada–Driss and Ikram Guizani
Laboratoire d'Epidemiologie et d'Ecologie Parasitaire / Epidémiologie Moléculaire et Pathologi Expérimentale Appliquée (Leishmania Genomics and Genetics Program), Institut Pasteur de Tunis, Université Tunis el Manar, Tunisia

Index

9 781639 873401